THE MEDICAL CLINICS OF NORTH AMERICA

VOLUME 56 / NUMBER 2
MARCH 1972

SYMPOSIUM ON
CLINICAL IMMUNOLOGY

Jules Harris, M.D., *Guest Editor*

W. B. SAUNDERS COMPANY — Philadelphia · London · Toronto

W. B. Saunders Company: West Washington Square
                           Philadelphia, Pa.   19105

                           12 Dyott Street
                           London, WC1A   1DB

                           1835 Yonge Street
                           Toronto 7, Ontario

The Medical Clinics are also published in other languages,
by the following:

Spanish   Nueva Editorial Interamericana, S. A. de C. V., Cedro 512,
                Apartado 26370, Mexico 4, D.F., Mexico

Italian   Piccin Editore, Via Porciglia, 10,
                35100 Padua, Italy

Portuguese   Editora Guanabara Koogan, S.A., Rua do Ouvidor,
                132 ZC 21, Rio de Janeiro, Brazil

Greek   John Mihalopoulos and Son,
                Thessaloniki, Greece

THE MEDICAL CLINICS OF NORTH AMERICA
March 1972   Volume 56 – Number 2

The Medical Clinic of North America is published every other month by W. B. Saunders Company, West Washington Square, Philadelphia, Pennsylvania 19105, at Hampton Road, Cherry Hill, New Jersey 08034. Subscription price is $21.00 per year. Second class postage paid at Cherry Hill, New Jersey 08034.
This issue is Volume 56, Number 2.
The editor of this publication is Albert E. Meier, W. B. Saunders Company, West Washington Square, Philadelphia, Pennsylvania 19105.

Library of Congress catalog card number 17-28505

Contributors

DAVID ALGOM, M.D., Instructor, Internal Medicine, Tel Aviv University Medical School, Tel Aviv; Senior Resident, Beilinson Hospital, Petah Tikva, Israel.

R. M. ARMSTRONG, M.D., Associate, Department of Medicine (Neurology), and Lecturer, Department of Pathology (Neuropathology), Faculty of Medicine, University of Toronto; Attending Physician, Toronto General Hospital, Toronto, Ontario, Canada.

RAMESH C. BAGAI, Ph.D., Research Fellow, Laboratory of Immunology, Division of Oncology, Faculty of Medicine, University of Ottawa, Canada.

JOHN BIENENSTOCK, M.D., Department of Medicine, McMaster University, Hamilton, Ontario, Canada; Medical Research Council Scholar.

I. BRODER, M.D., Associate Professor of Medicine, University of Toronto; Medical Research Associate, Medical Research Council of Canada.

D. H. COWAN, M.D., F.R.C.P.(C), Assistant Professor, Department of Medicine, University of Toronto; Physician, Princess Margaret Hospital in the Ontario Cancer Institute, Toronto, Ontario, Canada.

FRITZ DAGUILLARD, M.D., Ph.D., Director, Immunobiology Laboratory, Hôpital du Saint-Sacrement; Assistant Professor of Medicine, Université Laval, Québec, Canada.

PETER B. DENT, M.D., Assistant Professor, Department of Pediatrics, McMaster University, Hamilton, Ontario, Canada.

ERWIN DIENER, Ph.D., Professor of Pathology, Co-Director, MRC-Transplantation Unit, Faculty of Medicine, University of Alberta, Edmonton, Alberta, Canada.

STANISLAW DUBISKI, M.D., Ph.D., Associate Professor, Departments of Pathological Chemistry and Medicine; Member, Institute of Immunology, University of Toronto; Head, Laboratory of Immunology, The Toronto Western Hospital, Toronto, Ontario, Canada.

J. A. FALK, B.Sc., Director, Tissue Typing Laboratory, Toronto Western Hospital, Toronto, Ontario, Canada.

R. E. FALK, M.D., F.R.C.S.(C), Assistant Professor, Department of Surgery, and Institute of Immunology, University of Toronto; Staff Surgeon, Toronto General Hospital, Toronto, Ontario, Canada

D. A. GORDON, M.D., Assistant Professor of Medicine, University of Toronto Rheumatic Disease Unit, The Wellesley Hospital, Toronto, Ontario, Canada.

JULIUS GORDON, Ph.D., Associate Professor, Department of Experimental Surgery, McGill University, Montreal; Research Associate of the Medical Research Council of Canada.

JULES HARRIS, M.D., F.R.C.P.(C), F.A.C.P., Assistant Professor of Medicine, Division of Oncology, Faculty of Medicine, University of Ottawa, Canada.

DENNIS JIRSCH, M.D., Resident in Thoracic and Cardiovascular Surgery, and Fellow, Medical Research Council of Canada, Faculty of Medicine, University of Alberta, Edmonton, Alberta, Canada.

R. P. BRYCE LARKE, M.D., D.Cl.Sc., Assistant Professor, Departments of Pediatrics and Pathology, McMaster University, Hamilton, Ontario, Canada.

MARTIN G. LEWIS, M.D., M.R.C.Path., Professor and Chairman, Department of Pathology, Memorial University of Newfoundland, St. John's, Newfoundland, Canada.

W. H. MARSHALL, M.D., Ph.D., Professor of Immunology, Faculty of Medicine, Memorial University of Newfoundland, St. John's, Newfoundland, Canada.

HENRY Z. MOVAT, M.D., Ph.D., F.R.C.P.(C), Professor and Division Head, Faculty of Medicine, University of Toronto, Toronto, Ontario, Canada.

M. A. OGRYZLO, M.D., F.R.C.P.(C), Professor of Medicine, University of Toronto; Director, University of Toronto Rheumatic Disease Unit, The Wellesley Hospital, Toronto, Ontario, Canada.

DAVID OSOBA, M.D., F.R.C.P.(C), Associate Professor, Department of Medicine, University of Toronto; Associate of the Medical Research Council of Canada.

DANIEL Y. E. PEREY, M.D., Department of Pathology, McMaster University, Hamilton, Ontario, Canada; Queen Elizabeth II Scientist.

R. A. PHILLIPS, Ph.D., Associate Professor, Department of Medical Biophysics, University of Toronto; Division of Biological Research, Ontario Cancer Institute, Toronto, Ontario, Canada.

W. PRUZANSKI, M.D., F.R.C.P.(C), F.A.C.P., Assistant Professor of Medicine, University of Toronto; Director, Immunoproteins Research Laboratory, University of Toronto Rheumatic Disease Unit, The Wellesley Hospital, Toronto, Ontario, Canada.

MAXWELL RICHTER, Ph.D., M.D., Associate Professor, Department of Experimental Medicine, McGill University; Associated Scientist, Royal Victoria Hospital, Montreal, Canada.

HAROLD E. TAYLOR, M.D., F.R.C.P. (Can., Edin.), Director, Antilymphocyte Serum Program and Personnel Support Programs, Medical Research Council of Canada; Professor, Department of Pathology, University of Ottawa, Ontario, Canada.

M. B. UROWITZ, M.D., Associate, Department of Medicine, University of Toronto Rheumatic Disease Unit, The Wellesley Hospital, Toronto, Ontario, Canada.

Contents

Recent studies provide an understanding of the immunologic significance of the in vitro stimulation of lymphocytes by various mitogens. The capacity of these in vitro tests to detect and characterize immunologic deficiency states is evaluated.

The role of the lymphocyte in the evolution of a variety of disease states, such as autoimmune and immunodeficiency disorders, and in immune responses, either beneficial or detrimental to the host, such as tumor immunity and graft rejection.

Current concepts about the development and differentiation of the immunologic system form a basis for a discussion of the pathogenesis of immunologic deficiency disorders and autoimmune diseases. The immunodeficiency disorders are classified according to the cellular stage of development which appears to be affected in each condition. The development of autoreactive antibodies is considered as an epi-

phenomenon caused by the action of environmental
pathogens in an immunologically deficient milieu.

Julius Gordon

Mechanism of the mixed leukocyte culture reaction
and its application in histocompatibility matching and
the detection of immunocompetent cells.

Peter B. Dent and R. P. Bryce Larke

The basic principles of virus biology and mechanisms
of host resistance are reviewed with respect to their
relevance in clinical situations. Host-virus relationships in various syndromes of current interest are
discussed.

W. Pruzanski and M. A. Ogryzlo

The early detection of M components, utilizing sensitive immunochemical techniques, makes it possible to
institute treatment at an early stage in diseases such
as multiple myeloma, macroglobulinemia, primary
systemic amyloidosis, and heavy chain diseases.

John Bienenstock and Daniel Y. E. Perey

Information about the normal physiologic mechanisms
for maintaining the integrity of the organism at the
mucous membrane level has only been explored systematically in the last decade. While the importance
of apparently non-immunologic factors is acknowledged, this article deals primarily with the question
of immunologic mechanisms at this level, and implications for the clinical application of the concept of
local immunity.

J. A. Falk and R. E. Falk

Studies have shown that rejection of various types of
organ and tissue grafts can be reduced or prevented by
selecting donor-recipient combinations that are
matched as nearly as possible for transplantation antigens. A consistent and specific technique for monitor-

ing and characterizing the immune responses during allograft rejection needs to be developed. Three in vitro methods of detecting sensitization to transplantation antigens are discussed.

Harold E. Taylor

The clinical use of ALG is still experimental, and more information must be obtained by carefully controlled clinical trials before its precise role as a therapeutic agent can be defined. Potential hazards are discussed, as well as aspects of its use in organ transplants and autoimmune disorders.

R. A. Phillips and D. H. Cowan

A potentially useful procedure, bone marrow transplantation still remains a high-risk, experimental procedure that should be attempted only in selected patients. This article reviews major conceptual and procedural advances made since 1969, particularly with respect to aplastic anemias, acute leukemias, and congenital immunologic deficency disorders.

Erwin Diener and Dennis Jirsch

Research is aiming toward the goal of providing the practicing physician with a technique which will specifically block the transplant recipient's immune response to grafted tissue, yet maintain those mechanisms necessary to combat infections. Investigations are focussed upon the mechanisms which govern the immune reaction at the cellular and molecular levels, so that subsequent manipulation of these reactions may become possible.

W. H. Marshall

Transfer of cells or cell extracts may be used in immunodeficiency diseases, where the aim is to reconstitute the immune mechanism; in infectious disease, where transfer has been used to destroy an invading microorganism; and in tumors, based upon the discovery that a tumor may be antigenic to the host in which it grows.

Tumor-specific antibodies have been demonstrated
in a variety of human tumors, and their relevance to
the clinical stage of disease has been emphasized. It
is suggested that circulating humoral antibodies are
important at some stage in the natural history of malignancy in preventing rapid dissemination of disease.
The first clues to the role of immunity in malignancy
have come from careful clinical observation. Now
laboratory tests are adding to our understanding of
tumor-specific antibodies and antigens.

Unique patterns of immunologic impairment characterize chronic lymphocytic leukemia, multiple
myeloma, and acute leukemia. Cell-mediated immunity appears to be affected earlier in the course of
malignant illness than humoral immunity. With the
development of disseminated disease, both these
components are depressed.

Exploration of the relationship of clinical diseases to
experimental allergic encephalomyelitis and neuritis.
Immunologic mechanisms in myasthenia gravis.

The nature of immune complexes and the type of
injury they may produce; experimental and naturally
occurring models of the concept of immune complex
disease; evidence for the role of immunologic mechanisms in the pathogenesis of rheumatoid arthritis.

Vasoactive amines, plasma proteases and polypeptides,
slow-reacting substances, and neutrophil leukocyte
lysosomes and their role in the acute inflammatory
reaction.

Stanislaw Dubiski

One of the main difficulties in research into the area of antibody formation is the vast heterogeneity of immunoglobulin molecules in terms of their antibody-combining sites. This discussion is confined to a limited number of genetic markers of immunoglobulin molecules, known as allotypes or allotypic specificities.

RECENT SYMPOSIA

May 1971
MEDICAL ASPECTS OF CANCER

July 1971
DIABETES MELLITUS

September 1971
INTENSIVE CARE UNITS

November 1971
MODERN CONCEPTS IN RENAL DISEASE

January 1972
HEMORRHAGIC DISORDERS

FORTHCOMING SYMPOSIA

May 1972
THERAPEUTIC PROBLEMS
HENRY M. ZELLMANN, M.D., *Guest Editor*

July 1972
ENDOCRINE DISEASE
RAYMOND V. RANDALL, M.D., *Guest Editor*

September 1972
VENEREAL DISEASES
BRUCE WEBSTER, M.D., *Guest Editor*

November 1972
CLINICAL NEUROLOGY
MELVIN D. YAHR, M.D., *Guest Editor*

January 1973
CORONARY HEART DISEASE
LEON RESNEKOV, M.D., *Guest Editor*

Foreword

This number of the *Medical Clinics of North America* represents its first "all-Canadian" issue. It is appropriate under these circumstances that the volume deal with medical problems of an immunological nature. The past decade has seen an impressive expansion in departments of immunology associated with each of the Canadian medical schools. This has in part been due to generous and forward looking grant support provided by the Medical Research Council of Canada and due also to the increasing importance that each of the schools attaches to the study of immunology and its relationship to major areas of medical investigation. This has led, among other developments, to the establishment of the Transplantation Unit in the University of Alberta's Edmonton branch, to the organization of the University of Toronto's Institute of Immunology, and to the rapid growth of the University of Ottawa's Division of Immunology.

The papers selected for this Symposium were chosen to illustrate the range of interests and the scope of activity among immunologists across Canada. Taken together they provide a "primer of modern immunology" with presentations of both basic immunological theory and detailed accounts of specific problem areas. They offer the reader a sound introduction to many of the recently shaped immunological concepts which will influence the direction of clinical and laboratory studies in the coming years.

The major difficulty in the organization of this issue arose from the need to edit it to fit the standard size of individual *Medical Clinics of North America* issues. This has led to some minor deletions in individual papers and has required that one major contribution, "The Future of Tumor Immunology," by Dr. Bernhard Cinader, be reserved for a later volume.

JULES E. HARRIS, M.D.
Guest Editor

Faculty of Medicine
University of Ottawa
Ottawa, Ontario
Canada

Immunologic Significance of In Vitro Lymphocyte Responses

*Fritz Daguillard, M.D., Ph.D.**

The purpose of this paper is to review recent studies which provide an understanding of the immunologic significance of the in vitro stimulation of lymphocytes by several reagents and to determine the capacity of these in vitro tests to detect and characterize immunologic deficiency states.

Special attention will be paid to the proliferative response of lymphocytes in the presence of mitogens and antigens. Mention will also be made of the production of effector molecules by the stimulated cells. Finally, we will indicate certain discrepancies between the results obtained with in vitro and in vivo tests.

In accordance with the present concept of a two component division of the immune system, attempts will be made to assess the capacity of each test to determine a defect of either the T or the B lymphocyte.[39] It is now accepted that both types of lymphocytes originate from the bone marrow as stem cells.[39] The T lymphocyte (TL) or T cell, thymus-derived or thymus-dependent, develops under the influence of the thymus and engages in cell-mediated immune functions (graft rejection, delayed skin hypersensitivity, protection against viruses, fungi, pneumocystis).[39] T cells act either directly or through the release of soluble factors, some of which may be cytotoxic per se, or help to recruit more noncommited cells for the reaction. B lymphocytes (BL) or B cells seem to develop independently from the thymus and eventually become antibody-producing cells.[39] There are indications however that cooperation between B and T cells may be necessary for a full scale production of antibody to certain antigens.[17, 72]

THE IN VITRO PROLIFERATIVE RESPONSE OF LYMPHOCYTES

Several substances are known to stimulate lymphocytes in vitro.[62, 76] We will discuss here the immunologic significance of the in vitro

*Director, Immunobiology Laboratory, Hôpital du Saint-Sacrement; Assistant Professor of Medicine, Université Laval, Québec

response to some of these substances, namely phytohemagglutinin (PHA), pokeweed (PWM), anti-immunoglobulin serum (AGS), allogeneic leukocytes, and antigens (Ag). Antigens, unlike the other mitogens, require prior specific sensitization.

Numerous changes, both biochemical and morphologic, take place within the lymphocytes stimulated by mitogens. The determination of some of these changes, i.e., transformation to blast-like cells, mitosis, and DNA, RNA, and protein synthesis, permits the study of the action of most of the mitogens.[62, 76]

The mechanism whereby mitogens stimulate lymphocytes is considered to involve the interaction with cell membrane receptors.[22, 62, 76] The receptor for antigen and AGS is most probably an antibody-like membrane component.[28, 47, 59, 74, 93, 102, 103] The receptor for the other mitogens are less well characterized.[27, 61] However the attractive concept that functionally different lymphocytes might carry membrane-bound receptors which interact with different mitogens is the object of active investigations. In this section we will try to determine if the response of lymphocytes to mitogens can characterize B and T cells.

The Proliferative Response of Lymphocytes to PHA and Allogeneic Leukocytes

The capacity to respond in vitro to PHA and allogeneic leukocytes is thought to be the property of the T lymphocyte. Thymectomized animals exhibit a diminished capacity to respond to PHA and allogeneic leucocytes.[37, 46, 69, 70, 104] However the decreased PHA response in thymectomized mice can be restored to normal levels by thymus grafting.[100] In fact most of the lymphocytes, in the peripheral blood of reconstituted mice and rats responding to PHA and/or allogeneic leukocytes, bear the chromosome marker of the thymus graft.[31, 51]

Recent studies have indicated that the early precursor of the PHA-responsive cell is an hemopoietic stem cell which requires traffic through the thymus for the expression of its proliferative capacity.[34, 100] There is no indication that the capacity to respond to PHA may be acquired under the humoral influence of the thymus gland. However in a recent study, the combination of normal thymus and marrow cell suspensions in vitro resulted in a synergistic activity in response to PHA.[105]

By and large, the capacity of lymphocytes to respond to PHA and allogeneic leukocytes was found to be greatly decreased in the case of a primary developmental defect of the thymus gland itself (DiGeorge's syndrome, thymic aplasia)[18, 33, 54] or in the case of an involution of this gland deriving from a stem cell defect (Swiss type agammaglobulinemia, congenital thymic dysplasia).[7, 44, 49, 67] The capacity to respond to PHA was restored in the first case by implantation of foetal thymus[5, 6, 18] and in the second case by grafting of bone marrow with or without foetal thymus.[4, 41, 53]

There are however notable exceptions to the rule that the responses to PHA and allogeneic leukocytes are always affected in instances of thymus deficiency:

Differing Responses of T Cells to PHA and Allogeneic Leukocytes. Although the capacity to respond to PHA and allogeneic leukocytes seems to be the property of T cells, certain studies suggest that T lymphocytes may be differently affected in their capacity to respond to PHA and allogeneic leukocytes. Cells of 2 patients with congenital thymic dysplasia have been found to respond consistently to stimulation with allogeneic leukocytes, although the response to PHA was impaired.[48, 67] A similar dissociation of responsiveness to PHA and allogeneic leukocytes has been observed with lymphocytes of an adult patient.[7] These findings correlate well with certain experimental studies in which thymocytes responsive to PHA and allogeneic leukocytes were separated on a density gradient.[19] A possible explanation is that the response to these mitogens may constitute various steps in the differentiation of the T cell. Failure to develop beyond an early stage would impair the capacity to respond to PHA, while the capacity to respond to allogeneic leukocytes, already acquired, would persist.

NORMAL PHA RESPONSE IN THYMUS-DEFICIENT STATES. Despite the numerous clinical and experimental observations which establish the thymus dependency of the PHA response, cases have been reported of normal PHA responses in the presence of an obvious thymic defect.

The lymphocytes of a 12 year old boy[89] having the features of congenital thymic aplasia were found to transform normally in response to PHA. Similarly, the lymphocytes of 1 patient with Swiss type agammaglobulinemia could be stimulated with PHA, as well as those of a normal control, following removal of phagocytes prior to cultivation.[50] However there were no indications that the capacity of the lymphocytes of these 2 patients to respond to previously encountered antigens was intact. These findings nonetheless suggest that the capacity to respond to PHA is not the final stage in the differentiation of the T lymphocyte and does not reflect its ability to mediate all the in vivo cellular immune functions.

PHA-RESPONSIVE B LYMPHOCYTES. The majority of investigators have reported that in the case of selective B cell defects (such as impairment of humoral immunity, or primary agammaglobulinemia, congenital or acquired) the lymphocytes incubated with PHA show a degree of blast transformation and mitosis comparable to normal.[7, 14, 21, 40, 44, 60, 86, 87] However Tormey et al.[101] have found a decreased synthesis of RNA and DNA in PHA-stimulated agammaglobulinemia lymphocytes. Also, a recent experimental work indicates that in the mouse, certain B lymphocytes respond to PHA.[12] However the contribution of B cells to the total PHA response seems minimal and unlikely to serve as a valid assessment of B cell defect.

The Proliferative Response of Lymphocytes to Antigen

There has been some controversy as to whether the specific transformation of lymphocytes by antigen is a reflection of cellular or humoral immunity. Lymphocytes of animals exhibiting delayed hypersensitivity in the absence of circulating antibodies can be stimulated with the specific antigen in vitro.[73, 77] Similarly, lymphocytes obtained from guinea pigs immunized intravenously, which did not subsequently show delayed skin reactivity, did not undergo blastogenesis in the presence of antigen in vitro.[73] However several investigators have shown that the stimulation of lymphocytes by antigen in vitro may occur in the absence of demonstrable cellular sensitivity to that antigen in vivo, and may at times correlate with antibody production.[9, 38, 43]

However, despite one report to the contrary,[56] there seems to be no indication that a large proportion of blast cells stimulated by Ag in vitro engage in active antibody production.[42, 97] This makes the majority of these cells resemble antigen-reactive cells (ARC) which, in the mouse, are mostly thymus-derived and proliferate following challenge with antigen, but do not produce antibodies.[30, 32] The mode of interaction between this antigen-reactive cell and the actual antibody forming cell (AFC) is not clear.[30] However there exist indications that not all ARC are thymus-derived. Indeed, in the chicken, bursectomy or thymectomy, which both cause a selective defect of either humoral or cellular immunity,[20, 68] both depress the capacity of lymphocytes to proliferate in the presence of antigen in vitro and in vivo,[1, 3] demonstrating that in this species, both thymus-dependent and thymus-independent lymphocytes are activated by antigen. Whether such a situation exists in man is not certain.

In one case of complete absence of the thymus (thymic aplasia, DiGeorge's syndrome) the transformation of human lymphocytes by antigen was found greatly decreased.[33] Moreover, despite normal immunoglobulin levels, this patient was able to produce only small amounts of antibodies to some antigens and produced no antibodies to other antigens.[33] This was used as an argument for a role for the thymus in the humoral response of man to certain antigens.[63] In the mouse, this role is well established[17, 72] and a clear pattern of thymus-dependent and thymus-independent antigens is now emerging.[75] In congenital thymic dysplasia (stem cell defect), in which both cellular and humoral immune functions are absent, lymphocytes respond poorly to antigen.[7, 49, 58, 67]

The proliferative response of agammaglobulinemia lymphocytes to specific antigens has been the subject of numerous and contradictory reports. Fudenberg and Hirschhorn[40] studied the lymphocytes of 5 patients with agammaglobulinemia (2 had "typical" sex-linked agammaglobulinemia, and 3 the "acquired" form of the disease): the lymphocytes of all of the patients failed to differentiate or produce gamma globulin when challenged in culture by the immunizing antigen. Similarly, Bach et al.[7] challenged the lymphocytes of numerous agammaglobulinemic patients with antigen in vitro: out of 7 patients with Bruton-type disease, 5 did not respond and 1 gave a borderline response; the cells of 3 patients with late-onset (acquired) agammaglobulinemia responded to at least some of the antigens. On the other hand, recent studies[21, 44] indicate that circulating lymphocytes from patients with congenital X-linked or acquired agammaglobulinemia proliferate in a normal manner following stimulation with a specific antigen. Furthermore, the lymphocytes of some of these patients produced in vitro a quantity of IgG similar in amount to that found in normal cell cultures.[21]

It is therefore obvious that in these patients there exists a variety of lymphocyte abnormalities which can be detected by in vitro culture: the lymphocytes of some patients react to antigens, the lymphocytes of other patients do not. This may indicate that the defect leading to a decreased production of antibodies could be situated at two different levels: when the response to Ag is intact, the ARC is present and the defect is more likely situated at the level of the AFC. In case of no response to Ag, the ARC is most probably defective.

The Proliferative Response of Lymphocytes to Anti-Immunoglobulin Serum (AGS)

A few experimental studies have indicated that B lymphocytes are those which respond mainly to AGS. The arguments in favor of this suggestion are that bursectomy of the chicken decreases the capacity of their lymphocytes to respond to AGS[2] and that thymocytes are not stimulated by anti-immunoglobulin serum.[27] However there are indications that T cells carry light-chain determinants[45] and may respond weakly to anti-light chain sera in vitro,[96] although most evidence favors the exclusive presence of immunoglobulin determinants on B lymphocytes.[27, 78, 80, 82, 83]

The capacity to respond to AGS should be considered as a test for the ARC in view of the studies indicating that an immunoglobulin receptor on the membrane of lymphocytes seem to mediate the recognition of antigens.[28, 47, 59, 66, 74, 103] The capacity to respond to AGS was found either intact or decreased in several cases of agammaglobulinemia or hypogammaglobulinemia.[24] As in the case of the response to Ag, the response to AGS suggested that the lymphocyte defect of these patients was located at the level of either the ARC or the AFC.[24]

The Proliferative Response of Lymphocytes to Pokeweed Mitogen (PWM)

Studies based on the morphologic appearance of lymphoblasts following stimulation with PWM have suggested that B lymphocytes respond to PWM: the blast cells formed by PWM are more differentiated than those resulting from the action of PHA and in many respects are similar to plasma cells and plasmablasts.[8, 35] A recent report also indicates that the response of mouse lymphoid cells to PWM is less thymus-dependent than the responses to PHA.[99] However thymectomy significantly reduced the capacity of rat lymphocytes to respond to PWM.[70] This, together with the observation that rabbit[25] and rat[25, 98] thymocytes can be stimulated in vitro with PWM, suggests that both B and T cells respond to PWM in vitro.

THE LIBERATION OF BIOLOGICALLY ACTIVE MOLECULES BY STIMULATED LYMPHOCYTES

The interaction of lymphocytes in vitro with Ag or mitogens results in the release of a family of molecules capable of affecting in one way or another large populations of cells. Some of these factors prevent the migration of cells introduced into capillary tubes,[13, 29] others directly induce lymphocytes to proliferate[52, 65] or make them susceptible to the action of specific antigens.[57] Finally, some display cytotoxicity for target cells in different experimental models.[79]

The migration inhibitory factor (MIF) which impedes capillary migration of guinea pig macrophages has been the most thoroughly investigated, and several of its properties are now characterized.[13, 29, 81, 85] It is produced following the interaction of either sensitized lymphocytes with Ag[13, 29] or normal lymphocytes with nonspecific mitogens.[55, 81, 84] A recent study suggests that the inability to produce MIF may be a reliable indication of T cell defect.[89] Lymphocytes of patients lacking cellular immune functions failed to produce MIF. Following a thymic transplant one of these patients (congenital thymic aplasia) produced the factor.[89]

The relation of the other molecules with the T lymphocyte has not been established as clearly as in the above experiment of nature. However several experimental models do indicate that the production of most of these factors is defective in situations displaying an impairment of the cellular branch of immunity.[13, 29, 57]

CORRELATION BETWEEN IN VITRO AND IN VIVO TESTS

Comparison between the delayed hypersensitivity skin reaction and the two in vitro correlates of cellular immunity (MIF and blastogenesis) has been the subject of recent studies. Several reports have stressed the presence of an intact proliferative response of lymphocytes to PHA and/or antigens in the absence of delayed skin reaction to antigens.[11, 16, 23, 24, 92] Instances have also been reported of normal MIF production by lymphocytes from anergic patients or animals.[88, 91] But, by and large, the production of MIF was found to be a better correlate of in vivo cellular immune functions than the proliferative response to antigens.[90] This result may be explained on the basis of difference in sensitivity of the techniques. Indeed there are indications that these tests may be differently affected by the molecular size of an antigen.[15]

However there is evidence, already mentioned in a previous section, that the capacity to proliferate in the presence of Ag in vitro can be related to both B and T lymphocytes.[9, 38, 43,] As only T lymphocytes seem capable of producing MIF,[89] this would make this property the best in vitro test of their integrity.

The lack of delayed skin hypersensitivity in patients capable of producing MIF could be explained by the fact that the in vivo reaction does require, in addition to antigen-reactive T cells, other types of cells which participate in the local inflammatory reaction.[64] It is important that the fate of these different cell populations as well as the production of serum inhibitors of their expression, during a state of cutaneous anergy, be better understood.

CONCLUSION

In this paper evidence for differing in vitro behavior of B and T lymphocytes was reviewed. It is established that the capacity to produce

MIF or respond in vitro to allogeneic leukocytes and PHA are properties of T lymphocytes. Whether these properties always imply fully mature and immunocompetent T cells is somewhat doubtful. Indeed, examples were given of patients possessing lymphocytes capable of proliferating in vitro in the presence of PHA or allogeneic leukocytes, and yet unable to manifest in vivo cellular immune functions.[48, 50, 67, 89]

The in vitro assessment of B lymphocytes is an area of active research. Although certain studies indicate that T cells may carry light-chain determinants on their membrane,[45] most evidence favors the exclusive presence of heavy chains (if not, in fact, immunoglobulin in general) on the membrane of B lymphocytes.[27, 78, 80, 82, 83] There are also indications that BL carry exclusively a receptor for the third component of complement, which make them capable of binding antigen-antibody-complement complexes.[10, 36, 71] These cells were termed complement receptor lymphocytes (CRL).[10] Receptors for complement and immunoglobulin determinants were found in identical populations of cells in the mouse.[10] The same was true in the spleen of the rabbit.[26] However there is a notable exception to this rule: rabbit peripheral blood lymphocytes which respond very well to in vitro stimulation with anti-heavy chain immunoglobulin serum[94, 95] are surprisingly poor in CRL.[26]

It seems therefore that both B and T lymphocytes constitute heterogeneous populations of cells displaying diverse properties at different stages of their differentiation. The attempts to correlate already known in vitro properties as well as newly discovered ones with a given functional state of the cell constitute a vast area for rewarding experimental and clinical research.

REFERENCES

1. Alm, G. V.: The in vivo spleen response to sheep erythrocytes in bursectomized-irradiated chickens. Acta Path. Microbiol. Scand. 78:641, 1970.
2. Alm, G. V., and Peterson, R. D. A.: Antibody and immunoglobulin production at the cellular level in bursectomized-irradiated chickens. J. Exper. Med., 129:1247, 1969.
3. Alm, G. V., and Peterson, R. D. A.: Effect of thymectomy and bursectomy on the in vitro response of chick spleen cells to PHA, sheep erythrocytes (SRBC) and allogeneic cells. Fed. Proc., 29:430, 1970.
4. Ammann, A. J., Meuwissen, H. J., Good, R. A., and Hong, R.: Successful bone marrow transplantation in a patient with humoral and cellular immunity deficiency. Clin. Exper. Immunol., 7:343, 1970.
5. August, C. S., Berkel, A. I., Levey, R. H., and Rosen, F. S.: Establishment of immunological competence in a child with congenital thymic aplasia by a graft of fetal thymus. Lancet, 1:1080, 1970.
6. August, C. S., Rosen, F. S., Filler, R. M., Janeway, C. A., Markowski, B., and Kay, H. E. M.: Implantation of a foetal thymus restoring immunological competence in a patient with thymic aplasia (DiGeorge's syndrome), Lancet, 2:1210, 1968.
7. Bach, F. H., Meuwissen, H. J., Albertini, R. J., and Good, R. A.: Agammaglobulinemic leucocytes—Their in vitro reactivity, In W. O. Rieke, Ed.: Proceedings of the Third Leucocyte Culture Conference. New York, Appleton-Century-Crofts, 1969.
8. Barker, B. E., Lutzner, M. A., and Farnes, P.: Ultrastructural properties of pokeweed stimulated leucocyte in vivo and in vitro, In W. O. Rieke, Ed.: Proceedings of the Third Leucocyte Culture Conference. New York, Appleton-Century-Crofts, 1969.
9. Benezra, D., Gery, I., and Davies, A. M.: The relationship between lymphocyte transformation and immune response. II. Correlation between transformation and humoral and cellular immune responses, Clin. Exper. Immunol., 5:155, 1969.
10. Bianco, C., Patrick, R., and Nussenzweig, V.: A population of lymphocytes bearing a membrane receptor for antigen-antibody-complement complexes. J. Exper. Med., 132:702, 1970.

11. Blaese, M., Brown, R. S., Strober, W., and Waldmann, T. A.: The Wiscott-Aldrich syndrome: A disorder with a possible defect in antigen processing or recognition. Lancet, 1:1056, 1968.

12. Blomgren, H., and Svedmyr, E.: Evidence for thymic dependence of PHA-reactive cells in spleen and lymph nodes and independence in bone marrow. J. Immunol., 106:835, 1971.

13. Bloom, B. R., and Bennett, B.: Macrophages and delayed type hypersensitivity. Seminars Hematol., 7:215, 1970.

14. Bradley, J., and Oppenheim, J. J.: The in vitro proliferation of lymphocytes from patients with hypogammaglobulinemia. Clin. Exper. Immunol., 2:549, 1967.

15. Chaparas, S. D., Thor, D. E., and Hedrick, S. R.: Comparison of lymphocyte transformation, inhibition of macrophage migration and skin tests using dialyzable and non-dialyzable tuberculin fractions from mycobacterium bovis (BCG). J. Immunol., 107:149, 1971.

16. Chilgren, R. A., Meuwissen, H. J., Quie, P. G., and Hong, R.: Chronic mucocutaneous candidiasis, deficiency of delayed hypersensitivity, and selective local antibody defect. Lancet, 2:688, 1967.

17. Claman, H. N., and Chaperon, E. A.: Immunological complementation between thymus and marrow cells-A model for the two-cell theory of immunocompetence. Transplant. Rev., 1:92, 1969.

18. Cleveland, W. M., Fogel, B. J., Brown, W. T., and Kay, H. E. M.: Foetal thymic transplant in a case of DiGeorge's syndrome. Lancet, 2:1211, 1968.

19. Colley, D. G., Shih Wu, A. Y., and Waksman, B. H.: Cellular differentiation in the thymus. III. Surface properties of rat thymus and lymph node cells separated on density gradients, J. Exper. Med., 132:1107, 1970.

20. Cooper, M. D., Gabrielsen, A. E., and Good, R. A.: Role of the thymus and other central lymphoid tissues in immunological disease. Ann. Rev. Med., 18:113, 1967.

21. Cooperband, S. R., Rosen, F. S., and Kibrick, S.: Studies on the in vitro behavior of agammaglobulinemic lymphocytes. J. Clin. Invest., 47:836, 1968.

22. Coulson, A. S.: Recognition pathway in lymphocytes. J. Theoret. Biol., 25:127, 1969.

23. Daguillard, F.: Heterogenéité de l'atteinte du lymphocyte dans les syndromes de carence immunitaire. L'Union Med. du Canada, 99:1068, 1970.

24. Daguillard, F., Heiner, D. C., Richter, M., and Rose, B.: The response of leucocytes of agammaglobulinemia subjects to phytohemagglutinin and anti-immunoglobulin antiserum. Clin. Exper. Immunol., 4:203, 1969.

25. Daguillard, F., and Prochazkova, E.: Manuscript in preparation.

26. Daguillard, F., and Prochazkova, E.: Separation of lymphocytes responsive to phytohemagglutinin and anti-immunoglobulin serum. In Schwarz, M. R., ed.: Proceedings of the Sixth Leucocyte Culture Conference. New York, Academic Press, in press.

27. Daguillard, F., and Richter, M.: Cells involved in the immune response. XII. The differing responses of normal rabbit lymphoid cells to phytohemagglutinin, goat anti-rabbit immunoglobulin antiserum and allogeneic and xenogeneic lymphocytes, J. Exper. Med., 130:1187, 1969.

28. Daguillard, F., and Richter, M.: Cells involved in the immune response. XVI. The response of immune rabbit cells to phytohemagglutinin, antigen and goat anti-rabbit immunoglobulin antiserum. J. Exper. Med., 131:119, 1970.

29. David, J. R.: Macrophage migration. Fed. Proc., 27:6, 1968.

30. Davies, A. J. S.: The thymus and the cellular basis of immunity. Transplant. Rev., 1:43, 1969.

31. Davies, A. J. S. Festenstein, H., Leuchars, E., Wallis, V. S., and Doenhoff, M. J.: A thymic origin for some peripheral blood lymphocytes. Lancet, 1:183, 1968.

32. Davies, A. J. S., Leuchars, E., Wallis, V., Marchant, R., and Elliot, E. V.: The failure of thymus-derived cells to produce antibodies. Transplantation, 5:222, 1967.

33. DiGeorge, A. M.: Congenital absence of the thymus and its immunologic consequences: Concurrence with congenital hypoparathyroidism. Birth Defects (Orig. Art. Series), 4:116, 1968.

34. Doenhoff, M. J., and Davies, A. J. S.: Reconstitution of the T-cell pool after irradiation of mice. Cell. Immunol., 2:82, 1971.

35. Douglas, S. D., and Fudenberg, H. H.: In vitro development of plasma cells from lymphocytes following pokeweed mitogen stimulation: a fine structural study, Exper. Cell. Res., 54:277, 1969.

36. Dukor, P., Bianco, C., and Nussenzweig, V.: Tissue localization of lymphocytes bearing a membrane receptor for antigen-antibody-complement complexes. Proc. Nat. Acad. Sci., U. S. A., 67:991, 1970.

37. Dukor, P., and Dietrich, F. M.: Impairment of phytohemagglutinin induced blastic transformation in lymph nodes from thymectomized mice. Int. Arch. Allergy Appl. Immunol., 32:521, 1967.

38. Fellner, M. J., Baer, R. L., Ripps, C. S., and Hirschhorn, K.: Response of lymphocytes to

Penicillin: Comparison with skin tests and circulating antibodies in man. Nature, 216:803, 1967.

39. Fudenberg, H., Good, R. A., Goodman, H. C., Hitzig, W., Kunkel, H. G., Roitt, I. M., Rosen, F. S., Rowe, D. S., Seligmann, M., and Soothill, S. R.: Primary immunodeficiencies. Report of a World Health Organization Committee. Pediatrics, 47:927, 1971.

40. Fudenberg, H. H., and Hirschhorn, K.: Agammaglobulinemia: the fundamental defect. Science, 145:611, 1964.

41. Gatti, R., Allen, H. D., Meuwissen, H. J. Hong, R., and Good, R. A.: Immunological reconstitution of sex-linked lymphopenic immunological deficiency. Lancet, 2:1366, 1968.

42. Gery, I., Benezra, D., and Davies, A. M.: The relationship between lymphocyte transformation and immune response. I. Ratio of transforming cells to antibody forming cells. Immunology, 16:381, 1969.

43. Girard, J. P., Rose, N. R., Kunz, M. L., Kobayashi, S., and Arbesman, C. E.: In vitro lymphocyte transformation in atopic patients: Induced by antigens. J. Allergy, 39:65, 1967.

44. Gotoff, S. P.: Lymphocytes in congenital immunological deficiency diseases. Clin. Exper. Immunol., 3:843, 1968.

45. Greaves, M. F.: Biological effects of anti-immunoglobulins, Transplant. Rev., 5:45, 1970.

46. Greaves, M. F., Roitt, I. M., and Rose, M. E.: Effect of bursectomy and thymectomy on the responses of chicken peripheral blood lymphocytes to phytohemagglutinin. Nature, 220:293, 1968.

47. Greaves, M. F., Torrigiani, G., and Roitt, I. M.: Blocking of the lymphocyte receptor site for cell mediated hypersensitivity and transplantation reactions by anti-light chain sera. Nature, 222:825, 1969.

48. Greenberg, A. H., Ray, M., and Tsai, Y. T.: Thymic alymphoplasia and dysgammaglobulinemia type I. J. Pediat., 75:95, 1969.

49. Hitzig, W. H.: The Swiss type of agammaglobulinemia. Birth Defects (Orig. Art. Series), 4:82, 1968.

50. Hitzig, W. H., Landolt, R., Müller, G., and Bodmer, P.: Heterogeneity of phenotypic expression in a family with Swiss-type agammaglobulinemia: Observations on the acquisition of agammaglobulinemia. J. Pediat., 78:968, 1971.

51. Johnston, J. M., and Wilson, D. B.: Origin of immunoreactive lymphocytes in rats. Cell. Immunol., 1:430, 1970.

52. Kasakura, S.: Heterogeneity of blastogenic factors produced in vitro by antigenically stimulated and unstimulated leucocytes. J. Immunol., 105:1162, 1970.

53. de Koning, J., Dooren, L. J., van Bekkum, D. W., van Rood, J. J., and Radl. J.: Transplantation of bone-marrow cells and fetal thymus in an infant with lymphopenic immunological deficiency. Lancet, 1:1223, 1970.

54. Kretschmer, R., Lay, B., Brown, D., and Rosen, F. S.: Congenital aplasia of the thymus gland (DiGeorge's syndrome). New Eng. J. Med., 279:1295, 1968.

55. Lamelin, J. P., and Vassali, P.: Inhibition of macrophage migration by a soluble factor from lymphocytes stimulated with PHA or ALS. Nature, 229:426, 1971.

56. Lamvik, J. O.: Antibody synthesis by blastoid cells transformed in vitro from rabbit blood lymphocytes. Scand. J. Haematol., 5:171, 1968.

57. Lawrence, H. S.: Transfer factor-an initiator of cellular immunity and its relation to effector molecules. Harris, J., Ed.: In Proceedings of the Fifth Leucocyte Culture Conference. New York, Academic Press, 1970.

58. Leikin, S., Purugganan, G., and Chandra, R.: Thymic dysplasia. J. Pediat., 75:229, 1969.

59. Lesley, J., and Dutton, R. W.: Evidence for antigen receptor molecules, Fed. Proc., 29:697, 1970.

60. Lieber, E., Hirschhorn, K., and Fudenberg, H. H.: Response of agammaglobulinemic lymphocytes in mixed lymphocyte culture. Clin. Exper. Immunol., 4:83, 1969.

61. Lindahl-Kiessling, K., and Peterson, R. D. A.: The mechanism of phytohemagglutinin (PHA) action. II. The effect of certain enzymes and sugars. Exper. Cell. Res., 55:81, 1969.

62. Ling, N. R.: Lymphocyte Stimulation. Amsterdam, North Holland Publishing Co., 1968.

63. Lischner, H. W., and DiGeorge, A. M.: Role of the thymus in humoral immunity. Lancet, 2:1044, 1969.

64. Lubaroff, D. M., and Waksman, B. H.: Bone marrow as source of cells in reactions of cellular hypersensitivity. II. Identification of allogeneic or hybrid cells by immunofluorescence in passively transferred tuberculin reactions, J. Exper. Med., 128:1438, 1968.

65. Maini, R. N., Bryceson, A. D. M., Wolstencroft, R. A., and Dumonde, D. C.: Lymphocyte mitogenic factor in man. Nature, 224:43, 1969.

66. Mason, S., and Warner, N. L.: The immunoglobulin nature of the antigen recognition site on cells mediating transplantation immunity and delayed hypersensitivity. J. Immunol., 104:762, 1970.

67. Meuwissen, H. J., Bach, F. H., Hong, R., and Good, R. A.: Lymphocyte studies in congenital thymic dysplasia: the one-way stimulation test. J. Pediat., 72:177, 1968.

68. Meuwissen, H. J., Stutman, O., and Good, R. A.: Functions of the lymphocytes. Seminars Hematol., 6:28, 1969.
69. Meuwissen, H. J., Van Alten, P. J., Bach, F. H., and Good, R. A.: Influence of thymus and bursa on in vitro lymphocyte function. Birth Defects (Orig. Art. Series), 4:253, 1968.
70. Meuwissen, H. J., Van Alten, P. J., and Good, R. A.: Decreased lymphoid cell multiplication in the post thymectomy state. Transplantation, 7:1, 1969.
71. Michlmayr, G., and Huber, H.: Receptor sites for complement on certain human peripheral blood lymphocytes. J. Immunol., 105:670, 1970.
72. Miller, J. F. A. P., and Mitchell, G. F.: Thymus and antigen-reactive cells. Transplant. Rev., 1:3, 1969.
73. Mills, J. A.: The immunologic significance of antigen induced lymphocyte transformation in vitro. J. Immunol., 97:239, 1966.
74. Mitchison, N. A.: Antigen recognition responsible for the induction in vitro of the secondary response. Cold Spring Harbor Symp. Quant. Biol., 32:431, 1967.
75. Moller, G.: Immunocompetent cells in graft rejection. Trans. Proc., 3:15, 1971.
76. Naspitz, C. K., and Richter, M.: The action of phytohemagglutinin in vivo and in vitro. A Review. Progr. Allergy, 12:1, 1968.
77. Oppenheim, J. J.: Relationship of in vitro lymphocyte transformation to delayed hypersensitivity in guinea pigs and man. Fed. Proc., 27:21, 1968.
78. Paraskevas, F., Lee, S-T., and Israels, L. G.: Cell surface associated gammaglobulins in lymphocytes. J. Immunol., 106:160, 1971.
79. Perlmann, P., and Holm, G.: Cytotoxic effects of lymphoid cells in vitro. Advanc. Immunol., 11:117, 1969.
80. Pernis, B., Forni, L., and Amante, L.: Immunoglobulin spots on the surface of rabbit lymphocytes. J. Exper. Med., 132:1001, 1970.
81. Pick, E., Brostoff, J., Krejci, J., and Turk, J. L.: Interaction between sensitized lymphocytes and antigen in vitro. II. Mitogen-induced release of skin reactive and macrophage migration inhibitory factors. Cell. Immunol., 1:92, 1970.
82. Rabellino, E., Colon, S., Grey, H. M., and Unanue, E. R.: Immunoglobulins on the surface of lymphocytes. I. Distribution and quantitation. J. Exper. Med., 133:156, 1971.
83. Raff, M. C., Sternberg, M., and Taylor, R. B.: Immunoglobulin determinants on the surface of mouse lymphoid cells. Nature, 225:553, 1970.
84. Remold, H. G., and David, J. R.: Cellular immunity: Characterization of migration inhibitory factor (MIF) from guinea pig lymphocytes stimulated with concavalian A. In Schwartz, M. R., Ed.: Proceedings of the Sixth Leucocyte Culture Conference. New York, Academic Press, in press.
85. Remold, H. G., Katz, A. B., Haber, E., and David, J. R.: Studies on migration inhibitory factor (MIF): Recovery of MIF activity after purification by gel filtration and disc electrophoresis. Cell. Immunol., 1:133, 1970.
86. Ripps, C. S., and Hirschhorn, K.: The production of immunoglobulins by human peripheral blood lymphocytes in vitro. Clin. Exper. Immunol., 2:377, 1967.
87. Robbins, J. H.: Human peripheral blood in tissue culture and the action of phytohemagglutinin. Experientia, 20:1, 1964.
88. Rocklin, R. E., Reardon, G., Sheffer, A., Churchill, W. H., and David, J. R.: Dissociation between two in vitro correlates of delayed hypersensitivity: Absence of migration inhibitory factor (MIF) in the presence of antigen-induced incorporation of 3H-Thymidine, In Harris, J., Ed.: Proceedings of the Fifth Leucocyte Culture Conference. New York, Academic Press, 1970.
89. Rocklin, R. E., Rosen, F. S., and David, J. R.: In vitro lymphocyte response of patients with immunologic deficiency diseases. New Eng. J. Med., 282:1340, 1970.
90. Rocklin, R. E., Sheffer, A., and David, J. R.: Sarcoidosis: A clinical and in vitro immunologic study. In Schwarz, M. R., Ed.: Proceedings of the Sixth Leucocyte Culture Conference. New York, Academic Press, in press.
91. Salvin, S. B., Nishio, J., and Gribik, M.: Lymphoid cells in delayed hypersensitivity. I. In vitro vs. in vivo responses. Cell. Immunol., 1:62, 1970.
92. Seeger, R. C., Ammann, A. J., Good, R. A., and Hong, R.: Progressive lymphoid system deterioration: A new familial lymphopenic immunological deficiency disease. Clin. Exper. Immunol., 6:169, 1970.
93. Sell, S.: Development of restrictions in the expression of immunoglobulin specificities by lymphoid cells. Transplant. Rev., 5:19, 1970.
94. Sell, S.: Studies on rabbit lymphocytes in vitro. V. The induction of blast transformation with sheep antisera to rabbit IgG subunits, J. Exper. Med., 125:289, 1967.
95. Sell, S.: Studies on rabbit lymphocytes in vitro. VI. The induction of blast transformation with sheep antisera to rabbit IgA and IgM, J. Exper. Med., 125:393, 1967.
96. Sell, S., Hughes, S. J., and Mascari, R. A.: In vitro stimulation of rabbit peripheral blood, thymus, spleen and peritoneal exudate cells with phytohemagglutinin, staphylococcal

filtrate, concavalian A, anti-lymphocytic, anti-immunoglobulin and anti-allotypic sera. *In* Harris, J., Ed.: Proceedings of the Fifth Leucocyte Culture Conference. New York, Academic Press, 1970.

97. Simons, M. J., and Fitzgerald, M. G.: Apparent dissociation of antigen responsiveness and antibody production by human small lymphocytes in culture. Clin. Exper. Immunol., 4:55, 1969.
98. Stayner, L., and Schwarz, M. R.: The response of long and short-lived small lymphocytes of the rat to pokeweed mitogen. J. Immunol., 102:1260, 1969.
99. Stockman, G. D., Gallagher, M. T., Heim, L. R., South, M. A., and Trentin, J. J.: Differential stimulation of mouse lymphoid cells by phytohemagglutinin and pokeweed mitogen. Proc. Soc. Exper. Biol. Med., 136:980, 1971.
100. Stutman, O.: Hemopoietic origin of cells responding to Phytohemagglutinin in mouse lymph nodes. *In* Harris, J., Ed.: Proceedings of the Fifth Leucocyte Culture Conference. New York, Academic Press, 1970.
101. Tormey, D. C., Kamin, R., and Fudenberg, H. H.: Quantitative studies of phytohemagglutinin-induced DNA and RNA synthesis in normal and agammaglobulinemic leukocytes. J. Exper. Med., 125:863, 1967.
102. Walters, C. S., and Wigzell, H.: Demonstration of heavy and light chain antigenic determinants on the cell-bound receptor for antigen. J. Exper. Med., 132:1233, 1970.
103. Warner, N. L., Byrt, P., and Ada, G. L.: Blocking of the lymphocyte antigen receptor site with anti-immunoglobulin sera in vitro. Nature, 226:942, 1970.
104. Wilson, D. B., Silvers, W. K., and Nowell, P. C.: Quantitative studies on the mixed lymphocyte interaction in rats. II. Relationship of the proliferative response to the immunologic status of the donors. J. Exper. Med., 126:655, 1967.
105. Winkelstein, A.: Augmentation of PHA responsiveness in mixed thymus-marrow cultures. J. Immunol., 107:195, 1971.

Hôpital du Saint-Sacrement
Quebec City, Quebec
Canada

The Heterogeneity of Lymphocytes

A Consideration of Future Developments and Their Impact on Clinical Medicine

Maxwell Richter, Ph.D., M.D.,* and David Algom, M.D.**

The past two decades have been witness to a remarkable shift in the conceptualization and understanding of the role of the lymphocyte, from the secure position of viewing the lymphocyte as a single type of cell with constant and unchanging morphology and function, to that of viewing it as a multi- or toti-potent cell. Its capacities to generate or transform into other cell types appear to be unlimited, and its heterogeneous nature is today taken for granted. Whether there exists a single or multiple precursors of the mature lymphocyte is for the moment an academic question. This review is not concerned with the ontogenic development of the lymphocytes during embryogenesis and the immediate postnatal period, but will focus on the situation as it exists in the adult, immunologically mature individual. It is the intention of the authors to relate the concept of lymphocyte diversity with the cell mechanisms involved in the immune response, both humoral and cell-mediated. The approach presented is a pragmatic one which we feel will be appreciated by clinicians whose interest in the lymphocytes is dictated by the role which this cell plays in (a) the evolution of a variety of diseased states, such as autoimmune diseases and the various immunodeficiency states, the etiology and pathogenesis of which are still only vaguely understood, and (b) immune responses, either beneficial or detrimental to the host, such as tumor immunity and graft rejection, respectively.

The concept of the heterogeneity of the lymphocyte is a recent one, having been accepted only in the past 20 years. Until recently, the lymphocytes were considered to constitute a relatively homogeneous population of cells in the animal body, albeit segregated into the different

From the Harry Webster Thorp Laboratories, Division of Immunochemistry and Allergy, McGill University Clinic, Royal Victoria Hospital, Montreal, Quebec, Canada

*Associate Professor, Department of Experimental Medicine, McGill University; Associated Scientist, Royal Victoria Hospital
**Instructor, Internal Medicine, Tel Aviv University Medical School, Tel Aviv; Senior Resident, Beilinson Hospital, Petah Tikva, Israel

parenchymal lymphoid organs. It must be remembered that the role of the lymphocyte in immunity was not recognized until the late 1930's[21–23, 34, 35, 42, 43] and therefore an understanding of its functions was based solely on conjecture and was considered to be a single and uniform one to tie in with its constant morphology. The morphologists' rather simplistic picture of the lymphocyte, with its relatively large nucleus and thin rim of cytoplasm, appears to have impressed upon the immunologist and lymphologist a desire to paint a similar simple picture with respect to the function of these cells in the immune response. The result was that up to the mid 1960's the prevailing view held that antibody synthesis was the function of a single type of lymphocyte, which as a result of antigenic stimulation, underwent a series of morphologic changes and mitotic divisions to give rise to identical progeny endowed with the faculty to synthesize antibody molecules.[37, 40, 66, 67] However, three findings during the past decade have necessitated a re-evaluation of this view:

1. The demonstration of a division of the lymphoid system immunologically and nonimmunologically into central and peripheral lymphoid organs.[15, 20, 24, 34, 41, 46, 54] A central lymphoid organ is one whose extirpation, either in utero or in the early postnatal period, results in an alteration of the normal histology in any other lymphoid organ. Both the thymus and the avian bursa of Fabricius have been shown to satisfy this criterion. Fortuitously, these organs also appear to possess a central role immunologically. It has been demonstrated that extirpation of the thymus results in a diminished capacity to manifest cell-mediated immunity,[36, 39, 44, 46] while excision of the bursa results in a profound diminution of humoral antibody formation.[4, 31, 70, 71]

2. The demonstration that the interaction of at least two types of morphologically identical lymphocytes are required in order to facilitate the humoral immune response.[1, 11, 17, 45, 51, 68] These cells are functionally different in that the initial cell, referred to as the antigen reactive cell (ARC), is capable of interacting with the antigen but is unable to transform into or give rise to the second type of cell, the antibody-forming cell (AFC), which appears to arise from a different clone or line of cells.

3. The recognition of the immunodeficiency syndromes and the realization that spontaneously occurring immunodeficiency states in man and similar conditions induced in animals, as a result of extirpation of either the thymus or the bursa of Fabricius, are characterized by a loss of function attributed to one or other of the functionally different types of lymphocytes.[5, 29, 30–32, 61]

These three basic findings set the stage for a large series of investigations concerned with other than immunologic properties of the lymphocytes. The results of these investigations have wrought a fundamental change in our consideration of the lymphocyte, the unequivocal abandonment of the concept of lymphocyte homogeneity. These studies can be broadly categorized on the basis of specific critera. These properties will be enumerated rather than discussed since the references given provide for extensive discussion and review of the subjects listed.

NONIMMUNOLOGIC CRITERIA

Studies Which Demonstrate the Physicochemical Heterogeneity of the Lymphocytes

Centrifugation of lymphocytes in a density gradient results in the separation of the lymphocytes into 3 to 5 fractions, the cells of which display varying degrees of reactivity to nonspecific mitogenic agents and of immunocompetence.[3, 6, 16, 47] Passage of lymphocytes through columns of glass beads facilitates their separation on the basis of size.[50, 52, 55] However, the beads have a tendency to retain a large fraction of the lymphocytes applied originally to the column.

Studies Which Demonstrate Differences in the Behavioral Patterns of the Lymphocyte

DIFFERENCES IN THE MIGRATION PATHWAYS OF THE CELLS IN VIVO, UNDER A NUMBER OF DIFFERENT EXPERIMENTAL CONDITIONS. It has been demonstrated, for example, that bone marrow lymphocytes enter the thymus more readily than other lymphocytes,[27] that thoracic duct cells do not enter the thymus,[28] and that the recirculating cell, which is probably a thymus-derived or thymus-dependent cell,[20, 28, 31] segregates mostly to the lymph nodes.[73] This subject is extensively covered in references 20, 25, 26, 28, 31, and 54.

DIFFERENCES IN THE ORGAN DEPENDENCY OF THE CELLS. Certain lymphocytes localized to one lymphoid organ are dependent on the influence of a second organ in order to remain viable and to proliferate. Examples are the thymus-dependent cells and the bursal or bone marrow-dependent cells in the lymph node and spleen[15, 20, 24, 31, 41, 46, 54] (Fig. 1).

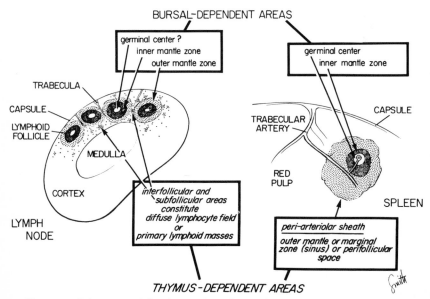

Figure 1. Delineation of the thymus-dependent and bursal-dependent lymphoid compartments in the lymph node and spleen.

These lymphocytes appear to be confluent with other lymphocytes with which they share identical morphology. However, they disappear from their normal sites following extirpation of either the thymus or the bursa of Fabricius in the chicken or the SAPP organs (sacculus rotundus, appendix and Peyer's patches) in the rabbit, which appear to constitute the bursal homologue in this animal.[31]

Table 1 presents a summary of the different lymphoid cell compartments already alluded to, as well as those which we may anticipate will soon be demonstrated to constitute unique lymphoid cell compartments. For the present, these latter are presented with question marks in the table. The demonstrations of such compartments will provide the opportunity to analyze the role of each of the lymphoid organs in the maintenance of the general lymphocyte pool and in the mediation of humoral and cellular immunity.

DIFFERENCES IN THE LIFE-SPANS OF THE CELLS. Lymphocytes can be differentiated into short-lived (4 to 8 days) and long-lived (weeks to months) cells.[10, 25, 26, 31, 50, 54] Results of recent investigations suggest that, although the thymocyte itself is a short-lived cell, nevertheless the progeny of these cells, referred to as thymus-derived or T-cells, are long-lived[54] (Fig. 2). The relationship between the longevity of the cell and its organ dependency remains to be determined.

DIFFERENCES IN THE SENSITIVITY OF LYMPHOCYTES TO STEROIDS AND IMMUNOSUPPRESSANT DRUGS. Sahiar and Schwartz[62] observed that the germinal centers of follicles in the lymph node tend to hypertrophy whereas those in the spleen involute as a result of 6-mercaptopurine injection. The thymus involutes dramatically in response to cortisone administration,[9, 13] but it is interesting to note that the small residual population of thymocytes which are steroid resistant are immunocompetent, both in humoral[12, 13] and cell-mediated[9] immunity. Bone marrow lympho-

Table 1. *Organ of Origin, Derivation, and Dependency of Lymphoid Cells*

ORGAN OF ORIGIN	ORGAN OF DERIVATION	ORGAN OF DEPENDENCY
Bone marrow lymphocytes	Bone marrow-derived lymphocytes	Bone marrow-dependent lymphocytes
Thymus lymphocytes	Thymus-derived lymphocytes	Thymus-dependent lymphocytes
Bursal lymphocytes	Bursal-derived lymphocytes	Bursal-dependent lymphocytes
Lymph node lymphocytes	Lymph node-derived lymphocytes ?	Lymph node-dependent lymphocytes ?
Spleen lympocytes	Spleen-derived lymphocytes ?	Spleen-dependent lymphocytes ?
Appendix lymphocytes	Appendix-derived lymphocytes ?	Appendix-dependent lymphocytes ?
Sacculous rotundus lymphocytes	Sacculus rotundus-derived lymphocytes ?	Sacculus rotundus-derived lymphocytes ?
Peyer's patches lymphocytes	Peyer's patches-derived lymphocytes ?	Peyer's patches-dependent lymphocytes ?
Circulating lymphocytes	–	–

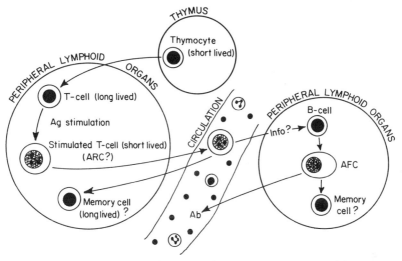

Figure 2.   Relation between the lifespan of the thymus lymphocytes and their role in the humoral immune response. In the mouse, the ARC and AFC are considered to be of thymic and bone marrow origin, respectively (see text). The T-cell or thymic dependent cell is long lived, unlike the thymocyte itself which is short lived.[54]

cytes, especially those participating in the immune response, are resistant to the lytic action of corticosteroids.[13]

Studies Which Demonstrate Antigenic Differences Among Lymphocytes

In a series of beautifully executed experiments, Raff and his colleagues[56] have demonstrated that the thymus-derived cells (T-lymphocytes) in the mouse possess a surface antigen, called theta, not detected on the surface of other unrelated lymphocytes. This observation has since been confirmed by other investigators.[14, 53, 57, 63, 69, 72] This same group of investigators[56, 57] has also observed that the bone marrow-derived lymphocyte (B-lymphocytes) may be characterized by the presence on its surface of a specific antigen which differentiates this cell from the other lymphocytes in the lymphoid cell pool. Findings of a similar nature have been observed with rabbit lymphoid cells. Rabbit thymus cells can be characterized by the presence of a specific antigen not found on the surface of lymphocytes in any of the other lymphoid organs.[49] Results of current investigation, of a preliminary nature, suggest that the rabbit bone marrow and appendix possess organ specific antigens as well.[49]

Studies Which Permit Differentiation of Lymphocytes on the Basis of Their Response to Mitogenic Agents in Vitro

The response of the lymphocytes of the different lymphoid organs of the rabbit to stimulation with phytohemagglutinin (PHA) was investigated in an in vitro system. It was observed that the cells of the different organs could be characterized on the basis of (a) the speed of response to PHA, (b) the extent of the response, (c) the duration of the response, (d) the concentration of the cells in culture required to facilitate an optimal response and (e) the sensitivity of the cells to PHA.[64] The cells of the different lymphoid organs presented with individualized profiles of response which permit their discrimination with respect to their organ source.[64]

IMMUNOLOGIC CRITERIA

Knowledge of the heterogeneity of the lymphocyte constitutes only a single dimension with respect to the study of the lymphocyte. As in other biologically oriented fields, the impetus which provides the direction of study is dictated largely by the clinical application of the potential or anticipated findings. The demonstration of the unique role of the lymphocyte in such unrelated areas as autoimmune disease, transplantation rejection, cancer immunity, and immunodeficiency disease has necessitated a more refined approach toward the lymphocyte other than the "all-or-none" approach of contemporary chemotherapy, i.e., total lymphocyte depletion afforded by the so-called immunosuppressive agents administered under the guise of chemotherapy. The demonstration of lymphocyte heterogeneity introduced a new equation into the problem, the resolution of which may reside in the finding that a specific family of lymphocytes may be singled out as the causative agent in the particular condition being investigated and that these lymphocytes may be eliminated or inactivated by specifically directed immunotherapeutic or chemotherapeutic agents in such a way as to inflict the least harm onto the bystander lymphocyte population. This should be the ultimate goal of the investigators concerned with lymphocyte heterogeneity.

There are a number of immunologic criteria which can be applied to further define lymphocyte heterogeneity.

Heterogeneity of the Cells Mediating the Humoral Immune Response

It has been shown that in both the mouse[11, 17, 45, 51, 68] and the rabbit[1, 58] at least two functionally distinct but morphologically identical types of lymphocytes are required to interact in order to facilitate antibody formation. These two cells are referred to as the antigen-reactive cell (ARC) and the antibody-forming cell (AFC). The ARC is characterized by its ability to interact with the antigen and undergo a proliferative response;[17, 19] however, this cell is unable to synthesize antibodies.[11, 17, 18, 45, 51, 68] The AFC is defined as the cell which synthesizes and releases antibody molecules into the circulation.[1] In the immunologically mature mouse, the organ sources of the ARC and AFC are the thymus and bone marrow, respectively[11, 17, 45, 51, 68] (Fig. 2). Whether the memory cell is of thymic or bone marrow origin has not as yet been unequivocally determined. The organ source of the ARC in the immunologically mature rabbit is the bone marrow,[1, 59] while the organ source of the AFC has not as yet been clearly defined (Table 2). Furthermore, in both of these animal species, the spleen constitutes the organ source of the memory cells. Whether the memory cell can be further dif-

Table 2.   *Organ Source(s) of the Cells Mediating*
Humoral Immunity in the Adult Animal

Organ source(s) of virgin antigen-reactive cells (ARC)
Bone marrow (rabbit)
Thymus   (mouse, rat)
Spleen ?   (mouse, rat)

Organ source(s) of virgin antibody-forming cells (AFC)
?   (rabbit)
Bone marrow (mouse, rat)

Organ source(s) of memory cells
Spleen   (rabbit)
Spleen   (mouse, rat)

In the *unimmunized* animal, the CIRCULATION is devoid of immunocompetent cells.

---

ferentiated from the virgin ARC and AFC by other criteria, such as antigenic specificity, remains to be determined.

Difference Between Cells Participating in Humoral and Cell-Mediated Immunity (CMI)

The organ sources of the cells participating in CMI are presented in Table 3 (reviewed in ref. 7). Through a variety of experimental procedures, it has been observed that a number of lymphoid organs serve as sources of these cells in the rabbit, mouse, and rat. It is of interest, however, that these organs do not overlap with those which serve as the sources of the cells participating in humoral immunity (Table 2).

The Probable Heterogeneity of Cells Participating in the Different Cell-Mediated Immune Responses

In view of the large number of different reactions considered to be representative of cell-mediated immunity (Table 4), it is quite probable that the cells participating in these different reactions are different.

Table 3.   *Organ Source(s) of Cells Participating in*
Cell-Mediated Immunity in the Adult Animal

Organ source of virgin effector cell
Circulation ⎫
Spleen   ⎪
Lymph node   ⎬   mouse and rat
Peyer's patches ⎭

Circulation   ⎫
Appendix   ⎪
Sacculus rotundus ⎬ rabbit
Peyer's patches   ⎪
(Spleen)   ⎪
(Lymph node)   ⎭

In the *unimmunized* animal, the CIRCULATION contains effector cell(s) in a state most highly susceptible to antigenic stimulation.

Table 4. *Cell-Mediated Immunity*

In Vivo
  Transplant rejection
  Autoimmune lesion
  Delayed hypersensitivity skin reaction
  Normal lymphocyte transfer reaction (NLTR)
  Inflammation following transfer under kidney capsule in homologous
      animal
  Tumor immunity

In Vitro
  Target cell lysis
  Blastogenic response to mitogenic agents (i.e., PHA)
  Graft-versus-graft (or cell-versus-cell) reaction
  Inhibition of migration
  Release of migration inhibitory factor following interaction of antigen
      and sensitized cells
  Mixed leukocyte culture (MLC) reaction; blastogenic response to allo-
      geneic lymphocyte stimulation

Heterogeneous Nature of the Immunocyte Pathways

Antigens can be differentiated on the basis of their being ARC-dependent and ARC-independent.[1] Thus, some antigens can by-pass the ARC and act directly on the AFC (Table 5). However, it is possible that the AFC stimulated directly by an ARC-independent antigen is different from the AFC which is stimulated by the ARC-dependent antigen. Similarly, recent investigations have disclosed that the mechanisms, and therefore probably the cells involved, in allogeneic and xenogeneic graft rejection are different[33, 39] (Table 5). It would appear that rejection of allogeneic cells is mediated by a single effector cell,[33] whereas rejection of xenogeneic cells requires the participation of two cells, the respondent and effector cells.[39]

Differences Between Cells Participating in Humoral and Cell-Mediated Immunity on the Basis of their Migration Pathways in Vivo

As can be seen in Figures 3 to 5, the migration pathways of the virgin ARCs, AFCs, memory cells, and effector cells are different. It is

Table 5. *Heterogeneity of the Cell Pathways in the Expression of the Immune Response*

TYPE OF IMMUNITY	STIMULANT	NUMBER OF CELL TYPES INVOLVED
Humoral	ARC-dependent antigen	2 (ARC and AFC)
	ARC-independent antigen	1 (AFC only)
Cell-mediated	Allogenic cell rejection	1 (effector cell only)
	Xenogeneic cell rejection	2 (respondent and effector cells)

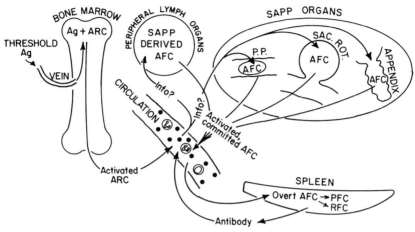

Figure 3. The organ sources and migration pathway of the virgin ARC and AFC in the immunologically mature rabbit following immunization with antigen in threshold concentration. Ag = antigen; ARC = antigen-reactive cell; AFC = antibody-forming cell; RFC = rosette-forming cell; PFC = plaque-forming cell

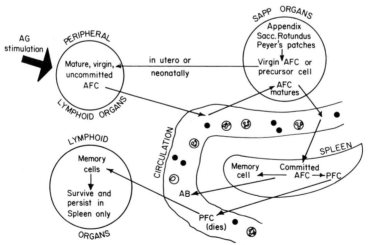

Figure 4. The relationship between the virgin antibody-forming cells and the memory cells. Their ontogenic origin and migration pathways following immunization with antigen in threshold concentration.

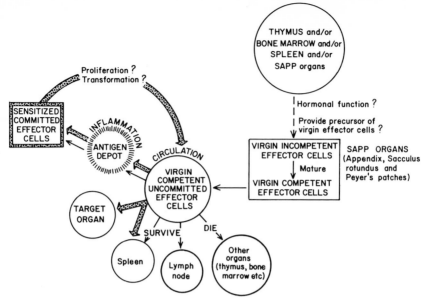

Figure 5.   The organ source of the virgin immunocompetent effector cells mediating the cellular immune reaction. A schematic representation.

suggested that these differences can be translated into functional or behavioral differences of the cell types involved, since the predisposition of a cell to home in on a particular organ must be predicted by specific properties of the cells concerned. It has been observed that, in the rabbit, the ARC vacates the bone marrow following antigenic stimulation.[1, 2, 65] However, its destination is still to be determined. The source of the virgin AFC is not known, but at least one of the organs to which it migrates during its maturation stage is the Peyer's patches.[8] From there, it migrates to the spleen, where it matures into the overt AFC.[8] The migration pathway of the antigen-stimulated immunocompetent cells in the mouse and rat has not been investigated to date.

As will surely be appreciated by the reader, the subject matter covered in this short review is only now beginning to emerge from its state of infancy. Newer techniques of labelling the lymphocytes, the anticipated discovery of more antigens specific to particular populations of lymphocytes, and more sophisticated approaches to the study of the migration of lymphocytes, especially immunocytes, should soon lead to a veritable explosion in our knowledge concerning the delicate interrelationships which the different families of lymphocytes have with each other. Progress in this area cannot but provide a basis for a better understanding of the manner whereby lymphocyte activity manifests itself as a pathologic lesion. The elucidation of the different immunodeficiency states will be categorized in terms of the specific types of lymphocytes affected rather than only in terms of symptoms and laboratory diagnosis. The establishment of cause and effect relationships with respect to certain lymphocyte types will stimulate studies into methods for altering the normal situation with respect to these effector, but not other, lymphocytes. Thus will probably emerge a new field concerned with the biomanipulation of lymphocyte populations, directed toward the elimination of those lymphocytes which are involved in the pathogenesis of the specific disease and their replacement by lymphocytes of a more inocuous type. Although we cannot predict with certainty the future developments in this field, we may rest assured that they will usher in a new mode of therapy of the diseases characterized by a malfunction of or inappropriate activity by the lymphocyte.

REFERENCES

1. Abdou, N. I., and Richter, M.: The role of the bone marrow in the immune response. Adv. Immunol., 12:201, 1970.
2. Abdou, N. I., and Richter, M.: Cells involved in the immune response. VI. The immune response to red blood cells in irradiated rabbits after administration of normal, primed or immune allogeneic rabbit bone marrow cells. J. Exper. Med., 129:757, 1969.
3. Adler, W. H., Peary, D., and Smith, R. T.: The effect of PHA, PPD, allogeneic cells and sheep erythrocytes on albumin gradient-fractionated mouse spleen cell populations. Cell Immunol., 1:78, 1970.
4. Alm, G. V.: In vitro studies of chicken lymphoid cells. II. The anamnestic response of spleen cells from control-irradiated and bursectomized-irradiated chickens to sheep erythrocytes. Int. Arch. Allergy, 40:643, 1971.
5. Arnason, B. G., Jankovic, B. D., Waksman, B. H., and Wennerstein, C.: Role of the thymus in immune reactions in rats. II. Suppressive effect of thymectomy at birth on reactions of delayed (cellular) hypersensitivity and the circulating small lymphocyte. J. Exper. Med., 116:177, 1962.
6. August, C. S., Merler, E., Lucas, D. O., and Janeway, C. A.: The response in vitro of human lymphocytes to phytohemagglutinin and to antigens after fractionation on discontinuous density gradients of albumin. Cell Immunol., 1:603, 1970.
7. Behelak, Y., and Richter, M.: Cells involved in cell-mediated and trasnplantation immunity. III. The organ source(s) of the cells in the normal rabbit which mediate a reaction of cellular immunity in vitro. Cell Immunol., in press.
8. Behelak, Y., and Richter, M.: Manuscript in preparation.
9. Blomgren, H., and Svedmyr, E.: In vitro stimulation of mouse thymus cells by PHA and allogeneic cells. Cell Immunol., 2:285, 1971.
10. Buckton, K. E., Court-Brown, W. M., and Smith, P. G.: Lymphocyte survival in man treated with x-rays for ankylosing spondylitis. Nature, 214:470, 1967.
11. Claman, H. N., and Chaperon, E. A.: Immunologic complementation between thymus and narrow cells – a model for the two-cell theory of immunocompetence. Transplant. Rev., 1:92, 1969.
12. Cohen, J. J., Fischbach, M., and Claman, H. N.: Hydrocortisone resistance of graft-versus-host activity in mouse thymus, spleen and bone marrow. Immunology, 105:1146, 1970.
13. Cohen, J. J., and Claman, H. N.: Thymus-marrow immunocompetence. V. Hydrocortisone-resistant cells and processes in the hemolytic antibody response of mice. J. Exper. Med., 133:1026, 1971.
14. Colley, D. G., Malakion, A., and Waksman, B. H.: Cellular differentiation in the thymus. II. Thymus-specific antigens in rat thymus and peripheral lymphoid cells. J. Immunol., 104:585, 1970.
15. Cooper, M. D., Peterson, R. D. A., Smith, M. D., and Good, R. A.: The functions of the thymus system and the bursa system in the chicken. J. Exper. Med., 123:75, 1966.
16. Cutts, J. H.: Cell Separation Methods in Hematology. New York, Academic Press, 1970.
17. Davies, A. J. S.: The thymus and the cellular basis of immunity. Transplant. Rev., 1:43, 1969.
18. Davies, A. J. S., Leuchars, E., Wallis, V., Marchant, R., and Elliot, E. V.: The failure of thymus-derived cells to produce antibody. Transplantation, 5:222, 1967.
19. Davies, A. J. S., Leuchars, E., Wallis, V., and Koller, P. C.: The mitotic response of thymus-derived cells to antigen stimulation. Transplantation, 4:438, 1966.
20. Doenhoff, M. J., Davies, A. J. S., Leuchars, E., and Wallis, V.: The thymus and circulating lymphocytes of mice. Proc. Roy. Soc. Med., 176:69, 1970.
21. Dougherty, T. F., Chase, J. H., and White, A.: The demonstration of antibodies in lymphocytes. Proc. Soc. Exper. Biol., 57:295, 1944.

22. Ehrich, W. E., and Harris, T. N.: The formation of antibodies in the popliteal lymph node in rabbits. J. Exper. Med., 76:335, 1942.

23. Elves, M. W.: The Lymphocyte. Chicago, Illinois, Year Book Medical Publishers, 1967.

24. Everett, N. B., Rieke, W. O., and Caffrey, R. W.: The kinetics of small lymphocytes in the rat with special reference to those of thymic origin. *In* Good, R. A., and Gabrielson, A. E., eds.: The Thymus in Immunobiology. New York, Harper and Row, 1964.

25. Everett, N. B., Caffrey, R. W., and Rieke, W. O.: Recirculation of lymphocytes. Ann. N.Y. Acad. Sci., 113:887, 1964.

26. Everett, N. B., and Tyler, R. W.: Lymphopoiesis in the thymus and other tissues: Functional implications. Int. Rev. Cytol., 22:205, 1967.

27. Ford, C. E., and Micklem, H. S.: The thymus and lymph nodes in radiation chimaeras. Lancet, 1:359, 1963.

28. Ford, W. L., and Gowans, J. L.: The traffic of lymphocytes. Seminars Hematol., 6:67, 1969.

29. Freedman, S. O.: Clinical Immunology. New York, Harper and Row, 1971.

30. Fulginiti, V. A., Hathaway, W. E., Perlman, D. S., Blackburn, W. R., Githens, J. H., Claman, H. N., and Kempe, C. H.: Dissociation of delayed hypersensitivity and antibody-synthesizing capacity in man: Report of two sibships with thymic dyplasia, lymphoid tissue depletion and normal immunoglobulins. Lancet, 2:5, 1966.

31. Gatti, R. A., Stutman, O., and Good, R. A.: The lymphoid system. Ann. Rev. Physiol., 32:529, 1970.

32. Gatti, R. A., and Good, R. A.: The immunological deficiency diseases. Med. CLIN. N. AMER., 54:281, 1970.

33. Harding, B., Pudifin, D. J., Gotch, F., and MacLennan, I. C. M.: Cytotoxic lymphocytes from rats depleted of thymus processed cells. Nature New Biology, 232:80, 1971.

34. Harris, T. N., Grimm, E., Mortens, E., and Ehrich, W. E.: The role of the lymphocyte in antibody formation. J. Exper. Med., 81:73, 1945.

35. Harris, T. N., and Harris, S.: Biological and technical factors in the demonstration of antibody production by lymphatic tissues. J. Immunol., 64:45, 1950.

36. Hess, M. W.: Experimental Thymectomy, Possibilities and Limitations. Exper. Med., Path. Klinik. New York, Springer-Verlag, Publishers, 1968, vol. 25.

37. Jerne, N. J.: Summary: Waiting for the end. Symp. Quant. Biol., 32:591, 1967.

38. Levine, M. A., and Claman, H. N.: Bone marrow and spleen, dissociation of immunologic properties by cortisone. Science, 167:1515, 1970.

39. MacLennan, I. C. M., and Harding, B.: The role of immunoglobulins in lymphocyte-mediated cell damage in vitro. II. The mechanism of target cell damage by lymphoid cells from immunized rats. Immunol., 18:405, 1970.

40. Makela, O., Cross, A. M., and Ruoslahti, E.: Similarities between the cellular receptor antibody and the secreted antibody. *In* Smith, R. T., and Good, R. A., eds.: Cellular Recognition. New York, Appleton-Century-Crofts, 1969.

41. McKneally, M. F., Sutherland, D. E. R., and Good, R. A.: The central lymphoid tissues of rabbits. II. Functional and morphological studies in adult animals. Surgery, 69:345, 1971.

42. McMaster, P. D.: Sites of antibody formation. *In* pappenheimer, A. M., Jr., ed.: The Nature and Significance of the Antibody Response. New York, Columbia University Press, 1953.

43. McMaster, P. D., and Hudack, S. S.: The formation of agglutinins within lymph nodes. J. Exper. Med., 61:783, 1935.

44. Metcalf, D.: The Thymus. Recent Results in Cancer Research, New York, Springer-Verlag, vol. 5, 1966.

45. Miller, J. F. A. P., and Mitchell, G. F.: Thymus and antigen-reactive cells. Transplant. Rev., 1:3, 1969.

46. Miller, J. F. A. P., and Osoba, D.: Current concepts of the immunological function of the thymus. Physiol. Rev., 47:437, 1967.

47. Mishell, R. I., Dutton, R. W., and Raidt, D. J.: Cell components in the immune response. I. Gradient separation of immune cells. Cell Immunol., 1:175, 1970.

48. Nossal, G. J. V., Shortman, K. D., Miller, J. F. A. P., Mitchell, G. F., and Haskill, J. S.: The target cell in the induction of immunity and tolerance. Symp. Quant. Biol., 32:369, 1967.

49. de la Noue, H. C., Koperstych, S., and Richter, M.: In preparation.

50. Oppenheim, J. T., Leventhal, B. G., and Hersh, E. M.: The transformation of column-purified lymphocytes with non-specific and specific antigenic stimuli. J. Immunol., 101:262, 1968.

51. Playfair, J. H. L.: Cell Cooperation in the immune response. Clin. Exper. Immunol., 8:839, 1971.

52. Plotz, P. H., and Talal, N.: Fractionation of splenic antibody-forming cells on glass bead columns. J. Immunol., 99:1236, 1967.

53. Potworoswski, E. F., and Nairn, R. C.: Origin and fate of a thymocyte-specific antigen. Immunol., 13:597, 1967.

54. Parrot, D. M. V., and de Sousa, M.: Thymus-dependent and thymus-independent populations: origin, migratory patterns and lifespan. Clin. Exper. Immunol., 8:663, 1971.
55. Rabinowitz, Y.: Separation of lymphocytes, polymorphonuclear leukcocytes and monocytes on glass bead columns, including tissue culture observations. Blood, 23:811, 1964.
56. Raff, M. C.: Surface antigenic markers for distinguishing T and B lymphocytes in mice. Transplant. Rev., 6:52, 1971.
57. Raff, M. C., Nase, S., and Mitchison, N. A.: Mouse specific bone marrow-derived lymphocyte antigen as a marker for thymus-independent lymphocytes. Nature, 230:50, 1971.
58. Richter, M., and Abdou, N. I.: Cells involved in the immune response. VII. The demonstration, using allotype markers, of antibody formation by radioresistant cells of irradiated rabbits injected with normal allogeneic bone marrow cells and sheep erythrocytes. J. Exper. Med., 129:1261, 1969.
59. Richter, M., Rose, B., and Abdou, N. I.: Cells involved in the immune response. XV. The organ source of the antigen-reactive cell (ARC) in the normal rabbit. Int. Arch. Allergy, 28:269, 1970.
60. Robinson, S. H., Brecker, G., Laurie, I. S., and Haley, J. E.: Leukocyte labelling in rats during and after continuous infusion of tritiated thymidine: Implications for lymphocyte longevity and DNA reutilization. Blood, 26:281, 1965.
61. Rosen, F. A.: The thymus gland and the immune deficiency syndrome. In Samter, M., ed.: Immunological diseases. Boston, Little, Brown and Co., 1971.
62. Sahiar, K., and Schwartz, R. S.: The immunoglobulin sequence. II. Histological effects of the suppression of M and G antibody synthesis. Int. Arch. Allergy, 29:52, 1966.
63. Schlesinger, M., and Yron, I.: Antigenic changes in lymph node cells after administration of antiserum to thymus cells. Science, 164:1412, 1969.
64. Singhal, S. K., Daguillard, F., and Richter, M.: Cells involved in the immune response. II. The response of normal rabbit hemopoietic and lymphopoietic cells to phytohemagglutinin in vitro. Int. Arch. Allergy, 34:119, 1968.
65. Singhal, S. K., and Richter, M.: Cells involved in the immune response. IV. The response of normal and immune rabbit bone marrow and lymphoid tissue lymphocytes to antigens in vitro. J. Exper. Med., 128:1099, 1968.
66. Siskind, G. W., and Benacerraf, B.: Cell selection by antigen in the immune response. Adv. Immunol., 10:1, 1969.
67. Starzl, J., and Silverstein, A. M.: Developmental aspects of immunity. Adv. Immunol., 6:337, 1967.
68. Taylor, R. B.: Cellular cooperation in the antibody response of mice to two serum albumins: Soecific function of thymus cells. Transplant. Rev., 1:114, 1969.
69. Waksman, B. H.: Study of functional lymphocyte populations with heterologous antisera. Transplant. Rev., 6:30, 1971.
70. Warner, N. L., Ovary, Z., and Kantor, F. S.: Delayed hypersensitivity reactions in normal and bursectomized chickens. Int. Arch. Allergy, 40:719, 1971.
71. Warner, N. L., Uhr, J. W., Thorbecke, G. J., and Ovary, Z.: Immunoglobulins, antibodies and the bursa of Fabricius: induction of agammaglobulinemia and the loss of antibody-forming capacity by hormonal bursectomy. J. Immunol., 103:1317, 1969.
72. Williams, R. M., Chanana, A. D., Cronkite, E. P., and Waskman, B. H.: Antigenic markers on cells leaving calf thymus by way of the efferent lymph and venous blood. J. Immunol., 106:1143, 1971.
73. Zatz, M. M., and Lance, E. M.: The distribution of chromium-31 labelled lymphoid cells in the mouse. A survey of anatomical compartments. Cell Immunol., 1:3, 1970.

Royal Victoria Hospital
687 Pine Avenue
Montreal, Quebec
Canada

Thymic Function, Immunologic Deficiency, and Autoimmunity

David Osoba, M.D., F.R.C.P.(C)*

There has been a rapid expansion of knowledge relating to the functions of the thymus since the demonstration, 10 years ago, that the thymus plays an important role in immunity.[88, 100] From experiments in mice[18, 61, 109] and in cell culture systems,[70, 108, 112, 139] it is now evident that the formation of 19S hemolytic antibodies to sheep erythrocytes is dependent upon interactions between at least three separate classes of cells. These classes of cells, found in the spleen and lymph nodes, are "helper" T cells (derived from the thymus), B cells (probably derived from the bone marrow in mammals and from the bursa of Fabricius in birds), and A cells. Cell-mediated immune responses are dependent upon effector cells arising from thymus-derived T cells[16] that are probably different than the "helper" T cells involved in antibody formation.[84] The roles of these cells will be considered more fully in the sections dealing with humoral and cell-mediated immunity. From the study of immunologic deficiency diseases in man it has become evident that these diseases can be explained on the basis of knowledge derived from experimental animal models. This knowledge will lead to therapeutic strategies capable of curing, or at least controlling, most of these diseases in the near future. My purpose in this paper is to suggest a view of the pathogenesis of immunologic deficiency and autoimmune diseases, based upon current concepts of the development and differentiation of the immunologic system.

DEVELOPMENT OF THE IMMUNOLOGIC SYSTEM

In the human being, the epithelial rudiment of the thymus develops from clusters of cells in the foregut endoderm of the third and fourth

*Assistant Professor, Department of Medicine, University of Toronto; Associate of the Medical Research Council of Canada

Portions of the work cited were supported by the Medical Research Council of Canada (MA-1609) and the Ontario Cancer Treatment and Research Foundation (Project No. 203).

pharyngeal pouches[67] at about the sixth week of gestation.[46] Initially, the primordia for the thymus, parathyroids, and great vessels are in close proximity, but by the eighth week the thymus begins to descend into the superior mediastinum. By the tenth week lymphocytes appear in the epithelial rudiment. Although the source of these first thymic lymphocytes in man is unknown, in chicken embryos they are derived from blood-borne cells[106] which probably originate in the blood islands.

Lymphocytic colonization of the thymus, with development of the characteristic medulla and cortex, proceeds rapidly during the next few weeks. Lymphocytes appear in the blood,[117] and thereafter lymphoid development of the spleen and lymph nodes occurs. Sequestration of stem cells by the thymus probably continues throughout fetal and neonatal life and, if experimental evidence in mice[38, 68] is also true for man, the thymus continues to receive stem cells from the bone marrow even during adult life.

In the mouse, cells colonizing the thymus are closely related to stem cells (colony-forming cells) responsible for the development of the myeloid component of the hematopoietic system.[145] Indeed, both may be the progeny of a single class of stem cells capable of giving rise to the entire myeloid and lymphoid systems. That a similar situation exists in man can be inferred from some diseases which affect these stem cells.

The thymus is the site of unusually active cellular proliferation,[96] probably under the control of genetic and thymic humoral factors,[101] since the rate of proliferation is independent of antigenic stimulation.[62] Apparently, most of the cells born in the thymus also die there, since only a small proportion leave the thymus.[95] The reasons for the high death rate are unknown, but this observation has contributed to a hypothesis that the thymus is a "mutant-breeding organ".[79]

Jerne postulates that the thymus, and perhaps the bone marrow (in mammals) and the bursa of Fabricius (in birds) are sites for the proliferation of clones of cells capable of reacting with environmental (exogenous) antigens, as well as with histocompatibility antigens of other members of the same species. These clones develop from precursor cells carrying genes coding for self-antigens, but as they proliferate in the thymus, some cells will sustain random somatic mutations rendering them no longer capable of self-reactivity. Such cells will now be capable of reacting with environmental antigens, and will be allowed to survive, but those that do not sustain mutations will be suppressed and die in the thymus. The surviving cells eventually migrate to and populate the peripheral lymphoid organs.

As yet, this hypothesis has not been adequately tested, but it provides an explanation for the development of tolerance to self-antigens at the same time as the development of diversity of immune reactivity to foreign histocompatibility antigens and to exogenous antigens. In addition, a failure of the mechanism for suppressing clones of cells with self-reactivity might explain the development of autoimmune diseases.

In mice, the lymphocytes in the thymus bear a specific alloantigen, called θ.[120] This marker also identifies thymus-derived lymphocytes (T cells) in the peripheral lymphoid organs. About 35 per cent of the cells in the spleen and Peyer's patches and 65 per cent of cells in the lymph nodes are θ-positive.[114, 119] As yet, a similar marker has not been demonstrated on human thymic lymphocytes.

The first indication that immunologic responsiveness in higher animals depends upon more than one class of cells arising in diverse anatomic structures came from experiments in chickens.[24, 49, 143] In addition to the thymus, chickens have a second structure, the bursa of Fabricius, necessary for full development of immune responsiveness. The bursa develops from the epithelial endoderm of the hindgut associated with the cloaca. The bursal lymphocytes are derived from blood-borne stem cells.[105] Cells leaving the bursa populate areas of the spleen and lymph nodes anatomically distinct from those populated by thymus-derived cells.[24, 77, 114] Although the equivalent of the bursa in rabbits may be the sacculus rotundus and Peyer's patches,[23] the bursal equivalent in most mammals, including man, is unknown. However, there is indirect evidence from experiments in mice[18, 109] and from experience with immunologic deficiency diseases in man[45] to suggest that the bone marrow itself has this function.

In mice, cells derived from the bone marrow (B cells) also bear a specific antigenic marker called MBLA (mouse-specific B lymphocyte antigen).[118] Thymus cells do not have this antigen, but approximately 40 per cent of the cells in the bone marrow are MBLA-positive. Peyer's patches, spleen, and lymph nodes also contain MBLA-positive cells (70, 55, and 30 per cent, respectively).

Although T and B cells develop in separate anatomical areas, it is likely that they are the progeny of a single class of stem cells capable of populating the entire lymphoid system.[33]

A third class of cells (A, or accessory cells) also participates in humoral antibody production.[50, 61, 107, 112, 125, 131] These cells are found in the spleen and lymph nodes and are probably derived from precursors present in bone marrow.[61, 113] Whether A-cell precursors are related to the precursors of T and B cells is unknown. The roles of B, T, and A cells in the two major types of immune response will now be considered more fully.

HUMORAL IMMUNE RESPONSES

Circulating antibodies are produced in response to immunization with soluble antigens, e.g. foreign erythrocytes. In mice, the response to foreign erythrocytes is dependent upon an interaction between B, "helper" T, and A cells (see references 110 and 124 for brief reviews). B cells bear specific surface receptors capable of binding antigens.[9, 60, 112] These receptors have some of the characteristics of light (κ and λ) and heavy chains (μ).[63, 64] Before antigenic stimulation, B cells do not produce significant quantities of antibody,[18, 102] but after stimulation they proliferate and mature into antibody-forming cells.[109] Thus, B cells are the immediate precursors of antibody-forming cells. Each clone of B cells is restricted with respect to the number of specific antigens to which it can respond.[1, 32, 102, 111, 112, 116] It is still uncertain whether or not a clone of B cells is class-restricted, even though its progeny produce antibody molecules of only a single class of immunoglobulin at any given time.[15, 66, 87]

"Helper" T cells also appear to bear specific receptors for antigens,[9, 65] but thus far these receptors have been shown only to have the characteristics of κ chains.[64] "Helper" T cells do not mature into antibody-forming cells.[109] Their exact function in the interaction with B cells in humoral responses is still unclear, but from secondary responses there is evidence that when antigens are composed of hapten-carrier moieties, "helper" T cells react with the carrier portion and B cells with the hapten portion of the immunogenic molecule.[11, 103]

In contrast to B and "helper" T cells, A cells need not proliferate during an immune response.[50, 61, 125] It has been suggested that they may play a role in "processing" certain antigens, rendering these antigens more immunogenic, but may not be necessary in the immune response to all antigens.[131] If A cells do play a role in processing antigen, then it is likely that they function during the first stage of an immune response. Presumably, "helper" T and B cells are triggered at later stages.

CELL-MEDIATED IMMUNE RESPONSES

Cell-mediated responses are characteristic of delayed hypersensitivity, homograft immunity, and graft-versus-host reactions. The effector ("killer") cells are found in the circulation, thoracic duct, spleen, and lymph nodes. The mechanism by which "killer" cells destroy allogeneic cells is unknown. Up to the present time, they have not been found to secrete any known class of immunoglobulin. The "killer" cells are derived from precursors originating in the thymus and proliferate in response to foreign histocompatibility antigens.[16] It is likely that the precursors of the "killer" cells are not identical to the "helper" T cells participating in humoral immune responses, since cells having these two functions appear to have different physical properties following separation on equilibrium density gradients.[84] It is still unclear whether or not the T-cell precursors of "killer" cells bear specific surface receptors for antigens or whether the "killer" function is specific. However, they do have surface receptors which combine with anti-light-chain antisera.[63] There is growing evidence that cell-cell interactions[73, 122, 129] or interactions with the products of other cells[6] may be required for the transition of T cells into "killer" cells.

A SUMMARY OF THE CELLULAR BASIS OF IMMUNOLOGICAL RESPONSIVENESS

The cells of the immunologic system can be considered to pass through three stages of differentiation during development (Fig. 1). Cellular proliferation is an important part of all of these stages. During the first stage, pluripotential stem cells give rise to cells capable of

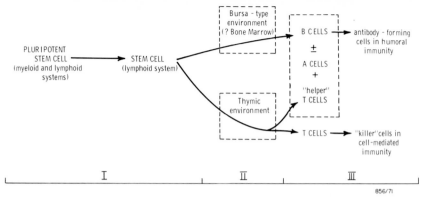

Figure 1.   A schematic representation of a model depicting cellular differentiation in the development of the immunological system. The numerals I, II, and III refer to three distinct stages in the differentiation process.

populating the lymphoid system, and these migrate to the thymus and perhaps the marrow (the equivalent of the avian bursa). Under the influence of the thymic environment and the bursa-like environment in the marrow, cells in the thymus differentiate into T cells, and those in the marrow into B cells. Each clone of B cells is restricted in its capacity to react with a variety of antigens. Thus, these cells may be considered to be immunologically committed. Whether or not T cells are restricted in their capacity to react with a variety of antigens is still unclear. The third stage is the formation of effector cells.

In cell-mediated immune responses T cells having the capacity to react with histocompatibility antigens become "killer" cells. In humoral responses to environmental antigens, "helper" T cells interact with A cells and B cells, and the B cells mature into antibody-forming cells. T cells with "killer" potential and "helper" T cells are probably not identical. Whereas the proliferation in the first two stages is independent of antigen, that in the third stage is triggered by antigen, and therefore is antigen dependent.

TESTS OF IMMUNOLOGIC FUNCTION IN MAN

Immunologic responses in man, as in animals, are classified as being humoral and cell-mediated in type. However, both the identification of the number of classes of cells involved in each kind of response, and the characterization of these cells, beyond their general morphologic identification as lymphocytes, still require much further investigation. Studies of humoral immunity in man would be aided greatly by the development of cell culture systems for the generation of antibody-forming cells. At present, it is necessary to directly challenge a patient with antigens to determine if the capacity to form a primary humoral response is present. Although such tests are useful, they require a lengthy time interval between challenge and determination of serum antibody levels, and they do not give information about the number of cells producing a specific antibody at a given time, nor about the number of precursors and possible cell-cell interactions necessary for antibody production.

On the other hand, cell culture systems which test the capacity of lymphocytes to proliferate and to participate in cell-mediated immune responses are available. The addition of phytohemagglutinin (PHA) to peripheral blood cells stimulates lymphocytes to proliferate. It is likely that it is the T cells which undergo proliferation.[17, 27] The cells of patients[83] and mice[35] with congenital absence of the thymus usually do not respond to PHA. Although the PHA response is useful for determining whether or not thymus-derived cells capable of proliferation are present in the circulation, there is little evidence that this test gives any indication of the capacity of these cells to function immunologically. This latter information is given by the one-way mixed leukocyte reaction.[7] In this test, the peripheral blood lymphocytes of the individual to be tested are cultured in the presence of allogeneic cells which have been rendered incapable of proliferation by pretreatment with appropriate drugs or irradiation. It is likely that this test detects the presence of functional T cells capable of recognizing foreign histocompatibility antigens. The cells of patients and mice[35] with congenital absence of the thymus fail to respond. Tests of cellular migration out of capillary tubes in the presence or absence of antigen show promise of being useful,[26, 36] but at present it is still unclear just what functions these procedures are testing.

Finally, skin tests of delayed hypersensitivity to a variety of antigens are also useful, but again they suffer from the defects that they must be done directly on the patient, are time consuming, and do not give information about the cellular basis of these responses. At present, there do not seem to be any known tests of A-cell function in man. In spite of the lack of sufficient specific tests of the immunologic system in man, clinical experience from immunologic deficiency diseases correlated with knowledge obtained from animal experimental systems has allowed an inference of the cellular basis of many of these diseases.

IMMUNOLOGIC DEFICIENCY DISEASES

In the past it has been conventional to classify immunologic deficiency diseases into two broad groups – those which are probably genetically determined (primary) and those which are either associated with malignancy or are the result of immunosuppression (secondary). However, an alternative method of classifying these diseases (Table 1) is based upon a consideration of the cellular stage of development which appears to be affected in each condition. This latter method has the advantage of providing a functional basis for discussing these diseases, although it is still uncertain in some cases what the exact nature of the lesion is, or the exact stage which is affected. A recent article by Gatti and Good[44] provides an excellent review of the clinical features of these diseases.

Diseases Resulting from Defects in Stem Cells

In *reticular dysgenesis*[28, 48] both the myeloid and lymphoid systems fail to develop. Although this failure of development is probably the

Table 1.   *Examples of Immunological Deficiency Diseases Reflecting Defects at Different Stages of Development of the Immunological System*

I. Defects in the Function of Stem Cells
   A. Stem cells of both the myeloid and lymphoid systems
      1. Reticular dysgenesis
   B. Stem cells of the lymphoid system
      1. Combined immunodeficiency syndromes (Swiss-type agammaglobulinemia, sex-linked lymphopenic agammaglobulinemia)

II. Defects in the Function of Thymic and Bursal-type (Bone Marrow) Environments
   A. Thymic environment
      1. III-IV pharyngeal pouch syndrome of diGeorge
      2. Ataxia telangiectasia
   B. Bursal-type environment
      1. Sex-linked agammaglobulinemia (Bruton-type)
      2. Late-onset agammaglobulinemia ("acquired")

III. Defects in the Function of B, T and A Cells
   A. Temporary
      1. After immunosuppressive therapy
      2. Associated with viral infections
   B. Persistent
      1. Associated with lymphoreticular malignancy (e.g., Hodgkin's disease, multiple myeloma, chronic lymphocytic leukemia)
      2. Deficiencies of single immunoglobulin classes
      3. Wiskott-Aldrich syndrome

---

result of an absence of pluripotent stem cells, it is conceivable that such stem cells are present but fail to differentiate because of a defect in their environment. (An example of the latter possibility, in the myeloid system, is the hereditary anemia of $S1/S1^d$ mice. These mice have stem cells of the myeloid system, but they fail to function normally in the $S1/S1^d$ environment. When transplanted into irradiated wild-type recipients, the $S1/S1^d$ stem cells can fully repopulate the myeloid system.)[90] Only a few patients with reticular dysgenesis have been described, and all have died early in neonatal life, so that studies of their immune systems have not been possible. However, in addition to anemia and neutropenia, absence of the thymus and marked lymphopenia have also been present.

    Combined immunodeficiency diseases include both *Swiss-type agammaglobulinemia*[20, 31, 71, 75, 77, 126] and *sex-linked lymphopenic agammaglobulinemia.*[47, 77, 127] These are probably variants of the same disease. Both are transmitted in a recessive fashion; the former is autosomal, affecting both males and females, and the latter is sex-linked, with expression in male infants. The adjective "combined" indicates that the end result of the lesion in these conditions is a loss of both T-cell and B-cell functions. Thus, affected children show a profound deficiency of both cell-mediated and humoral immune responses.

    Although the lesion responsible for these defects could conceivably be affecting precursors of both T and B cells during their development in the thymic and bursal-type environments, it is more likely that the lesion is at an earlier stage of development, affecting stem cells responsible for development of the lymphoid system. Supporting this argument is the fact that some of these children have been treated successfully, with complete restoration of immunological functions, by grafts of histocompatible bone marrow.[45, 97] These results suggest that the thymic environment in these children is capable of giving rise to functioning T cells once it has been provided with the appropriate stem cells.

(An analogous situation in mice is found in the myeloid system of the W/W^v strain. These mice lack normal myeloid stem cells, and their bone marrow is unable to repopulate the myeloid system of irradiated wild-type recipients. However, the environment necessary for differentiation of myeloid stem cells is normal in W/W^v mice since the myeloid system in these mice can be restored by transplants of wild-type bone marrow.)[89]

Diseases Resulting from Defects in the Thymic and Bursal-type Environments

The *III-IV pharyngeal pouch syndrome of diGeorge*[30, 69, 81] is an example of a disease in which the thymic environment responsible for differentiation of stem cells into T cells is defective. In this condition, a lesion early in embryonic life affects the development of the epithelial anlage of the thymus, parathyroids, and great vessels. Consequently, these children exhibit a lack of functional T cells (with the concomitant inability to mount cell-mediated immune responses), hypoparathyroidism with tetany and, often, anomalies of the great vessels. Immunoglobulin levels are normal in these children, and they can form antibodies in response to some antigens.

An important result of the lack of T-cell functions in these children is that they are prone to graft-versus-host disease caused by viable allogeneic lymphocytes in fresh blood transfusions. Stem cells of the lymphoid system are presumably normal in these children, because these patients do exhibit normal B-cell functions, and because they can be treated successfully by a thymic graft and do not require a bone-marrow transplant.[5, 19] This situation in man is paralleled by the results of experiments in neonatally thymectomized mice.[101] These mice are unable to reject skin grafts, and their cells cannot give rise to graft-versus-host disease because their lymphoid organs lack T cells.

Ataxia telangiectasia[34, 37, 115] also appears to be a disease in which the thymic environment is faulty. However, the deficiency of T-cell function in these children does not become clinically evident until a few years after birth. Furthermore, although B-cell functions are apparently normal for a time, most of them eventually develop IgA and IgE[3] deficiency as well. Whether the immunoglobulin deficiencies are the result of a lack of "helper" T cells involved in antibody responses, or whether there is a separate lesion affecting B cells, is unknown. The latter situation is conceivable since the genetic defect in these children is pleomorphic, affecting blood vessels as well as the immune system.

It is noteworthy that these children are unusually prone to developing malignant tumors,[43] an association that, in conjunction with the results of experiments in neonatally thymectomized mice,[101] has been used as evidence to suggest that T cells may have a surveillance function in suppressing clones of malignant cells.[13]

The evidence that *sex-linked agammaglobulinemia*[12, 44, 56, 57, 59] represents the lack of a normal bursal-type environment is based primarily upon the results of bursectomy (surgical and hormonal) in chickens.[24, 49, 143] Chickens lacking a bursa are hypogammaglobulinemic and do not form antibodies, but cell-mediated immune responses dependent upon T cells remain intact. Boys affected with this disease are hypogammaglobulinemic, with subnormal or absent levels of all major classes of immunoglobulins, but they do have the capacity to produce delayed hypersensitivity reactions and can reject skin grafts. Furthermore, if untreated, they suffer almost entirely from bacterial rather than viral and fungal infections. Therapy with gamma globulin injections and antibiotics is simple and reasonably effective, and thus marrow transplants have not been attempted in these children.

Late-onset agammaglobulinemia[44, 58, 128, 144] has many of the hallmarks of the sex-linked variety of agammaglobulinemia, but the onset is usually in adult life. Since the relatives of many of these patients display various defects of the immune system, it is thought that the lesion is genetically-determined. T-cell functions are usually normal, and therapy with gamma globulin appears to be effective in decreasing the frequency and severity of further infections. If this condition is attributable to a failure of the bursal-type environment, then this failure occurs later in life, perhaps in some manner analogous to that of adult-onset diabetes mellitus.

Diseases Resulting from Defects in the Function of B, T, and A Cells

To classify a disease as representing either an absence or abnormal function of B, T or A cells, it is necessary to be certain that a normal lymphoid stem cell population is present and that the thymic and marrow environments function normally. Immunodeficiencies resulting from the use of *immunosuppressive therapy*[42, 121, 130, 132] and those associated with *viral infections*[133, 136, 142] fit into this category. During immunosuppressive therapy it is likely that the obligatory requirement of T and B cells to proliferate in response to antigens is suppressed. The antiproliferative effect of immunosuppressive agents is well known, and forms the basis for their use in allotransplantation. The chemotherapy of malignant diseases also produces the inadvertent side-effect of suppressing the normal immune response.

During certain viral infections, such as rubeola and rubella, the capacity to initiate immune responses requiring T cells is deficient, e.g. individuals with skin tests previously positive to PPD show negative skin tests. The addition of rubella virus to cells exposed in culture to PHA or allogeneic cells suppresses the response. Thus, it is likely that T cells are either temporarily absent or incapable of responding to antigens. This temporary deficiency is probably not the explanation for the high IgM levels found in neonates with congenital viral infections.[137]

In *lymphoreticular malignancies*[2, 21, 55, 74, 91, 99, 141] and *deficiencies of a single immunoglobulin class*,[4, 8, 134, 135] such as IgA, the exact stage of development affected is open to argument. In some lymphoreticular malignancies, e.g. Hodgkin's disease,[2, 55, 141] the defect seems to primarily affect T-cell functions, leaving B-cell functions intact. In others, e.g. multiple myeloma,[21, 91] the reverse situation is seen, while in chronic lymphocytic leukemia[21] both B-cell and T-cell functions are affected. However, the nature of these defects is not clear. T and B cells may develop normally, but replacement of the lymphoid tissues by malignant tissue might alter the environment in which these cells function. Another possibility is that T and B cells fail to develop normally because the malignancy affects the thymic or bursa-like environments. It is also possible that A-cell function may be abnormal.

Similarly, deficiencies of a single immunoglobulin class could arise as a result of defects at more than one stage of the development of the class of cells affected. It is still uncertain whether precursors of IgA-secreting cells are restricted to maturing only into IgA-secreting cells, or whether a switch-over from production of one immunoglobulin to another can occur within a single cell. If the former is true, then the most likely defect is a failure of differentiation in the IgA-cell line; if the latter, then a fault in the switch-over mechanism could account for isolated immunoglobulin class deficiencies.

Abnormal A-cell function may be the basis of the immunologic deficiency seen in the *Wiskott-Aldrich syndrome*.[22] Some of the patients studied have shown a deficiency in their capacity to process pneumococcal polysaccharide and Vi antigens and have low IgM, with high IgA, and normal or high IgG levels in the serum. In keeping with the postulate that A-cell function is abnormal, thus affecting the production of IgM antibodies, is the discovery that A cells are required for immune responses giving rise to at least some IgM antibodies in mice.[61, 112]

In these diseases, as in all the immunodeficiency diseases, investigations would be aided greatly by specific markers for B, T, and A cells and by precise quantitative assays capable of testing the function of each class of cells in cell culture.

AUTOIMMUNE REACTIVITY

The presence of autoimmune reactivity has been associated frequently with well documented cases of immunologic deficiency, e.g. isolated IgA deficiency[4, 39, 76] and late-onset agammaglobulinemia.[40, 41] There is reason to think that the development of autoreactive antibodies in these patients is an epiphenomenon caused by the action of environmental pathogens in an immunologically deficient milieu.

Mice that are thymectomized at birth and raised in a conventional environment frequently develop a "wasting disease," characterized by weight loss, diarrhea, and infections.[92] They are also predisposed to develop autoimmune manifestations such as dermatitis and Coombs-positive hemolytic anemia, as well as renal and hepatic lesions similar to those found in systemic lupus erythematosus.[29] However, neonatally thymectomized mice raised in a germ-free environment do not develop any of these manifestations until after they are placed in a conventional environment.[92] Thus, the exposure of such mice to environmental pathogens is almost certainly responsible for the development of "wasting disease."

It has been suggested that environmental pathogens also may be responsible for the development of autoimmune disease in immunologically deficient mice.[92] Furthermore, it is likely that viruses may be the etiologic agents responsible for the development of autoimmune hemolytic anemia, LE cells and immune-complex nephritis, as has been suggested in at least one experimental animal model, New Zealand mice.[93, 94, 138]

In humans, viral infections have often been associated with the subsequent development of autoimmune hemolytic disease.[25] It follows that the development of autoimmune reactivity in immunologically deficient patients could well be secondary to their inability to resist environmental pathogens.

It would seem reasonable to think that autoimmune reactivity in the diseases associated with "hyperplasia" of the thymus and with thymomas[52, 78] (Table 2) must have a different pathogenesis than does the development of autoimmune reactivity associated with known immunologic deficiency. At least two different mechanisms may be responsible in these diseases. In some, the autoimmune manifestations are probably secondary to immunologic deficiency, e.g. the hypogammaglobulinemia associated with thymoma.[52, 54, 86] These patients initially demonstrate deficient humoral antibody formation, but many subsequently also have deficient cell-mediated responses.[44, 140] The association of autoimmune reactivity with immunologic deficiency in the presence of a thymoma[104, 123] raises the question of whether or not some of the other autoimmune diseases associated with thymoma or "hyperplasia", such as rheumatoid arthritis, systemic lupus erythematosus, and autoimmune hemolytic anemia also may be epiphenomena superimposed on a background of immunologic deficiency. Rheumatoid arthritis has been associated with hypogammaglobulinemia in some patients. Autoimmune hemolytic anemia is known to occur in patients with chronic lymphocytic leukemia and Hodgkin's disease, both of which are frequently accom-

Table 2. *Diseases Associated with the Presence of Thymic Tumors and "Hyperplasia" of the Thymus*

Frequent Associations
  Hypogammaglobulinemia
  Myasthenia gravis
  Erythroid hypoplasia (pure red cell agenesis)

Rare Associations
  Systemic lupus erythematosus
  Rheumatoid arthritis
  Dermatomyositis, myositis and myocarditis
  Scleroderma
  Sjögren's syndrome
  Hyperglobulinemic purpura
  Cushing's syndrome
  Bullous dermatitis
  Autoimmune hemolytic anemia

---

panied by immunological deficiency. In New Zealand mice, aberrations in antibody formation and defects in cell-mediated immunity are present before the autoimmune manifestations appear.[14, 82, 138]

Whether or not heretofore unrecognized immunologic deficiency or other immunologic abnormalities play a role in the pathogenesis of rheumatoid arthritis, systemic lupus erythematosus, and autoimmune hemolytic anemia requires reappraisal. An indirect argument in support of this possibility is that relatives of patients with immunologic deficiency diseases have a very high frequency of autoimmune disease.[40] This suggests that a genetic lesion, perhaps one that predisposes to deficiencies of the immune system, may underlie all of these diseases.[39a]

Another mechanism operating in autoimmunity associated with morphological alterations in the thymus is exemplified by myasthenia gravis, and perhaps erythroid hypoplasia.[52] Evidence from experiments in guinea pigs suggests that a thymitis, induced by injections of autologous or heterologous striated muscle or thymus cells, results in the release of an agent capable of blocking neuromuscular transmission.[51, 53, 80] The experimental thymitis is probably caused by antibodies that react with myoid fibers normally present in the thymus. It has been suggested that a similar mechanism may operate in myasthenia gravis when a thymoma is present, since the thymic tissue surrounding a thymoma frequently shows the presence of lymphoid follicles and plasma cells.[52] Thus, in these conditions the thymus appears to be the target of antibodies with self-reactive properties.

Neither of the above mechanisms explains how clones of cells with self-reactive properties arise in the first place. The prevailing hypothesis is that during development and differentiation such clones have survived because of a failure in a suppressive mechanism whose function is to eliminate cells with potential for reactivity with self-antigens.[79]

Thus, the pathogenesis of autoimmune diseases, whether associated with abnormal thymic morphology or not, is still largely enigmatic, and further work is required to clarify the situation.

In the consideration of autoimmunity two further notes of caution are required. The first is the necessity to distinguish between autoantibodies capable of producing tissue injury and autoantibodies capable of combining with normal tissue but not producing any apparent injury. The former may truly result in autoimmune disease, while the latter may only reflect previous tissue damage.

The second is that it is not always clear whether or not so-called "hyperplasia" of the thymus is a pathologic state. Usually, the term "hyperplasia" is used to refer to a thymus containing lymph follicles with germinal centers. It has been stated that lymph follicles do not occur in the normal human thymus at any age.[85] However, several studies show that lymph follicles with germinal center formation are present in such diverse conditions as congenital heart disease, bronchogenic carcinoma, and healthy individuals killed in road accidents.[10, 72, 98] However, Henry[72] suggests that the extent of lymph follicle formation may be greater in those conditions we commonly think of as being autoimmune in nature than in the normal thymus.

REFERENCES

1. Ada, G. L., and Byrt, P.: Specific inactivation of antigen-reactive cells with ^{125}I-labelled antigen. Nature, 222:1291, 1969.
2. Aisenberg, A. C.: Quantitative estimation of normal and Hodgkin's disease lymphocytes with thymidine-2 [14]C. Nature, 205:1233, 1965.
3. Ammann, A. J., Cain, W. A., Ishizaka, K., Hong, R., and Good, R. A.: Immunoglobulin E deficiency in ataxia-telangiectasia. New Eng. J. Med., 281:469, 1969.
4. Ammann, A. J., and Hong, R.: Selective IgA deficiency: Presentation of 30 cases and a review of the literature. Medicine, 50:223, 1971.
5. August, C. S., Rosen, F. S., Filler, R. M., Janeway, C. A., Markowski, B., and Kay, H. E. M.: Implantation of a foetal thymus, restoring immunological competence in a patient with thymic aplasia (DiGeorge's syndrome). Lancet, 2:1210, 1968.
6. Bach, F. H., Alter, B. J., Solliday, S., Zoschke, D. C., and Janis, M.: Lymphocyte reactivity *in vitro*. II. Soluble reconstituting factor permitting response of purified lymphocytes. Cell. Immunol., 1:219, 1970.
7. Bach, F. H., and Voynow, N. K.: One-way stimulation in mixed leucocyte cultures. Science, 153:545, 1966.
8. Bachman, R.: Studies on serum γA-globulin level. III. Frequency of a-γA-globulinemia. Scand. J. Clin. Lab. Invest., 17:316, 1965.
9. Basten, A., Miller, J. F. A. P., Warner, N. L., and Pye, J.: Specific inactivation of thymus-derived (T) and non-thymus-derived (B) lymphocytes by ^{125}I-labelled antigen. Nature, 231:104, 1971.
10. Bhathal, P. S., and Campbell, P. E.: Eosinophil leucocytes in the child's thymus. Austral. Ann. Med., 14:210, 1965.
11. Boak, J. L., Mitchison, N. A., and Pattison, P. H.: The carrier effect in the secondary response to hapten-protein conjugates. III. The anatomical distribution of helper cells and antibody-forming-cell-precursors. European J. Immunol., 1:63, 1971.
12. Bruton, O. C.: Agammaglobulinemia. Pediatrics, 9:722, 1952.
13. Burnet, F. M.: Immunological Surveillance. Sydney, Pergamon Press (Australia) Ltd., 1970.
14. Cantor, H., Asofsky, R., and Talal, N.: Synergy among lymphoid cells mediating the graft-vs-host response. I. Synergy in graft-vs-host reactions produced by cells from NZB/B1 mice. J. Exper. Med., 131:223, 1970.
15. Cebra, J. J., Colberg, J. E., and Dray, S.: Rabbit lymphoid cells differentiated with respect to alpha, gamma, and mu heavy polypeptide chains and to allotypic markers Aa1 and Aa2. J. Exper. Med., 123:547, 1966.
16. Cerottini, J.-C., Nordin, A. A., and Brunner, K. T.: Specific *in vitro* cytotoxicity of thymus-derived lymphocytes sensitized to alloantigens. Nature, 228:1308, 1970.
17. Claman, H. N., and Brunstetter, F. H.: The response of cultured human thymus cells to phytohemagglutinin. J. Immunol., 100:1127, 1968.
18. Claman, H. N., Chaperon, E. A., and Triplett, R. F.: Thymus-marrow cell combinations. Synergism in antibody production. Proc. Soc. Exper. Biol. Med., 122:1167, 1966.
19. Cleveland, W. W., Fogel, B. J., Brown, W. T., and Kay, H. E. M.: Foetal thymic transplant in a case of DiGeorge's syndrome. Lancet, 2:1211, 1968.
20. Cole, R. B., D'Sousa, A., Good, R. A., Gatti, R. A., and Hoyer, J.: Lymphopenic agammaglobulinemia (Swiss type) in Chicago. Autosomal recessive form. Amer. J. Dis. Child., 17:22, 1961.
21. Cone, L., and Uhr, J. W.: Immunological deficiency disorders associated with chronic lymphocytic leukemia and multiple myeloma. J. Clin. Invest., 43:2241, 1964.
22. Cooper, M. D., Chase, H. P., Lowman, J., Krivit, W., and Good, R. A.: Wiskott-Aldrich syndrome – an immunologic deficiency disease involving the afferent limb of immunity. Amer. J. Med., 44:499, 1968.
23. Cooper, M. D., Perey, D. Y., McKneally, M. F., Gabrielsen, A. E., Sutherland, D. E. R., and Good, R. A.: A mammalian equivalent of the avian bursa of Fabricius. Lancet, 2:1388, 1966.
24. Cooper, M. D., Peterson, R. D. A., and Good, R. A.: Delineation of the thymic and bursal lymphoid systems in the chicken. Nature, 205:143, 1965.
25. Dacie, J. V.: III. Haemolytic anaemia following or associated with known virus infections. *In* The Haemolytic Anaemias. Part II. The Autoimmune Haemolytic Anaemias, 2nd ed., London, Churchill, 1965, p. 525.
26. David, J. R.: Macrophage migration. Fed. Proc., 27:6, 1968.
27. Davies, A. J. S., Festenstein, H., Leuchars, E., Wallis, V. J., and Doenhoff, M. J.: A thymic origin for some peripheral-blood lymphocytes. Lancet, 1:183, 1968.
28. DeVaal, O. M., and Seynhaeve, V.: Reticular dysgenesis. Lancet, 2:1123, 1959.
29. DeVries, M. J., van Putten, L. M., Balner, H., and van Bekkum, D. W.: Lésions suggérant une réactivité autoimmune chez des souris atteintes de la "runt disease" apres thymectomie néonatale. Rev. Franç. Etud. Clin. Biol., 9:381, 1964.

30. DiGeorge, A. M.: Congenital absence of the thymus and its immunologic consequences: Concurrence with congenital hypoparathyroidism. *In* Good, R. A., and Bergsma, D., eds.: Immunologic Deficiency Diseases in Man. Birth Defects Original Article Series, Vol. 4. New York, National Foundation Press, 1968, p. 116.
31. Donohue, W. L.: Alymphocytosis. Pediatrics, *11*:129, 1953.
32. Dutton, R. W., and Mishell, R. I.: Cell populations and cell proliferation in the in vitro response of normal mouse spleen to heterologous erythrocytes. J. Exper. Med., *126*:443, 1967.
33. Edwards, G. E., Miller, R. G., and Phillips, R. A.: Differentiation of rosette-forming cells from myeloid stem cells. J. Immunol., *105*:719, 1970.
34. Eisen, A. H., Karpati, G., Laszlo, T., Andermann, F., Robb, J. P., and Bacal, H. L.: Immunologic deficiency in ataxia-telangiectasia. New Eng. J. Med., 272:18, 1965.
35. El-Arini, M. O., and Osoba, D.: Unpublished observations.
36. Falk, R. E., Falk, J. A., and Zabriskie, J. B.: Reactivity of nonsensitized thymocytes to antigen: Release of specific lymphocyte-activating substances. Transpl. Proc., *3*:841, 1971.
37. Fireman, P., Boesman, M., and Gillen, D.: Ataxis telangiectasia: A dysgammaglobulinemia with deficient gamma$_{1A}$ - (B$_2$A) - globulin. Lancet, *1*:1193, 1964.
38. Ford, C. E., Micklem, H. S., Evans, E. P., Gray, J. G., and Ogden, D. A.: The inflow of bone marrow cells to the thymus: Studies with part-body irradiated mice, injected with chromosome-marked bone marrow and subjected to antigenic stimulation. Ann. N.Y. Acad. Sci., *129*:283, 1966.
39. Fraser, K. J.: IgA immunoglobulins and autoimmunity. Lancet, 2:804, 1969.
39a.Fudenberg, H. H.: Genetically determined immune deficiency as the predisposing cause of "autoimmunity" and lymphoid neoplasia. Amer. J. Med., *51*:295, 1971.
40. Fudenberg, H. H., German, J. J., III, and Kunkel, H. G.: The occurrence of rheumatoid factor and other abnormalities in families of patients with agammaglobulinemia. Arth. Rheum., 5:565, 1962.
41. Fudenberg, H. H., and Hirschhorn, K.: Agammaglobulinemia: Some current concepts. MED. CLIN. N. AMER., *49*:1533, 1965.
42. Gabrielson, A. E., and Good, R. A.: Chemical suppression of adaptive immunity. Adv. Immunol., 6:92, 1967.
43. Gatti, R. A., and Good, R. A.: Occurrence of malignancy in immunodeficiency diseases: A literature review. Cancer, 28:89, 1971.
44. Gatti, R. A., and Good, R. A.: The immunological deficiency diseases. MED. CLIN. N. AMER., 54:281, 1970.
45. Gatti, R. A., Meuwissen, H. J., Allen, H. D., Hong, R., and Good, R. A.: Immunologic reconstitution of sex-linked lymphopenic immunologic deficiency. Lancet, 2:1366, 1968.
46. Gilmour, J. R.: The embryology of the parathyroid glands, the thymus and certain associated rudiments. J. Path. Bact., *45*:507, 1937.
47. Gitlin, D., and Craig, J. M.: The thymus and other lymphoid tissues in congenital agammaglobulinemia. I. Thymic alymphoplasia and lymphocytic hypoplasia and their relation to infection. Pediatrics, 32:517, 1963.
48. Gitlin, D., Vawter, G., and Craig, J. M.: Thymic alymphoplasia and congenital aleukocytosis. Pediatrics, 33:184, 1964.
49. Glick, B., Chang, T. S., and Jaap, R. C.: The bursa of Fabricius and antibody production. Poultry Sci., 35:224, 1956.
50. Goldie, J. H., and Osoba, D.: Requirement of a nonproliferating class of cells for generation of immune responses in cell culture. Proc. Soc. Exper. Biol. Med., *133*:1265, 1970.
51. Goldstein, G.: The thymus and neuromuscular function: A substance in thymus which causes myositis and myasthenic neuromuscular block in guinea pigs. Lancet, 2:119, 1968.
52. Goldstein, G., and MacKay, I. R.: The Human Thymus. London, Wm. Heineman Medical Books Ltd., 1969.
53. Goldstein, G., and Whittingham, S.: Experimental autoimmune thymitis: An animal model for myasthenia gravis. Lancet, 2:315, 1966.
54. Good, R. A.: Agammaglobulinemia: A provocative experiment of nature. Bull. Univ. Minn. Hosp., 26:1, 1954.
55. Good, R. A., and Finstad, J.: The association of lymphoid malignancy and immunologic functions. *In* Zarafonetis, C., ed.: Proceedings of the International Conference on Leukemia-Lymphoma. Philadelphia, Lea and Febiger, 1968, p. 175.
56. Good, R. A., and Finstad, J.: The Gordon Wilson Lecture: The development and involution of the lymphoid system and immunologic capacity. Trans. Amer. Clin. Climatol. Assoc., 79:69, 1968.
57. Good, R. A., Kelly, W. D., Rotstein, J., and Varco, R. L.: Immunological deficiency diseases. Progr. Allergy, 6:187, 1962.
58. Good, R. A., and Varco, R. L.: A clinical and experimental study of agammaglobulinemia. J. Lancet, 75:245, 1955.

59. Good, R. A., and Zak, S. J.: Disturbances in gammaglobulin synthesis as experiments of nature. Pediatrics, *18*:109, 1956.
60. Gorczynski, R. M., Miller, R. G., and Phillips, R. A.: Identification by density separation of antigen-specific surface receptors on progenitors of antibody-producing cells. Immunol., *20*:693, 1971.
61. Gorczynski, R. M., Miller, R. G., and Phillips, R. A.: In vivo requirement for a radiation-resistant cell in the immune response to sheep erythrocytes. J. Exper. Med., in press.
62. Gordon, H. A.: Morphological and physiological characterization of germ-free life. Ann. N.Y. Acad. Sci., *78*:208, 1959.
63. Greaves, M. F.: Biological effects of anti-immunoglobulins: Evidence for immunoglobulin receptors on T and B lymphocytes. Transplant. Rev., *5*:45, 1970.
64. Greaves, M. F.: Personal communication.
65. Greaves, M. F., and Möller, E.: Studies on antigen binding cells. I. The origin of reactive cells. Cell. Immunol., *1*:372, 1970.
66. Green, I., Vassali, P., Nussenzweig, V., and Benacerraf, B.: Specificity of the antibodies produced by single cells following immunization with antigens bearing two types of antigenic determinants. J. Exper. Med., *125*:511, 1967.
67. Hammar, J. A.: Zur Histogenese und Involution der Thymusdrüse. Anat. Anz., *27*:23, 41, 1905.
68. Harris, J. E., Ford, C. E., Barnes, D. W. H., and Evans, E. P.: Cellular traffic of the thymus: Experiments with chromosome markers. Evidence from parabiosis for an afferent stream of cells. Nature, *201*:886, 1964.
69. Harvey, J. C., Dungan, W. T., Elders, M. J., and Hughes, E. R.: Third and fourth pharyngeal pouch syndrome, associated vascular anomalies and hypocalcemic seizures. Clin. Pediat., *9*:496, 1970.
70. Haskill, J. S., Byrt, P., and Marbrook, J.: *In vitro* and *in vivo* studies of the immune response to sheep erythrocytes using partially purified cell preparations. J. Exper. Med., *131*:57, 1970.
71. Haworth, J. C., Hoogstraten, J., and Taylor, H.: Thymic alymphoplasia. Arch. Dis. Child., *42*:40, 1967.
72. Henry, K.: The thymus in rheumatic heart disease. Clin. Exper. Immunol., *3*:509, 1968.
73. Hersh, E. M., and Harris, J. E.: Macrophage-lymphocyte interaction in the antigen-induced blastogenic response of human peripheral blood leukocytes. J. Immunol., *100*:1184, 1968.
74. Hirschhorn, K., Schreibman, R. R., Bach, F. H., and Sitzbach, L. E.: In vitro studies of lymphocytes from patients with sarcoidosis and lymphoproliferative disease. Lancet, *2*:842, 1964.
75. Hitzig, W. H., Biro, Z., Bosch, H., and Huser, H. J.: Agammaglobulinämie und Alymphocytose mit Schwund des lymphatischen Gewebes. Helv. Paediat. Acta, *13*:551, 1958.
76. Hobbs, J. R., Hepner, G. W., Douglas, A. P., Crabbé, P. A., and Johansson, S. G. O.: Immunological mystery of coeliac disease. Lancet, *2*:649, 1969.
77. Hoyer, J. R., Cooper, M. D., Gabrielsen, A. E., and Good, R. A.: Lymphopenic forms of congenital immunologic deficiency diseases. Medicine, *47*:201, 1968.
78. Irvine, W. J.: The thymus in autoimmune disease. Proc. Roy. Soc. Med., *63*:718, 1970.
79. Jerne, N. K.: The somatic generation of immune recognition. European J. Immunol., *1*:1, 1971.
80. Kalden, J. R., Williamson, W. G., Johnston, R. J., and Irvine, W. J.: Studies on experimental autoimmune thymitis in guinea-pigs. Clin. Exper. Immunol., *5*:319, 1969.
81. Kretschmer, R., Say, B., Brown, D., and Rosen, F. S.: Congenital aplasia of the thymus gland (DiGeorge syndrome). New Eng. J. Med., *279*:1295, 1968.
82. Leventhal, B. G., and Talal, N.: Response of NZB and NZB/NZW spleen cells to mitogenic agents. J. Immunol., *104*:918, 1970.
83. Lischner, H. W., Punnett, H. H., and DiGeorge, A. M.: Lymphocytes in congenital absence of the thymus. Nature, *214*:580, 1967.
84. MacDonald, H. R.: Personal communication.
85. MacKay, I. R.: Histopathology of the human thymus. In Wolstenholme, G. E. W., and Porter, R., eds.: The Thymus. London, Churchill, 1966, p. 449.
86. MacLean, L. D., Zak, S. J., Varco, R. L., and Good, R. A.: Thymic tumor and acquired immune agammaglobulinemia: Clinical and experimental study of immune response. Surgery, *40*:1010, 1956.
87. Mäkelä, O.: The specificity of antibodies produced by single cells. Cold Spring Harbor Symp. Quant. Biol., *32*:423, 1967.
88. Martinez, C., Kersey, J., Papermaster, B. W., and Good, R. A.: Skin homograft survival in thymectomized mice. Proc. Soc. Exper. Biol. Med., *109*:193, 1962.
89. McCulloch, E. A., Siminovitch, L., and Till, J. E.: Spleen-colony formation in anaemic mice of genotype W/W^v. Science, *144*:844, 1964.
90. McCulloch, E. A., Siminovitch, L., Till, J. E., Russell, E. S., and Bernstein, S. E.: The cellular basis of the genetically-determined hemopoietic defect in anaemic mice of genotype Sl/Sl^d. Blood, *26*:399, 1965.

91. McKelvey, E. M., and Fahey, J. L.: Immunoglobulin changes in disease; quantitation on the basis of heavy polypeptide chains IgG (gamma G), IgA (gamma A) and IgM (gamma M) and of light polypeptide chains type K (I) and type L (II). J. Clin. Invest., 44:1778, 1965.

92. McIntire, K. R., Sell, S., and Miller, J. F. A. P.: Pathogenesis of the post-neonatal thymectomy wasting syndrome. Nature, 204:151, 1964.

93. Mellors, R. C.: Autoimmune and immunoproliferative diseases of NZB/B1 mice and hybrids. Int. Rev. Exper. Pathol., 5:217, 1966.

94. Mellors, R. C.: Autoimmune disease and neoplasia of NZB mice: Experimental model and its implications. In Rose, N. R., and Milgrom, F., eds.: Immunology: Proceedings of the International Convocation on Immunology. New York, S. Karger, 1969, p. 222.

95. Metcalf, D.: Relation of the thymus to the formation of immunologically reactive cells. Cold Spring Harbor Symp. Quant. Biol., 32:583, 1967.

96. Metcalf, D.: The thymus and lymphopoiesis. In Good, R. A., and Gabrielson, A. E., eds.: The Thymus in Immunobiology, New York, Hoeber-Harper, 1964, p. 150.

97. Meuwissen, H. J., Gatti, R. A., Terasaki, P. I., Hong, R., and Good, R. A.: Treatment of lymphopenic hypogammaglobulinemia and bone marrow aplasia by transplantation of allogeneic marrow. New Eng. J. Med., 281:691, 1969.

98. Middleton, G.: The incidence of follicular structures in the human thymus at autopsy. Aust. J. Exper. Biol. Med. Sci., 45:189, 1967.

99. Miller, D. G., and Karnofsky, D. A.: Immunologic factors and resistance to infection in chronic lymphatic leukemia. Amer. J. Med., 31:748, 1961.

100. Miller, J. F. A. P.: Immunological function of the thymus. Lancet, 2:748, 1961.

101. Miller, J. F. A. P., and Osoba, D.: Current concepts of the immunological function of the thymus. Physiol. Rev., 47:437, 1967.

102. Miller, R. G., and Phillips, R. A.: Sedimentation analysis of the cells in mice required to initiate an in vivo immune response to sheep erythrocytes. Proc. Soc. Exper. Biol. Med., 135:63, 1970.

103. Mitchison, N. A.: The carrier effect in the secondary response to hapten-protein conjugates. II. Cellular cooperation. Eur. J. Immunol., 1:18, 1971.

104. Mongan, E. S., Kern, W. A., and Terry, R.: Hypogammaglobulinemia with thymoma, hemolytic anemia, and disseminated infection with cytomegalovirus. Ann. Int. Med., 65:548, 1966.

105. Moore, M. A. S., and Owen, J. J. T.: Chromosome marker studies on the development of the haemopoietic system in the chick embryo. Nature, 208:956, 1965.

106. Moore, M. A. S., and Owen, J. J. T.: Experimental studies on the development of the thymus. J. Exper. Med., 126:715, 1967.

107. Mosier, D. E.: A requirement for two cell types for antibody formation in vitro. Science, 158:1573, 1967.

108. Mosier, D. E., and Coppleson, L. W.: A three-cell interaction required for the induction of the primary immune response in vitro. Proc. Nat. Acad. Sci. U.S.A., 61:542, 1968.

109. Nossal, G. J. V., Cunningham, A., Mitchell, G. F., and Miller, J. F. A. P.: Cell to cell interaction in the immune response. III. Chromosomal marker analysis of single antibody-forming cells in reconstituted, irradiated, or thymectomized mice. J. Exper. Med., 128:839, 1968.

110. Osoba, D.: Cellular cooperation in the primary immune response – the need for a uniform terminology. European J. Clin. Biol. Res., 15:929, 1970.

111. Osoba, D.: Restriction of the capacity to respond to two antigens by single precursors of antibody-producing cells in culture. J. Exper. Med., 129:141, 1969.

112. Osoba, D.: Some physical and radiobiological properties of immunologically reactive mouse spleen cells. J. Exper. Med., 132:368, 1970.

113. Osoba, D.: Unpublished observations.

114. Parrott, D. M., deSousa, M. A. B., and East, J.: Thymus-dependent areas in the lymphoid organs of neonatally thymectomized mice. J. Exper. Med., 123:191, 1966.

115. Peterson, R. D. A., Cooper, M. D., and Good, R. A.: Lymphoid tissue abnormalities associated with ataxia-telangiectasia. Amer. J. Med., 41:342, 1966.

116. Playfair, J. H. L., Papermaster, B. W., and Cole, L. J.: Focal antibody production by transferred spleen cells in irradiated mice. Science, 149:998, 1965.

117. Playfair, J. H. L., Wolfendale, M. R., and Kay, H. E. M.: The leucocytes of peripheral blood in the human foetus. Brit. J. Haematol., 9:336, 1963.

118. Raff, M. C.: Surface antigenic markers for distinguishing T and B lymphocytes in mice. Transplant. Rev., 6:52, 1971.

119. Raff, M. C.: Theta isoantigen as a marker of thymus-derived lymphocytes in mice. Nature, 224:378, 1969.

120. Reif, A. E., and Allen, J. M. V.: The AKR thymic antigen and its distribution in leukemias and nervous tissues. J. Exper. Med., 120:413, 1964.

121. Revillard, J. P., and Brochier, J.: Selective deficiency of cell-mediated immunity in humans treated with antilymphocyte globulins. Transpl. Proc., 3:725, 1971.

122. Rode, H. N., and Gordon, J.: The mixed leukocyte culture: A three component system. J. Immunol., *104*:1453, 1970.
123. Rogers, H. G., Manaligod, J. R., and Blazek, W. V.: Thymoma associated with pancytopenia and hypogammaglobulinemia. Amer. J. Med., *44*:154, 1968.
124. Roitt, I. M., Greaves, M. F., Torrigiani, G., Brostoff, J., and Playfair, J. H. L.: The cellular basis of immunological responses. Lancet, 2:367, 1969.
125. Roseman, J. M.: The X-ray resistant cell required for the induction of *in vitro* antibody formation. Science, *165*:1125, 1969.
126. Rosen, F. S., Gitlin, D., and Janeway, C. A.: Alymphocytosis, agammaglobulinemia, homografts and delayed hypersensitivity: Study of a case. Lancet, 2:380, 1962.
127. Rosen, F. S., Gottoff, S. P., Craig, J. M., Ritchie, J., and Janeway, C. A.: Further observations on the Swiss type of agammaglobulinemia (alymphocytosis). The effect of syngeneic bone-marrow cells. New Eng. J. Med., *274*:18, 1966.
128. Sanford, J. P., Favour, C. B., and Tribeman, M. S.: Absence of serum gamma globulin in adults. New Eng. J. Med., *250*:1027, 1954.
129. Schechter, G. P., and McFarland, W.: Interaction of lymphocytes and a radioresistant cell in PPD-stimulated human leukocyte cultures. J. Immunol., *105*:661, 1970.
130. Schwartz, R. S.: Immunosuppressive drugs. Progr. Allergy, *9*:246, 1965.
131. Shortman, K., Diener, E., Russell, P., and Armstrong, W. D.: The role of nonlymphoid accessory cells in the immune response to different antigens. J. Exper. Med., *131*:461, 1970.
132. Simmons, R. L., Moberg, A. W., Gewurz, H., Soll, R., and Najarian, J. S.: Immunosuppression by antihuman lymphocyte globulin: correlation of human and animal assay systems with clinical results. Transpl. Proc., *3*:745, 1971.
133. Smithwick, E. M., and Berkovich, S.: The effect of measles virus on the *in vitro* lymphocyte response to tuberculin. *In* Smith, R. T., and Good, R. A., eds.: Cellular Recognition. New York, Appleton-Century-Crofts, 1969, p. 131.
134. South, M. A., Cooper, M. D., Hong, R., Wollheim, F. A., and Good, R. A.: Secretory IgA and the immunologic deficiency. *In* Good, R. A., and Bergsma, D., eds.: Immunologic Deficiency Diseases in Man. Birth Defects Original Article Series, Vol. 4. New York, National Foundation Press, 1968, p. 283.
135. South, M. A., Cooper, M. D., Wollheim, F. A., and Good, R. A.: The IgA system. II. The clinical significance of IgA deficiency. Amer. J. Med., *44*:168, 1968.
136. Starr, S., and Berkovich, S.: Effects of measles, gammaglobulin-modified measles and vaccine measles on the tuberculin test. New Eng. J. Med., *270*:386, 1964.
137. Stiehm, E. R., Ammann, A. J., and Cherry, J. D.: Elevated cord macroglobulins in the diagnosis of intrauterine infections. New Eng. J. Med., *275*:971, 1966.
138. Talal, N.: Immunologic and viral factors in the pathogenesis of systemic lupus erythematosus. Arth. Rheum., *13*:887, 1970.
139. Tan, T., and Gordon, J.: Participation of three cell types in the anti-sheep red blood cell response in vitro. J. Exper. Med., *133*:520, 1971.
140. te Velde, K., Huber, J., and Van der Slikke, L. B.: Primary acquired hypogammaglobulinemia, myasthenia and thymoma. Ann. Int. Med., *65*:554, 1966.
141. Thomas, J. W., Boldt, W., Horrocks, G., and Low, B.: Lymphocyte transformation by phytohemagglutinin: I. In Hodgkin's disease. Canad. Med. Assoc. J., *97*:832, 1967.
142. Thomas, J. W., Clements, D., and Naiman, S. C.: Lymphocyte transformation by phytohemagglutinin: IV. In acute upper respiratory infections. Canad. Med. Assoc. J., *99*:467, 1968.
143. Warner, N. L., Uhr, J. W., Thorbecke, G. J., and Ovary, Z.: Immunoglobulins, antibodies and the bursa of Fabricius: Induction of agammaglobulinemia and the loss of all antibody-forming capacity by hormonal bursectomy. J. Immunol., *103*:1317, 1969.
144. Wollheim, F. A., Belfrage, S., Coster, C., and Lindholm, H.: Primary "acquired" hypogammaglobulinemia. Clinical and genetic aspects of 9 cases. Acta Med. Scand., *176*:1, 1964.
145. Wu, A. M., Till, J. E., Siminovitch, L., and McCulloch, E. A.: Cytological evidence for a relationship between normal colony-forming cells and cells of the lymphoid system. J. Exper. Med., *127*:455, 1968.

Department of Medicine
Ontario Cancer Institute
500 Sherbourne Street
Toronto 284, Ontario
Canada

The Mixed Leukocyte Culture Reaction

Julius Gordon, Ph.D.[*]

I still remember my fascination when I first heard Barbara Bain describe her results on what we now call the mixed leukocyte culture reaction (MLCR), and my incredibility that this phenomenon represented an immune manifestation of some sort. This was in 1964.[23] In the same year Bach and Hirschhorn published similar data[9] indicating that when blood leukocytes of two individuals, other than identical twins, were incubated together for 5 to 7 days, some of the cells enlarged into blast cells which subsequently underwent cell division. Since these initial observations, contributions from numerous laboratories have established that the MLCR is an immune reaction, probably representing an in vitro correlate of cell-mediated immunity. The initial experiments carried out with human blood cells were extended and confirmed using cells from many species of experimental animals and opened up a new field of investigation, namely that of antigen-induced cell proliferation in vitro. In the case of the MLCR the antigens responsible for the elicitation of the reaction have been identified and correlated with the major transplantation antigens as defined and measured by serologic methods.

Lymphocytes are the cells which respond to stimulation by proliferation. They were identified morphologically in PHA-stimulated cultures by Carstairs[26, 27] and by isotopic labelling by Rubin et al.[34] They were shown to be the reactive cells in antigen-stimulated cultures by Coulson and Chalmers,[38] Mills,[122] and Marshall et al.[112] Lymphocytes were identified as the dividing cells in MLC by autoradiography by Bain et al.,[123] and by time lapse cinematography by McFarland and Heilman.[113] Experiments using thymectomized animals have suggested that reactivity in MLC may not be a property of all lymphocytes, but may be a function of only the thymus derived cells[86, 118, 138, 139, 181] This has been indeed directly demonstrated using chromosome markers by Johnston[81] in MLC and by Davies and Finklestein[39] in the reaction to PHA.

Lymphocytes perform a dual function in MLC. As well as being capable of responding, they can also provoke an MLC reaction. Recently Howe and Goldstein[74] proposed that in mice, stimulation of MLC may also be a sole function of the thymus derived lymphocytes. They found that spleen

[*]Associate Professor, Department of Experimental Surgery, McGill University, Montreal; Research Associate of the Medical Research Council of Canada

Medical Clinics of North America—Vol. 56, No. 2, March 1972

cells of neonatally thymectomized mice were unable to stimulate in MLC. Furthermore, this capacity to stimulate developed in mice at the age of 6 days, increased and disappeared after 75 days in parallel with their ability to respond in MLC.

Although lymphocytes are the cells which proliferate in MLC, when two highly purified populations of lymphocytes are cultured together, the MLC reaction does not take place.[5, 50, 95, 129, 140, 141, 169] This lack of reactivity is not due to cell damage incurred during purification. A wide variety of purification methods have been used, such as fractionation on columns of glass beads,[5] cotton,[50] nylon fibers,[129] and preferential destruction of cells other than lymphocytes.[140, 141] The reactivity of lymphocytes prepared by all these methods could be restored by the addition of glass-adherent cells or leukocytes subjected to 2000 r x-irradiation.[5, 50, 141] The latter preparations are unreactive by themselves in MLC.

The cell which participates in MLC with the lymphocytes is probably the monocyte or macrophage, into which it develops in culture. Monocytes do not appear to divide in MLC[23] and thus are not responsible for the proliferative reaction. They need only be present in MLC at a threshhold concentration of 1 to 2 per cent.[129, 141] Furthermore, their role in MLC is immunologically not specific. In "one-way" MLCR they can function equally well when derived from the responding or from the donor cell population.[5, 95, 147] Their function, or their precise role in MLC is not known. Bach et al.[13] have replaced them by a culture fluid derived from glass adherent cells. The nature of this material is not yet known, nor is it known whether it is in fact the mediator of the monocyte function in cultures of unfractionated cells.

The monocyte shares the quasi unique property of lymphocytes of being capable of turning on the MLC response.[111] This property is not shared by polymorphonuclear leukocytes, which are usually present in varying numbers in MLC.[142] The latter, according to a recent report, actually may suppress rather than stimulate.[80] Accordingly, three functions may be delineated in MLC. The proliferative response is a function of the lymphocyte or a subpopulation of lymphocytes. Stimulation can be elicited by all or only by some lymphocytes and monocytes. The third function, fulfilled by monocytes, may or may not be mediated by a soluble factor.

Elicitation of the MLC Response

Several as yet unexplained features characterize this facet of MLC. A correlation between disparity at the major histocompatibility locus and MLC reactivity has been established in several species.[8, 14, 43, 155, 164] Major transplantation antigens are expressed on all nucleated cells. Nevertheless, with one exception, only lymphocytes and monocytes were found to be capable of initiating an MLC response.[63, 147] The exception found so far is skin epithelium.[105] Fibroblasts do not stimulate[63] and epithelial cells do so only after vigorous trypsinization.[88]

This difference in the cells' ability to stimulate an MLC reaction may lie in differences in the quantity, distribution, and/or conformation of transplantation antigens on the cell surface. As far as lymphocytes are concerned, lymphoblasts from established cell lines trigger a more vigorous reaction than normal lymphocytes.[17, 158] Such lymphoblasts have indeed been shown to carry on their surface greater amounts of transplantation-antigens, and over a larger portion of their surface.[89]

This apparently unique feature of the lymphocyte may not be just an artifact of the MLC reaction. Sensitization of donor cells in graft-versus-host reactions appears to be due to host mononuclear cells.[44] Similarly, rat kidney transplants, freed of "passenger leukocytes," are much less able to provoke an allograft rejection and may survive longer.[59, 60]

The MLC reaction appears to reflect these phenomena in vitro. MLC reactivity appears to be restricted in man,[14, 17, 18, 148] in the rat,[33, 155] and in the mouse,[43] essentially to combinations where histocompatibility differences exist at the major locus. Colley and de Witt[33] found a small reactivity associated with a minor locus difference in the rat, while in the mouse multiple minor incompatibilities may provoke a reaction.[143, 148] A further interesting restriction is constituted by the fact that these very same antigens call forth a reaction only when confronting cells of the same species. For example, the reaction of rat lymphocytes to human cells is minimal;[179] so is the reaction of sheep to rat lymphocytes.[92] This reduced reactivity in xenogeneic combinations also parallels the in vivo graft versus host reaction.[92, 145]

Stimulation in MLC seems to require still another function besides the presentation of a major transplantation antigen of the species on the surface of a lymphocyte. Stimulation may require an intact metabolic function on the part of the stimulating cell. X-irradiated or mitomycin-C-treated cells can provoke a reaction comparable to untreated lymphocytes.[20, 85] In contrast, lymphocytes subjected to irradiation by ultraviolet light are completely without stimulating activity despite the fact that these cells appear intact by dye exclusion and possess transplantation antigens on their surface.[97] Similarly, cells treated with metabolic inhibitors[148] or subjected to heating[52, 148] are inactivated. Homogenates and sonicates of lymphocytes are also devoid of activity.[52, 63, 106]

A crude preparation of mouse transplantation antigens in the form of insoluble lipoproteins has been reported to be capable of eliciting MLC.[109] Two reports claim stimulation by soluble human transplantation antigens.[136, 174] However, we[142] and others[99] have been unable to obtain significant stimulatory activity with such preparations.

In our studies antigens were extracted by two methods,[40, 135] and were shown to contain transplantation antigens by serologic methods. More information is needed to clarify this important issue. Until then it would appear that on the whole, stimulation in MLC is restricted to major transplantation antigens of the species, presented on the surface of viable mononuclear cells. A further restriction might apply if not all but only thymus-derived lymphocytes could fulfill this function.[74]

The MLC Response

In antigen-induced proliferative reactions a relatively small number of cells respond initially by undergoing several cycles of cell division.[112] This number is small relative to that which can be activated by "nonspecific" mitogens such as phytohemagglutinin,[126] but it appears to be rather large to be compatible with the clonal selection hypothesis of immune responsiveness.[25] Bach et al., working with human peripheral cells,[16] and Wilson and co-workers with rat leukocytes,[177] estimated the number of initially responding cells in MLC to be about 2 per cent of the total population. This number also coincides with that found in graft-versus-host reactions by Nisbet, Simonsen, and Zaleski.[125] One may assume that these cells represent a subpopulation of lymphocytes which can react to any antigen, i.e., that they are totipotent or, alternatively, that a different subpopulation reacts to each and every antigen, i.e., that they are unipotent. Alternatively, each cell may only react to limited number of antigens, that is, they would be multipotent.

Several experiments militate against the first alternative. Zoschke and Bach[84, 183] have exposed leukocytes to allogeneic cells of one donor for 24 hours. The cells which responded were killed by several cycles of treatment with a DNA analogue, BUdR, activated by light. The remaining cell population no longer responded to cells of the same donor but reacted with full vigor against cells from a third individual. The experiment was repeated with similar results when the stimulating cells from the two donors were used in a reversed sequence. Essentially identical results were obtained by Salmon et al.[146] in experiments of the same type using high specific activity tritiated thymidine instead of BUdR in the first phase of the experiment.

These experiments clearly show that different populations of cells reacted to the two sets of antigens used in each experiment, and accordingly the cells responding in MLC would not be totipotent. However the data does not distinguish between unipotency and multipotency.

It has been suggested that all the initially responding cells may not be precommitted to the antigen but may be recruited in a nonspecific manner. Wilson et al.[179] in an ingenious experiment using rats found no evidence for such recruitment. They cultured cells from one parental strain of rats with F1 hybrid stimulating cells in the presence of leukocytes from the same parental strain of the opposite sex, previously rendered tolerant to the F1 hybrid. Cytologic analysis revealed that essentially all the responding cells were of one sex and none was derived from the tolerant animals.

In cultures of human leukocytes Kasakura et al.[83] and Gordon and MacLean[52] found a soluble substance in culture supernatants, termed blastogenic factor, which could induce blastogenesis when added to unrelated or autologous[77] cells. Although blastogenic factor (BF) could potentially be a recruiting agent, subsequent experiments have shown that BF can stimulate only a small subpopulation of lymphocytes and that this subpopulation could not account for the 2 per cent of cells activated in MLC.[30] Another factor, which apparently can only stimulate autologous cells, has been recently described by Powles et al.[133] Its role, if any, in the MLC reaction will have to be investigated.

If 2 per cent of the cells do respond specifically to one antigen and each cell is unipotent, then the response can cope with a total of only 50 antigens which clearly cannot be the case. One may consider however that the response to major transplantation antigens of the species, which is the MLC reaction, enjoys a very special status with a high frequency of responding cells and the frequency of responding cells to other antigens would be lower by several orders of magnitude. This may be the reason why reactions to xenogeneic cells or other antigens are seen only when cells from preimmunized animals are cultured.

Jerne has recently proposed a theory which can account for the high frequency of cells reacting to major transplantation antigens of the species.[79] According to this theory, germ line cells carry V genes for transplantation antigens of the species. Those cells which possess specificities directed against self, mutate to generate cells which recognize all foreign antigens. The others mature and become the cells which mediate reactions against allogeneic transplantation antigens.

The evidence reviewed in this chapter demonstrates that the MLC is a vigorous reaction restricted essentially to a response to the major transplantation antigens of the species. The results suggest that this reaction is the in vitro counterpart of an immune pathway for which the majority of the immunocompetent cells of the body appear to be reserved.

APPLICATION OF THE MLC

Histocompatibility Matching

Acceptance or rejection of allografts is governed by a major genetic locus in chickens,[36] mice,[157] rats,[132] dogs,[164] pigs,[170] and man.[14] It is currently held that in man this major locus, termed HL-A, consists of two subloci, each giving rise to a segregant series of alternative alleles, determining the HL-A transplantation antigens.[87] Each individual inherits two HL-A alleles from each parent and thus has four major transplantation antigens. If parents have alleles ab and cd, then their offspring will have alleles ac, ad, bc, or bd with a 25 per cent probability of being HL-A identical. The probability of HL-A identity in the population at large is much smaller, since the number of alleles so far detected is large: 8 for the sublocus "LA" and 13 for the sublocus "4".

Transplantation antigens are present on the surface of all nucleated cells and are customarily detected on leukocytes by isoantisera obtained from multiparous women, multitransfused patients or by antisera raised by deliberate immunization. With such sera the HL-A phenotypes, or when used for family studies, the HL-A genotype, of individuals may be determined.

That MLC is related to histocompatibility has been recognized by Bain and Lowenstein,[22] who have shown that cells from fraternal twins and siblings reacted less vigorously than those of unrelated individuals. Subsequently Bach has demonstrated that within families 29 per cent of the siblings failed to react to each other's cells in MLC suggesting that MLC reactivity was also determined by a single genetic locus.[10] Bach and Amos studied and compared the MLC reactivity and HL-A typing of several families and found that siblings who were HL-A identical by serotyping were also MLC identical, i.e., did not interact in MLC.[8, 14] This very important discovery suggesting that MLC reactivity was governed by the same locus or one closely linked with that determining HL-A antigens was confirmed by Schellekens et al.[148] and Sorensen and Kissmeyer-Nielsen.[160] Exceptions to this however were recently described by Yunis et al.[182]

JULIUS GORDON

The correlation between serotyping and MLC is not absolute. Whereas all MLC-identical individuals (with one exception, all siblings) were also HL-A identical, numerous unrelated HL-A identical pairs found were shown to interact in MLC.[15, 160, 168] Several reasons may account for this discrepancy. It may be that some HL-A antigens not yet defined remain undetected by typing, but can stimulate in MLC.

Since all four antigens of these individuals were detected, this explanation would hold only if another, third sublocus of HL-A existed. Some evidence for a third sublocus has been presented.[87] Another explanation may be that minor histocompatibility loci, other than HL-A, not measured by serotyping may stimulate in MLC. Indeed in mice, multiple minor loci incompatibilities can give rise to an MLC reaction[92, 143, 168] In man however-er, there is no evidence for non-HL-A participation in MLC.

Bach et al.[17] compared and found no difference in the capacity of cells of monozygotic twins and MLC-identical siblings either to respond to, or to stimulate, third party unrelated cells in MLC. Whereas the cells of the former should share all antigens, the latter would presumably differ at all loci except HL-A. In addition, antigens not related to HL-A, such as 5a, 5b, and 9a have been shown to be non-stimulatory in MLC.[11, 168, 172]

In view of the objections cited, neither explanation seems likely to account for the MLC stimulation between apparently HL-A identical pairs. It may well be that the HL-A identity is only apparent, and other specificities not shared are not revealed owing to inclusions, cross-reactivity of antigens, and unavailability of truly monovalent antisera.

Whatever the reason, it would seem that MLC matching within families is a more rigorous test of histocompatibility than serotyping, the demonstration and interpretation of the former not depending on extraneous reagents. This claim is supported by data comparing survival of skin grafts exchanged between unrelated, unrelated HL-A identical, and HL-A and MLC identical individuals. The mean graft survival in the three groups was found to be 10 ± 1.5, 13.1 ± 2.1, and 20 ± 4.2 days respectively.[166] In addition 6 groups of investigators found a correlation between MLC matching and the clinical course of kidney transplants.[11, 21, 61, 78, 124, 163] J. F. Bach et al.[21] found a better correlation with MLC than with serotyping.

MLC has also been used to select compatible bone marrow to repopulate stem cells in immunodeficient and leukemic children. Matching donors for bone marrow transfusion is more critical than for kidney transplantation since not only must the recipient accept the transplant for a successful engraftment, but the donor must also accept the recipient to avoid a graft-versus-host (GVH) disease. Four cases of successful bone marrow transplants have been reported in immunodeficient patients with little or moderate GVH reactions.[7, 12, 41, 117] In all instances MLC identical donors were used. The incidence of GVH reactions in leukemic patients given bone marrow was probably not higher, but several patients succumbed owing to recurrence of the malignancy.[56]

Clearly, MLC applies to matching within families by selecting MLC-identical siblings; what is its usefulness for selecting donors from the population at large? The prospects of finding unrelated MLC identical pairs don't seem very promising according to Bach,[11] who has not found any in 300 combinations. On the other hand, Van Rood et al.[172] were able to select four pairs of HL-A identical matches among 500 unrelated individuals, two of which were also MLC identical. If this is indeed a representative figure, then finding suitable donors becomes a logistic problem of serotyping large populations, selecting HL-A identical individuals by a computer program, and testing these in MLC.

Short of such an approach, can a selection be based on different degrees of responsiveness in MLC, and would it be meaningful? Bach et al.[10] and Sorensen and Kissmeyer-Nielsen[160] could clearly differentiate between siblings within families who differed from each other by one allele and those who differed at both. In the general population most individuals differ at both alleles. Among these, Bach et al.[19] find reactivities which may vary over a 30-fold range. The significance of this variation, and the bearing it may have on the prognosis of transplants carried out across a "strong" or a "weak" MLC barrier, must await the evaluation of the strength of different alleles in MLC and in clinical transplantation.

Detection of Immunocompetent Cells

Several attempts have been made to fractionate bone marrow in order to free the stem cells to be transplanted from immunocompetent cells, capable of mediating a graft-versus-host reaction. The MLC reaction has been one of the methods of assay used to monitor the immunocompetent cells in the various fractions.[16, 42] The theoretical basis for this application has been the demonstration that MLC, like the GVH reaction in vivo, measures a thymus-dependent, cell-mediated function.

Another application of MLC, based on the same consideration is the diagnosis of immunodeficient syndromes. The subject of immunologic deficiency diseases,[48] and the application of in vitro tests to their diagnosis have recently been reviewed.[137] MLC reactivity has been found to be absent in the Swiss type combined immunologic deficiencies,[18] and reduced in partial combined deficiencies such as ataxia telangiectasia[48, 66, 94, 128] and the Wiscott Aldrich syndrome.[110] Predictably, MLC reactivity was not demonstrable in patients with DiGeorge's syndrome which is the prototype of cell-mediated deficiency diseases,[90, 103, 115] whereas reactivity was normal[18, 35] or reduced[98] in diseases involving humoral immune mechanisms. An apparent dissociation between the reactivity of some patients' cells to allogeneic cells and to the nonspecific stimulant, PHA, would suggest that both tests should be performed at all times.[115]

MLC may also serve to evaluate the effectiveness of immunosuppressive therapy by studying the reactivity of the cells of patients during or after treatment.[55, 71, 116] Alternatively, immunosuppressive agents, such as antilymphocyte serum, may be tested directly by adding them to the cultures.[24, 150]

A lack of MLC reactivity may, under other specific circumstances, be an in vitro measure of tolerance.[149, 181] In fact this reaction may be useful in distinguishing between immunologic tolerance, a central failure of immune reactivity and a peripheral inhibition, such as enhancement. Cells from animals rendered tolerant by the injection of lymphoid cells neonatally are specifically unreactive against the donor-strain cells in MLC.

These animals also fail to reject skin allografts derived from the appropriate donor strain.

In contrast, cells from animals which have accepted kidney transplants permanently following the administration of donor bone marrow cells[60] or isoantisera directed against the graft,[104] or both,[162] do react fully in MLC against lymphoid cells derived from the kidney donors and can reject skin grafts from the same source. These animals are clearly not tolerant but are thought to retain the allogeneic kidney by virtue of enhancement. In one particular strain combination the majority of recipients accept a kidney transplant without pretreatment of any kind. These animals probably do become tolerant since they retain donor skin grafts and do not react against donor leukocytes in MLC.[144]

In some instances the MLC reaction may be negative while skin grafts may be rejected.[154] In such situations MLC reactivity may be the only indicator of a state of tolerance as the mechanism allowing the retention of an organ transplant.

The MLC may also be amenable to detecting serum factors which can mediate enhancement. Sera capable of inducing enhancement of heart transplants,[53] sera of dogs bearing kidney allografts,[120] and sera containing antibodies to HL-A antigens,[28] have all been shown to inhibit MLC reactions. Further investigation is required to find out whether this system can indeed detect and differentiate between different classes of antibodies which may mediate rejection and enhancement.

An entirely different application of MLC has been suggested by the experiments of Zoschke and Bach[184] and Salmon et al.[146] These authors have shown that lymphoid cell populations may be specifically depleted of cells reactive against one target (A) without essentially diminishing their reactivity against another (B). This was accomplished by exposing the cells to target A, and killing the cells which became activated by a thymidine analogue or by high specific activity tritiated thymidine. Bone marrow or other lymphoid cells exposed to antigens of the prospective recipient could be an excellent source for immunotherapy provided that this in vitro treatment is not lethal to stem cells.

Several applications of the MLC have been reviewed, and several others will no doubt be developed. In the application of MLC to matching donors and recipients for transplantation the most urgent need is the extension of the test to unrelated individuals. This may require considerable refinement in the technique.[151] Equally pressing is the need to reduce the time required for the test to make it applicable to transplantation of cadaveric organs. Probably the most promising potential of MLC is the one most recently described. It is the analysis of cells and sera of patients to reveal their specific immune status towards their transplant. Equally exciting is the prospect of being able to obtain through the MLC specifically depleted cell populations for transplantation. The next 5 years will hopefully fulfill these promises.

Pressure on space required deletion by the publisher of contributed material that justified the classification of the MLC reaction as an immune reaction (see references 2–4, 29, 33, 43, 45, 48, 51, 54, 61, 64, 67, 68, 73, 76, 96, 98, 103, 107, 108, 115, 119, 127–130, 143, 148, 149, 156, 158, 173, 175, and 178–181) and material that described the method of performing the MLC test as it is done in the author's laboratory (references 1, 9, 20, 32, 37, 46, 57, 58, 62, 65, 70, 75, 82, 84, 85, 93, 100, 102, 105, 112, 114, 123, 128, 131, 134, 141, 152, 153, 161, and 167). For recent reviews of the broad subject of lymphocyte stimulation, see the book by Ling[101] and the articles of Wilson and Billingham[176] and Valentine.[171]

REFERENCES

1. Adler, W. H., Peavy, D., and Smith, R. T.: The effect of PHA, PPD, allogeneic cells, and sheep erythrocytes on albumin gradient-separated mouse spleen cell populations. Cell. Immunol., 1:78–91, 1970.
2. Adler, W. H., Takiguchi, T., Marsh, B., and Smith, R. T.: Cellular recognition by mouse lymphocytes in vitro. II. Specific stimulation by histocompatibility antigens in mixed cell culture. J. Immunol., 105:984, 1000, 1970.
3. Albertini, R. J., and Bach, F. H.: Quantitative assay of antigenic disparity of HL-A – the major histocompatibility locus in man. J. Exper. Med., 128:639–651, 1968.
4. Alm, G. U., and Peterson, R. D. A.: Effect of thymectomy and bursectomy on the in vitro response of chick spleen cells to PHA, sheep erythrocytes (SRBC) and allogeneic cells. Fed. Proc., 29:430, 1970.
5. Alter, B. J., and Bach, F. H.: Lymphocyte reactivity in vitro. I. Cellular reconstitution of purified lymphocyte response. Cell. Immunol., 1:207–218, 1970.
6. Amato, D., Bergsagel, D. E., Clarysse, A. M., Cowan, D. H., Iscove, N. N., McCullogh, E. A., Miller, R. G., Philips, R. A., Ragab, A. M., and Senn, J. S.: Review of bone marrow transplants at the Ontario Cancer Institute. Transplant. Proc., III:397–399, 1971.
7. Ammann, A. J., Meuwissen, H. S., Good, R. A., and Hong, R.: Successful bone marrow transplantation in a patient with humoral and cellular immunity deficiency. Clin. Exper. Immunol., 7:343–353, 1970.
8. Amos, D. B., and Bach, F. H.: Phenotypic expressions of the major histocompatibility locus in man (HL-A): leukocyte antigens and mixed leukocyte culture reactivity. J. Exper. Med., 128:623–637, 1968.
9. Bach, F., and Hirschhorn, K.: Lymphocyte interaction: a potential histocompatibility test in vitro. Science, 143:813–814, 1964.
10. Bach, F. H.: Mixed leukocyte cultures – their assay and genetics. In In Vitro II. Baltimore, Maryland, Waverly Press, 1966.
11. Bach, F. H.: Transplantation: problems of histocompatibility testing. Science, 159:1196–1198, 1968.
12. Bach, F. H., Albertini, R. J., Joo, P., Anderson, J. L., and Bortin, M. M.: Bone-marrow transplantation in a patient with the Wiskott-Aldrich syndrome. The Lancet, 2:1364–1366, 1968.
13. Bach, F. H., Alter, B. J., Solliday, S., Zoschke, D. C., and Janis, M.: Lymphocyte reactivity in vitro. II. Soluble reconstituting factor permitting response of purified lymphocytes. Cell. Immunol., 1:219–227, 1970.
14. Bach, F. H., and Amos, D. B.: HU-1: Major histocompatibility locus in man. Science, 156:1506, 1967.
15. Bach, F. H., and Bach, M. L.: Mixed leukocyte cultures in histocompatibility testing. In Harris, J. E., ed.: Proceedings of the 5th Leukocyte Culture Conference. New York, Academic Press, 1970, pp. 287–297.
16. Bach, F. H., Bock, H., Graupner, K., Day, E., and Klostermann, H.: Cell kinetic studies in mixed leukocyte cultures: an in vitro model of homograft reactivity. Proc. Nat. Acad. Sci. (U.S.), 62:377–384, 1969.
17. Bach, F. H., Day, E., Lebrun, A., and Bach, M. L.: Histocompatibility matching. III. Phenotypic expression of HL-A: effect of other loci on stimulation by and the response to HL-A antigens. In Terasaki, P. I., ed.: Histocompatibility Testing. Copenhagen, Munksgaard, 1970, pp. 509–515.
18. Bach, F. H., Meuwissen, H. J., Albertini, R. J., and Good, R. A.: "Agammaglobulinemic leukocytes" – their in vitro reactivity. In Rieke, W. O., ed.: Proceedings of the Third Annual Leukocyte Culture Conference. New York, Appleton-Century-Crofts, 1969, pp. 709–723.
19. Bach, F. H., Segall, M., Day, E., and Bach, M. L.: Histocompatibility matching. II. Incompatibility strength of HL-A alleles. In Terasaki, P. I., ed.: Histocompatibility Testing. Copenhagen, Munksgaard, 1970, pp. 503–508.
20. Bach, F. H., and Voynow, N. K.: One-way stimulation in mixed leukocyte cultures. Science, 153:545, 547, 1966.
21. Bach, J. F., Debray-Sachs, M., Crosnier, J., Kreis, H., and Dormont, J.: Correlation between mixed lymphocyte culture performed before renal transplantation and kidney function. Clin. Exper. Immunol., 6:821–827, 1970.

22. Bain, B., and Lowenstein, L.: Genetic studies on the mixed leukocyte reaction. Science, *145*:1315–1316, 1964.

23. Bain, B., Vas, M. R., and Lowenstein, L.: The development of large immature mononuclear cells in mixed leukocyte culture. Blood, 23:108–116, 1964.

24. Brochier, J., and Revillard, J. P.: In vitro stimulation or inhibition of lymphocyte activation by anti-lymphocyte serum. Transplant. Proc., *3*:788–792, 1971.

25. Burnet, F. M.: The Clonal Selection Theory of Acquired Immunity. London, Cambridge University Press, 1959.

26. Carstairs, K.: Transformation of the small lymphocyte in culture. Lancet, 2:984, 1961.

27. Carstairs, K.: The human small lymphocyte: its possible pluripotential quality. Lancet, *1*:829–832, 1962.

28. Ceppellini, R., Bonnard, G. D., Coppo, F., Miggiano, V. C., Pospisit, M., Curtoni, E. S., and Pellegrino, M.: Mixed leukocyte cultures and HL-A antigens. II. Inhibition by anti-HL-A sera. Transplant. Proc., 3:63–70, 1971.

29. Cerottini, J. C., Nordin, A. A., and Brunner, K. T.: Cellular and humoral response to transplantation antigens. I. Development of alloantibody-forming cells and cytotoxic lymphocytes in the graft versus host reaction. J. Exper. Med., *131*:553–564, 1971.

30. Chan, E., and Gordon, J.: Stimulation of leukocytes by blastogenic factor: comparison with that provided by allogeneic cells. Cell. Immunol. (in press).

31. Chess, L., Bock, G. N., and Mardiney, M. R., Jr.: Reconstitution of the reactivity of frozen-stored human lymphocytes in the mixed lymphocyte reaction and in response to specific antigen. *In* Schwarz, M. R., ed.: Proceedings of the 6th Leukocyte Culture Conference. New York, Academic Press, in press.

32. Chessin, L. N., Borjeson, J., Welsh, P. D., Douglas, S. D., and Cooper, H. L.: Studies on human peripheral blood lymphocytes in vitro. J. Exper. Med., *124*:873–884, 1966.

33. Colley, D. G., and De Witt, C. W.: Mixed lymphocyte blastogenesis in response to multiple histocompatibility antigens. J. Immunol., *102*:107–116, 1969.

34. Cooper, E. H., Barkhan, P., and Hale, A. J.: Mitogenic activity of phytohemagglutinin. Lancet, 2:210, 1961.

35. Cooperband, S. R., Rosen, F. S., and Kibrick, S.: Studies on the in vitro behaviour of agammaglobulinemic lymphocytes. J. Clin. Invest., *47*:836–847, 1968.

36. Crittenden, L. B., Johnson, L. W., and Okazaki, W.: Histocompatibility and erythrocyte antigen variability within highly inbred lines of white leghorns. Transplantation, 2:362–374, 1964.

37. Coulson, A. S., and Chalmers, D. G.: Separation of viable lymphocytes from human blood. Lancet, *1*:468–469, 1964.

38. Coulson, A. S., and Chalmers, D. G.: Response of human blood lymphocytes to tuberculin PPD in tissue culture. Immunol., *12*:417, 1967.

39. Davies, A. J. S., Festenstein, H., Leuchars, E., Wallis, V. J., and Doenhoff, M. J.: The origin of some mouse peripheral blood lymphocytes. *In* Proceedings of the Second International Conference of Germinal Centers of Lymphatic Tissue, Padua, Italy, 1968.

40. Davies, D. A. L., Manstone, A. J., Viza, D. C., Colombani, J., and Dausset, J.: Human transplantation antigens: The HL-A (HU-1) system and its homology with the mouse H-2 system. Transplantation, 6:571–586, 1968.

41. de Koning, J., Dooren, L. J., van Bekkum, D. W., Van Rood, J. J., Dicke, K. A., and Radl, J.: Transplantation of bone marrow cells and fetal thymus in an infant with lymphogenic immunological deficiency. Lancet, *1*:1223, 1969.

42. Dicke, K. A., Tridente, G., and van Bekkum, D. W.: The selective elimination of immunologically competent cells from bone marrow and lymphocyte cell mixtures. III. In vitro test for detection of immunocompetent cells in fractionated mouse spleen suspensions and primate bone marrow suspensions. Transplantation, 8:422–434, 1969.

43. Dutton, R. W.: Spleen cell proliferation in response to homologous antigens studied in congenic resistant strains of mice. J. Exper. Med., *123*:665–671, 1966.

44. Elkins, W. L., and Guttmann, R. D.: Pathogenesis of a local graft host reaction: immunogenicity of circulating host leukocytes. Science, *159*:1250–1251, 1968.

45. Elves, L. W.: The mixed leukocyte reaction. An in vitro model for the homograft reaction. Transplantation, 8:44–50, 1969.

46. Elves, M. W.: The mixed leukocyte reaction in uremic subjects. Proc. Europe. Dialysis Transplant. Assoc., 2:165–172, 1965.

47. Fisher, D. B., and Mueller, G. C.: An early alteration in the phospholipid metabolism of lymphocytes by phytohemagglutinin. Proc. Nat. Acad. Sci., 60:1396–1402, 1968.

48. Gatti, R. A., and Good, R. A.: The immunological deficiency diseases. Med. Clin. N. Amer., 54:281–307, 1970.

49. Good, R. A., Dalmasso, A. P., Martinez, C., Archer, O. K., Pierce, J. C., and Papermaster, B. W.: The role of the thymus in development of immunologic capacity in rabbits and mice. J. Exper. Med., *116*:773–795, 1962.

50. Gordon, J.: Role of monocytes in the mixed leukocyte culture reaction. Proc. Soc. Exper. Biol. Med., *127*:30–33, 1968.

51. Gordon, J., David-Faridy, F., and MacLean, L. D.: Transfer of transplantation immunity by leukocytes sensitized in vitro. Transplantation, 5:1030–1039, 1967.
52. Gordon, J., and MacLean, L. D.: A lymphocyte-stimulating factor produced in vitro. Nature, 208:795–796, 1965.
53. Gordon, R. O., Stinson, E. B., Souther, S. G., and Oppenheim, J. J.: Mixed leukocyte reaction (MLR) as an assay for the presence of enhancing alloantiserum. In Schwarz, R. M., ed.: Proceedings of the Sixth Leukocyte Culture Conference. New York, Academic Press, in press.
54. Greaves, M. F., Roitt, I. M., and Rose, M. E.: Effect of bursectomy and thymectomy on the response of chicken peripheral blood lymphocytes to phytohemagglutinin. Nature (Lond.), 220:293–295, 1968.
55. Greaves, M. F., Roitt, I. M., Zamir, R., and Carnaghan, R. B. A.: Effect of anti-lymphocyte serum on responses of human peripheral-blood lymphocytes to specific and nonspecific stimulants in vitro. Lancet, 2:1317–1319, 1967.
56. Graw, R. G., Jr., and Santos, G. W.: Bone marrow transplantation in patients with leukemia. Transplantation, 11:197–199, 1971.
57. Greenwalt, T. J., Gajewski, M., and McKenna, J. L.: A new method for preparing buffy coat-poor blood. Transfusion, 2:221–229, 1961.
58. Grumet, F. C., and Leventhal, B. G.: Inhibition of the response in mixed leukocyte cultures by alloimmune plasma. Transplantation, 9:405–409, 1970.
59. Guttmann, R. D., and Lindquist, R. R.: Renal transplantation in the inbred rat. XI. Reduction of allograft immunogenicity by donor pretreatment with cytotoxic drugs. Transplantation, 8:490–495, 1969.
60. Guttmann, R. D., Lindquist, R. R., and Ockner, S. A.: Renal transplantation in the inbred rat. IX. Hematopoietic origin of an immunogenic stimulus of rejection. Transplantation, 8:472–484, 1969.
61. Hamburger, J., Crosnier, J., Descamps, B., and Rowinska, D.: The value of present methods used for the selection of organ donors. Transplant. Proc., 3:260–267, 1971.
62. Hardy, D. A., and Ling, N. R.: Effects of some cellular antigens on lymphocytes and the nature of the mixed leukocyte culture reaction. Nature (Lond.), 221:545–548, 1969.
63. Hardy, D. A., Knight, S., and Ling, N. R.: The interaction of normal lymphocytes and cells from lymphoid cell lines. I. The nature of the activation process. Immunol., 19:329–342, 1970.
64. Hardy, D. A., Wallin, J. M., and Ling, N. R.: Cytotoxic activity of human lymphocytes stimulated by x-irradiated cells from lymphoid cell lines. In Harris, J. E., ed.: Proceedings of the Fifth Leukocyte Culture Conference. New York, Academic Press, 1970, pp. 287–297.
65. Harris, R., and Ukaejiofo, E. O.: Rapid preparation of lymphocytes for tissue typing. Lancet, 2:327, 1970.
66. Hayakawa, M., and Kobayashi, N.: Blasts in ataxia-telangiectasia Lancet, 1:1279, 1967.
67. Hayry, P., and Defendi, V.: Mixed lymphocyte cultures produce effector cells: model in vitro for allograft rejection. Science, 168:133, 1970.
68. Hayry, P., and Defendi, V.: Allograft immunity in vitro: I. Cultivation conditions and mixed lymphocyte interaction of mouse peripheral lymphocytes. Clin. Exper. Immunol., 6:345–362, 1970.
69. Hayry, P., and Defendi, V.: Demonstration of the effector arm in the mixed lymphocyte interaction. In McIntyre, O. R., ed.: Proceedings of the Fourth Annual Leukocyte Culture Conference. New York, Appleton-Century-Crofts, 1971, pp. 449–455.
70. Hartzman, R. J., Segall, M., Bach, M. L., and Bach, F. H.: Histocompatibility matching. VI. Miniaturization of the mixed leukocyte culture test: a preliminary report. Transplantation, 11:268–273, 1971.
71. Hersh, E. N., and Oppenheim, J. T.: Inhibition of in vitro lymphocyte transformation during chemotherapy in man. Cancer Res., 27:98–105, 1967.
73. Hodes, R. J., and Svedmyr, E. A.: Specific cytotoxicity of H-2 incompatible mouse lymphocytes following mixed culture in vitro. Transplantation, 9:470–477, 1970.
74. Howe, M. L., and Goldstein, A. L.: Thymic influence on the stimulator cell in the mixed lymphocyte interaction (MLI). In Schwarz, M. R., ed.: Proceedings of the Sixth Leukocyte Culture Conference. New York, Academic Press, in press.
75. Huber, H., Pastner, D., Dittrich, P., and Braunsteiner, H.: In vitro reactivity of human lymphocytes in uremia—a comparison with the impairment of delayed hypersensitivity. Clin. Exper. Immunol., 5:75–82, 1969.
76. Huemer, R. P., Keller, L. S., and Lee, K. D.: Thymidine incorporation in mixed cultures of spleen cells from mice of differing H-2 types. Transplantation, 6:706–715, 1968.
77. Janis, M., and Bach, F. H.: Blastogenic factor production by PHA-stimulated leukocytes. In McIntyre, O. R., ed.: Proceedings of the Fourth Annual Leukocyte Culture Conference. New York, Appleton-Century-Crofts, 1971, pp. 335–345.
78. Jeannet, M.: Histocompatibility testing using leukocyte typing and mixed lymphocyte culture in kidney transplants. Helv. Med. Acta, 35:168–179, 1970.

79. Jerne, N. K.: The somatic generation of immune recognition. European J. Immunol., 1:1–9, 1971.
80. Johnson, M., Hattler, B., Alexander, J., and Currier, C.: Effect of granulocyte concentration of mixed lymphocyte culture. Fed. Proc., 30:1514, 1971.
81. Johnston, J. M.: Origin of immunoreactive lymphoid cells in the rat. In McIntyre, O. R., ed.: Proceedings of the Fourth Leukocyte Culture Conference. New York, Appleton-Century-Crofts, 1971, pp. 14–16.
82. Junge, U., Hoekstra, J., Wolfe, L., and Deinhardt, F.: Microtechnique for quantitative evaluation of in vitro lymphocyte transformation. Clin. Exper. Immunol., 7:431, 1970.
83. Kasakura, S., and Lowenstein, L.: A factor stimulating DNA synthesis derived from the medium of leukocyte cultures. Nature (Lond.), 208:794–795, 1965.
84. Kasakura, S., and Lowenstein, L.: The effect of uremic blood on mixed leukocyte reactions and on cultures of leukocytes with phytohemagglutinin. Transplantation, 5:283–289, 1967.
85. Kasakura, S., and Lowenstein, L.: Irradiated and preserved leukocytes in mixed leukocyte cultures. Proc. Soc. Exper. Biol. Med., 125:355–360, 1967.
86. Kisken, W. A., and Swenson, N. A.: Unresponsiveness of mixed leukocyte cultures from thymectomized adult dogs. Nature, 224:76–77, 1969.
87. Kissmeyer-Nielsen, F., and Thorsby, E.: Human transplantation antigens. Transplantation Rev., 4:17–29, 1970.
88. Kountz, S. L., Cochrum, K. C., and Main, R. K.: Five discrimination of antigenicity at the AgB locus by the mixed skin cell leukocyte reaction. In Schwarz, R. M., ed.: Proceedings of the Sixth Leukocyte Culture Conference. New York, Academic Press, in press.
89. Kourilsky, F. M., Silvestre, D., Lery, J. P., Dausset, J., Nicolai, M. G., and Senik, A.: Immunoferretin study of the distribution of HL-A antigens on human blood cells. J. Immunol., 106:454–466, 1971.
90. Kretschmer, R., Say, B., Brown, D., and Rosen, F. S.: Congenital aplasia of the thymus gland (DiGeorge's syndrome). New Eng. J. Med., 279:1295–1301, 1968.
91. Kuper, S. W. A., Bignall, J. R., and Luckcock, E. D.: A quantitative method for studying turnover cells in blood. Lancet, 1:852–853, 1966.
92. Lafferty, K. J., and Jones, A. S.: Reactions of the graft versus host (GVH) type. Austral. J. Exper. Biol. Med. Sci., 47:17–54, 1969.
93. Lamvik, J. O.: Separation of lymphocytes from human blood. Acta Haematol., 35:294, 1966.
94. Leiken, S. L., Bazelon, M., and Park, K. H.: In vitro lymphocyte transformation in ataxia-telangiectasia. J. Pediat., 68:477–479, 1966.
95. Levis, W. R., and Robbins, J. H.: Function of glass-adherent cells in human mixed lymphocyte cultures. Transplantation, 9:515–518, 1970.
96. Lindquist, R. R., and Guttmann, R. D.: Relevance of mixed lymphocyte reactions to renal allograft rejection mechanisms. Transplant. Proc., 3:879–887, 1971.
97. Lindahl-Kiessling, K. M.: Inability of UV-irradiated lymphocytes to stimulate allogeneic cells in MLC. In Schwarz, M. R., ed.: Proceedings of of the Sixth Leukocyte Culture Conference. New York, Academic Press, in press.
98. Lieber, E., Hirschhorn, K., and Fudenberg, H. H.: Response of agammaglobulinaemic lymphocytes in mixed lymphocyte cultures. Clin. Exper. Immunol., 4:83–91, 1969.
99. Ling, N. R.: Personal communications.
100. Ling, N. R.: Lymphocyte Stimulation, Amsterdam, North-Holland Publishing Co., 1968, p. 38.
101. Ling, N. R.: Lymphocyte Stimulation. Amsterdam, North Holland Publishing Co., 1968.
102. Ling, N. R., Acton, A. B., Roitt, I. M., and Doniach, D.: Interaction of lymphocytes from immunized hosts with thyroid and other cells in culture. Brit. J. Exper. Pathol., 46:348–359, 1965.
103. Lischner, H. W., Punnett, H. H., and Di George, A. M.: Lymphocytes in congenital absence of the thymus. Nature, 214:580–582, 1967.
104. Lucas, Z. J., Markley, J., and Travis, M.: Immunologic enhancement of renal allografts in the rat. I. Dissociation of graft survival and antibody response. Fed. Proc., 29:2041–2047, 1970.
105. Main, R. K., Cochrum, K. C., Jones, M. J., and Kountz, S. L.: Immunological potential of the in vitro mixed skin cell-leukocyte reaction. Nature New Biol., 229:89–91, 1971.
106. Main, R. K., and Jones, M. J.: Mixed leukocyte interaction involving mouse strains of strong and weak allogeneic specificities. Nature, 218:1251–1252, 1968.
107. Main, R. K., Cole, L. J., Jones, M. J., and Haire, H. M.: DNA synthesis in mixed cultures of dog leukocytes: differential effect of x-irradiation and freeze-thawing on cellular isoantigenicity. J. Immunol., 98:417–424, 1967.
108. Mangi, R. J., and Mardiney, M. R., Jr.: Transformation of mouse lymphocytes to allogeneic lymphocytes and phytohemagglutinin. J. Immunol., 105:90–97, 1970.
109. Manson, L. A., and Simmons, T.: Induction of the alloimmune response in mouse lymphocytes by cell-free transplantation antigens in vitro: enhancement of DNA synthesis and specific sensitization. Transplant. Proc., 1:498–501, 1969.

110. Marshall, W. C., Cope, W. A., Soothhill, J. F., and Dudgeon, J. A.: In vitro lymphocyte response in some immunity deficiency diseases and in intrauterine virus infections. Proc. Roy. Soc. Med., 63:351–355, 1970.
111. Marshall, W. H., Rigo, S. J., and Melman, S.: Lymphocyte transformation and mitosis in vitro initiated by homologous macrophages. Lancet, 1:730–732, 1966.
112. Marshall, W. H., Valentine, F. T., and Lawrence, H. S.: Cellular immunity in vitro. Clonal proliferation of antigen-stimulated lymphocytes. J. Exper. Med., 130:327–343, 1969.
113. McFarland, W., and Heilman, D. H.: Lymphocyte foot appendate: its role in lymphocyte function and in immunological reactions. Nature (Lond.), 205:887–888, 1965.
114. Mendelshon, J., Skinner, A., and Kornfeld, S.: Rapid induction of increased alpha-aminoisobutyric acid uptake by phytohemagglutinin stimulated lymphocytes. In Harris, J. E., ed.: Proceedings of the Fifth Leukocyte Culture Conference. New York, Academic Press, 1970, pp. 31–37.
115. Meuwissen, H. J., Bach, F. H., Hong, R., and Good, R. A.: Lymphocyte studies in congenital thymic dysplasia: the one-way stimulation test. J. Pediat., 72:177–185, 1968.
116. Meuwissen, H. J., Van Alten, P. A., and Good, R. A.: Decreased lymphoid cell multiplication in the post-thymectomy state. Transplantation, 7:1–11, 1969.
117. Meuwissen, H. J., Gatti, R. A., Terasaki, P. I., Hong, R., and Good, R. A.: Treatment of lymphopenic hypogamma globulinemia and bone marrow aplasia by transplantation of allogeneic marrow. New Eng. J. Med., 281:691–697, 1969.
118. Meuwissen, H. J., Van Alten, P. A., and Good, R. A.: Decreased lymphoid cell multiplication in the post-thymectomy state. Transplantation, 7:1–11, 1969.
119. Meuwissen, H. J., Van Alten, P. J., and Good, R. A.: Antigen-induced cell proliferation in cultures from antibody-deficient chickens. J. Immunol., 102:1079–1083, 1969.
120. Miller, J., Hattler, B., Davis, M., and Johnson, M. C.: Cellular and humoral factors governing canine mixed lymphocyte cultures after renal transplantation. I. Antibody. Transplantation, 12:65–76, 1971.
121. Miller, J. F. A. P., Marshall, A. H. E., and White, R. G.: The immunological significance of the thymus. Advances Immunol., 2:1962.
122. Mills, J. A.: The immunologic significance of antigen-induced lymphocyte transformation in vitro. J. Immunol., 97:239–247, 1966.
123. Moorhead, F. H., Connolly, J. J., and McFarland, W.: Factors affecting the reactivity of human lymphocytes in vitro. I. Cell number, duration of culture and surface area. J. Immunol., 99:413–419, 1967.
124. Nelson, S. D., Russel, P. S., and McGeown, M. G.: The lymphocyte transfer test and mixed cultures in kidney donor selection. Proc. Europ. Dialysis Transplant Assoc., 4:189, 1967.
125. Nisbet, N. W., Simonsen, M., and Zaleski, M.: The frequency of antigen-sensitive cells in tissue transplantation. A commentary on clonal selection. J. Exper. Med., 129:459–467, 1969.
126. Nowell, P. C.: Phytohemagglutinin. An initiator of mitosis in cultures of normal human leukocytes. Cancer Res., 20:462–466, 1960.
127. Oppenheim, J. J.: Relationship of in vitro lymphocyte transformation to delayed hypersensitivity in guinea pigs and man. Fed. Proc., 27:21–28, 1968.
128. Oppenheim, J. J., Barlow, M., Waldmann, T. A., and Block, J. B.: Impaired in vitro lymphocyte transformation in patients with ataxia-telangiectasia. Brit. Med. J., 2:330–333, 1966.
129. Oppenheim, J. J., Leventhal, B. G., and Hersh, E. M.: The transformation of column-purified lymphocytes with nonspecific and specific antigenic stimuli. J. Immunol., 101:262–270, 1968.
130. Oppenheim, J. J., Whang, J., and Frei, E., III: The effect of skin homograft rejection on recipient and donor mixed leukocyte cultures. J. Exper. Med., 122:651–664, 1965.
131. Ouastel, M. R., Dow, S. D., and Kaplan, J. G.: Stimulation of K-42 uptake into lymphocytes by phytohemagglutinin and role of intracellular K+ in lymphocyte transformation. In Harris, J. E., ed.: Proceedings of the Fifth Leukocyte Culture Conference. New York, Academic Press, 1970, pp. 97–123.
132. Palm, J.: Serological detection of histocompatibility antigens in two strains of rats. Transplantation, 2:603–612, 1964.
133. Powles, P., Balchin, L., Currie, G. A., and Alexander, P.: Specific autostimulatory factor released by lymphocytes. Nature, 231:161–164, 1971.
134. Rabinowitz, Y.: Separation of lymphocytes, polymorphonuclear leukocytes and monocytes on glass columns; including tissue culture observations. Blood, 23:811–828, 1964.
135. Reisfeld, R. A., Pellegrino, M. A., and Kahan, B. D.: Salt extraction of soluble HL-A antigens. Science, 172:1134–1136, 1971.
136. Reisfeld, R. A., and Kahan, B. D.: Biological and chemical characterisation of human histocompatibility antigens. Fed. Proc., 29:2034–2040, 1970.
137. Revillard, J. P.: Potential and actual clinical applications of in vitro tests for cell-mediated immunity. In Revillard, J. R., ed.: Cell Mediated Immunity. In Vitro Correlates. Baltimore, University Park Press, 1971, pp. 154–201.

138. Rieke, W. O.: Lymphocytes from thymectomized rats: immunologic, proliferative and metabolic properties. Science, 152:535–538, 1966.
139. Robson, L. G., and Schwarz, M. R.: The influence of adult thymectomy on immunological competence as measured by the mixed lymphocyte reaction. Transplantation, 11:465–470, 1971.
140. Rode, H. N., and Gordon, J.: Inhibition of the mixed leukocyte culture reaction (MLC) by pre-incubation of the leukocytes with sucrose. J. Immunol., 102:786–787, 1969.
141. Rode, H. N., and Gordon, J.: The mixed leukocyte culture: a three component system. J. Immunol., 104:1453–1457, 1970.
142. Rode, H. N., and Gordon, J.: Unpublished observations.
143. Rychlikova, L., and Ivanyi, P.: Mixed lymphocyte cultures and histocompatibility antigens in mice. Folio Biol., 15:126–135, 1969.
144. Salaman, J. P., Elves, M. W., and Festenstein, H.: Factors contributing to survival of rats transplanted with kidneys mismatched at major locus. Transplant. Proc., 3:577–579, 1971.
145. Saleh, W., MacLean, L. D., and Gordon, J.: A graft versus host reaction in a xenogeneic combination: the reaction of murine cells in rats. J. Immunol., 103:114, 1969.
146. Salmon, S. E., Krakauer, R. S., and Whitmore, W. F.: Lymphocyte stimulation: selective destruction of cells during blastogenic response to transplantation antigens. Science, 172:490–492, 1971.
147. Schellekens, P. Th. A., and Eijsvoogel, V. P.: Lymphocyte transformation in vitro. III. Mechanism of stimulation in the mixed lymphocyte culture. Clin. Exper. Immunol., 7:229–239, 1970.
148. Schellekens, P. Th. A., Vriesendorp, B., Eijsvoogel, N. P., Van Leeuwen, A. A. D., Van Rood, J. J., Miggiano, V., and Ceppellini, R.: Lymphocyte transformation in vitro. II. Mixed lymphocyte culture in relation to leukocyte antigens. Clin. Exper. Immunol., 7:241, 1970.
149. Schwarz, M. R.: The mixed lymphocyte reaction: an in vitro test for tolerance. J. Exper. Med., 127:879–890, 1968.
150. Schwarz, M. R., Tyler, R. W., and Everett, N. B.: Mixed lymphocyte reaction: an in vitro test for antilymphocytic serum activity. Science, 166:1014–1017, 1968.
151. Seigler, H. F., Ward, F. E., Amos, D. B., and Stickel, D. L.: Comparisons of mixed leukocyte reactions with skin graft survival in families genotyped for HL-A. Transplant. Proc., 3:115–147, 1971.
152. Senger, D. P. S., and Terasaki, I.: A semimicro mixed leukocyte culture test. Transplantation, 11:260–267, 1971.
153. Shortman, K.: The separation of different cell classes from lymphoid organs. I. The use of glass bead columns to separate small lymphocytes, remove damaged cells and fractionate cell suspensions. Austr. J. Exper. Biol. Med. Sci., 44:271–286, 1966.
154. Silvers, W. K., Lubaroff, D. M., Wilson, D. B., and Fox, D.: Mixed lymphocyte reactions and tissue transplantation tolerance. Science, 167:1264–1266, 1970.
155. Silvers, W. K., Wilson, D. B., and Palm, J.: Mixed leukocyte reactions and histocompatibility in rats. Science, 155:703–704, 1967.
156. Simonsen, M.: On the nature and measurement of antigenic strength. Transplant. Rev., 3:22–35, 1970.
157. Snell, G. D.: Methods for the study of histocompatibility genes. J. Genetics, 49:87–108, 1948.
158. Solliday, S., and Bach, F. H.: Cytotoxicity: specificity after in vitro sensitization. Science, 170:1406–1409, 1970.
159. Sørensen, S. F., Andersen, V., and Giese, J.: A rapid method for quantitation of the incorporation of 3H-thymidine by lymphocytes in vitro. Acta Path. Microbiol. Scand., 75:508–511, 1969.
160. Sørensen, S. F., and Kissmeyer-Nielsen, F.: Studies on the quantitation of the lymphocyte response in vitro. Acta Path. Microl. Scand., 77:117–133, 1969.
161. Spriggs, A. I., and Alexander, R. F.: An albumin gradient method for separating the different white cells of blood, applied to the concentration of circulating tumor cells. Nature, 188:863–864, 1960.
162. Stuart, F. P., Saitoh, T., and Fitch, F. W.: Rejection of renal allografts: specific immunological suppression. Science, 160:1463–1465, 1968.
163. Sullivan, C. E., Stevens, L. E., Main, R. K., Jones, M. J., and Reemtsma, K.: The correlation of mixed leukocyte culture responses with kidney allograft survival. Transplantation, 2:190–191, 1971.
164. Templeton, J. W., and Thomas, E. D.: Evidence for a major histocompatibility locus in the dog. Transplantation, 11:429–430, 1971.
165. Tennenbaum, J. I., St. Pierre, R. L., and Cerilli, G. J.: Evaluation of immunosuppressive therapy and clinical course in renal transplants by in vitro lymphocyte transformation. Transplantation, 6:986–990, 1968.
166. Thorsby, E.: Presented at Nato Advanced Study Institute on "Cellular Differentiation and Regulation of the Immune Response," Minaki Lodge, Ontario, Canada.

167. Tripodi, D., Lyons, S., Davies, D.: Separation of peripheral leukocytes by Ficoll density gradient centrifugation. Transplantation, 11:487–488, 1971.
168. Tridente, G., Cappuzzo, G. D., and Chieco-Bianchi, L.: Lymphocyte interaction in mixed mouse cultures. (A preliminary report). In Curtoni, E. S., ed.: Histocompatibility Testing. Copenhagen, Munksgaard, 1967, pp. 67–73.
169. Twomey, J. J., Sharkey, O., Jr., Brown, J. A., Laughter, A. H., and Jordon, P. H., Jr.: Cellular requirements for the mitotic response in allogeneic mixed leukocyte cultures. J. Immunol., 104:845–853, 1970.
170. Vaiman, M. V., Renard, C., LaFage, P., Ameteau, J., and Nizza, P.: Evidence for a histocompatibility system in swine (SL-A). Transplantation, 10:155–164, 1970.
171. Valentine, F. T.: The transformation and proliferation of lymphocytes in vitro. In Revillard, J. P., ed.: Cell Mediated Immunity. In vitro correlates. Baltimore, University Park Press, 1971, pp. 6–50.
172. Van Rood, J. J., and Eijsvoogel, V. P.: HL-A identical phenotypes and genotypes in unrelated individuals. Lancet, 1:698–700, 1970.
173. Virolainen, M., Hayry, P., and Defendi, V.: Effect of presensitization on the mixed lymphocyte reaction of rat spleen cell cultures. Transplantation, 8:179–188, 1969.
174. Viza, D. C., Degani, O., Dausset, J., and Davies, D. A. L.: Lymphocyte stimulation by soluble human HL-A transplantation antigens. Nature, 219:704–706, 1968.
175. Wilson, D. B.: Quantitative studies on the mixed lymphocyte interaction in rats. I. Conditions and parameters of response. J. Exper. Med., 126:625–654, 1967.
176. Wilson, D. B., and Billingham, R. E.: Lymphocytes in transplantation immunity. Advances Immunol., 7:189–273, 1967.
177. Wilson, D. B., Blyth, J. L., and Nowell, P. C.: Quantitative studies on the mixed lymphocyte interaction in rats. III. Kinetics of the response. J. Exper. Med., 128:1157–1181, 1968.
178. Wilson, D. B., and Elkins, W. L.: Proliferative interaction of lymphocytes in vitro and in vivo: manifestations of immunological competence. In Rieke, W. O., ed.: Third Annual Leukocyte Culture Conference. New York, Appleton-Century-Crofts, 1969, pp. 391–407.
179. Wilson, D. B., and Nowell, P. G.: Quantitative studies on the mixed lymphocyte interaction in rats. IV. Immunologic potentiality of the responding cells. J. Exper. Med., 131:391–407, 1970.
180. Wilson, D. B., and Nowell, P. C.: Quantitative studies on the mixed lymphocyte interaction in rats. J. Exper. Med., 133:442–453, 1971.
181. Wilson, D. B., Silvers, W. K., and Nowell, P. C.: Quantitative studies on the mixed lymphocyte interaction in rats. II. Relationship of the proliferative response to the immunologic status of the donors. J. Exper. Med., 126:655–665, 1967.
182. Yunis, E. J., Plate, J. M., Ward, F. E., Seigler, H. F., and Amos, D. B.: Anomalous MLR responsiveness among siblings. Transplant. Proc., 3:118–120, 1971.
183. Zoschke, D. C., and Bach, F. H.: Specificity of antigen recognition by human lymphocytes in vitro. Science, 170:1404–1406, 1970.
184. Zoschke, D. C., and Bach, F. H.: Lymphocyte reactivity in vitro. VIII. Specificity of allogeneic cell recognition in mixed leukocyte cultures. In Schwarz, M. R., ed.: Proceedings of the Sixth Leukocyte Culture Conference. New York, Academic Press, in press.

Department of Experimental Surgery
McGill University
Montreal, Quebec
Canada

Viral Infection and Immunity

Peter B. Dent, M.D.,* and R. P. Bryce Larke, M.D., D.Cl.Sc.**

A wide variety of undiagnosable and mostly benign symptom complexes have for many years been facilely explained as "viral infections," thereby assuaging the clinician's academic guilt and the patient's fears. Progress in our understanding of the biology of viruses and the pathogenesis of virus-induced diseases has revealed that many are not benign, though many are preventable by vaccination and some are amenable to therapy.[26] Furthermore, the possibility that some human disorders of unknown etiology may be caused by viruses or by the host response to the virus is now widely appreciated. While this new knowledge is only fragmentary some basic principles must be formulated in order to gain further clarification of the complex problems still unsolved. Such a formulation will be attempted in this review, bearing in mind that each virus species and each host is unique and thus extrapolation from one system to another is fraught with danger. The basic principles of virus biology and mechanisms of host resistance will be reviewed, emphasizing, where possible, relevance to clinical situations. The nature of host-virus relationships in syndromes of current interest will be briefly discussed. While reference is made in the text to a great number of individual studies and contributions in the area, where possible, the cited literature will consist of comprehensive reviews of the subject rather than original observations.

VIRUS-HOST CELL INTERACTIONS

In dealing with the complex problem of man's response to viral infection, it may be well to review briefly the various stages of the virus-host cell interaction and to look particularly at the ways in which the cells may manifest viral infection.[50] When a typical DNA virus (for example, a herpesvirus) comes into contact with a susceptible host cell, it first becomes

*Assistant Professor, Department of Pediatrics, McMaster University, Hamilton, Ontario

**Assistant Professor, Departments of Pediatrics and Pathology, McMaster University, Hamilton, Ontario

Supported in part by the Canadian Arthritis and Rheumatism Society, the Medical Research Council of Canada and Ontario Provincial Research Grants. P. B. D. is a Scholar of the Leukemia Society of America.

attached to receptor material on the cell membrane. The next stage is penetration of the virus particle into the cell cytoplasm, and in most instances the virus probably enters the cell in phagocytic vacuoles. This is followed by uncoating of the virus particle; that is, the protein coat becomes separated from the inner core of nucleic acid which then begins to redirect the biosynthetic mechanisms within the host cell. In the case of most DNA viruses, the viral genetic material enters the host cell nucleus where, over the next few hours, it regulates the synthesis of new viral proteins as well as replicas of its own genetic material. These newly formed protein and nucleic acid constituents are assembled in the cell nucleus into complete virus particles, which then make their way back through the cytoplasm to the cell membrane where they are released.

In the case of a typical RNA virus, such as poliovirus, the initial stages of the replicative cycle are essentially the same as for a DNA virus. As a rule, the RNA viruses do not directly involve the host cell nucleus, and the biosynthesis of new viral proteins and nucleic acid takes place in the cytoplasm. The protein and nucleic acid components are assembled into virus particles, which are then extruded through the cytoplasmic membrane of the host cell. Many of the RNA viruses, such as influenza virus, acquire a final coating or envelope as they bud out through the cytoplasmic membrane; in this way the virus acquires envelope antigens which are identical to host cell surface antigens.

The above outline of the replicative cycles of typical DNA and RNA viruses is greatly simplified and in no way reflects the vast scientific literature on the biochemical and morphologic events taking place within virus-infected cells. The important consideration here is an appreciation of the fact that viruses can reproduce themselves only by taking over the biosynthetic machinery of the host cells and exploiting it for their own purposes. This leads almost invariably to some adverse reaction within the host cell. Some viruses produce a cytocidal or lytic effect which can be recognized microscopically in cell cultures as a cytopathic effect. In other cells, a virus may establish a permissive infection in which cell function is not apparently disturbed although subtle alterations in cell biochemistry undoubtedly occur. Viruses, at least some of which may be present in incomplete forms, may establish long-term latent infections within host cells; such latent infections may be activated by other factors affecting the organism, such as fever or malignant disease.

Although evidence that viruses may induce malignant disease in man is only circumstantial, it has been well established that viruses are able to produce leukemia and solid tumours in various birds and experimental animals.[19] In the case of DNA tumour viruses, some of the viral genetic material becomes incorporated into the genome of the host cell, an event which apparently leads to breakdown of the normal control mechanisms within that cell. The cells undergo malignant transformation and proliferate unchecked, while the virus may direct the formation of unusual new host cell proteins both within the nucleus (T antigen) and on the surface of the transformed cell (transplantation antigen). It has been shown recently that RNA tumour viruses may induce malignant transformation through the action of a new DNA molecule, "provirus", which is transcribed from viral RNA by enzymes termed "reverse transcriptases."[51] It is this provirus which is then incorporated into the host cell genome, giving rise subsequently to malignant transformation. These concepts are mentioned here since they are important in understanding current knowledge of tumour immunology and provide a basis for devising new approaches to the therapy of malignant disease, ie. with specific enzyme inhibitors.

MECHANISMS OF HOST RESISTANCE TO VIRUSES

Various aspects of this subject have been reviewed in recent years.[2, 18, 45] It is useful to think of host resistance in terms of non-immunologic and immunologic factors, although in some instances it may be difficult to dissociate the two. Integrity of surface epithelia, local changes in oxygen tension and acidity, hormonal factors, and fever are nonspecific factors which play a role in host resistance to virus but will not be discussed here. Interferon is generally thought to be a non-immunological factor which plays an integral role in host resistance to virus and will be discussed in greater detail below. The immune responses to viruses will also be discussed in the following paragraphs in light of the current evidence that immunologic function involves a division of labour between antibody-mediated immunity and immunity mediated by lymphoid cells (cell-mediated immunity, CMI).[10]

The intact virion is a complex structure containing different antigenic groups and is in most cases a potent antigen. The immune response is directed in part to surface components of the virus, including virus-associated proteins with biological activity, such as enzymes or hemagglutinins. Antibodies to internal components of some viruses have also been described. Stimulated, perhaps, by the demonstration of changes in surface antigenicity of cells infected with oncogenic viruses, recent studies have suggested that cells infected with non-oncogenic viruses have new antigens on their surface which may be virus-specified but distinct from antigens present on the virus surface itself.[44, 55] The unique antigenicity of virus-infected cells may be a key factor in permitting the termination of virus infection by the host's immune response.

Humoral Immunity

The antibody response following virus infections is heterogeneous in terms of immunoglobulin class and biologic activity. The quantitative and qualitative implications of the antibody response are often as confusing to the clinician as they are to the immunologist or microbiologist. Teleologically, the most relevant type of antibody to a virus would be one which prevents it from causing infection; following most viral infections, immune sera can be shown to contain antibody which neutralizes viral infectivity. The mechanism of action of such antibody is as yet not well understood.[45] The combination of virus with specific antibody can inhibit adsorption to susceptible cells; in other situations adsorption and penetration are unaffected, but uncoating within the cytoplasm of the cell is prevented. In some systems addition of complement to virus-antibody mixtures enhances the neutralization of virus, however this can occur without destruction of the virus. There may be no involvement of terminal (and hence lytic) components of the complement sequence; furthermore, infectious virus can be recovered by dissociating the antibody and complement from the viral surface. In these instances, it is felt that the coating of the virus with antibody and complement in some way redirects the intracellular fate of the virus. The evidence that antiviral antibody and complement actually disrupt or kill viruses is meagre, although immune virolysis has been observed by electron microscopy[4] and by assessment of release of labelled nucleic acids from virus treated with antibody and complement.[39]

The fact that passively acquired neutralizing antibody can provide complete protection against primary viral infection is well documented, e.g., measles; however, it is less apparent how recovery from infection may be dependent on this type of antibody. Considerable evidence from clinical situations and experimental models has been brought to bear on this point, and the conclusions to be drawn are as follows. In most situations it is not possible to terminate a viral infection in vivo or in vitro by the administration of neutralizing antiviral antibody. On the other hand cessation of viremia is coincident with the appearance of circulating antibody and thereby the latter may serve to limit further dissemination of virus. Selective impairment of humoral or cellular immune function in most experimental models indicates that cellular immunity plays a greater role in recovery from viral infection;[18] however, data are conflicting probably because of the limitation of the experimental models and of the differing roles of the two types of immune function in infections with different viral agents.

It has recently been shown that immune serum in the presence of complement can destroy cells infected with virus.[38, 55] This antibody, reacting presumably with virus-dependent cell surface antigens, may play an important role in destroying virus-infected cells in the intact host. It may also contribute to the pathogenesis of tissue injury associated with virus infection.

In the assessment of humoral immunity to viruses serum antibody is most commonly measured. However, a significant part of the antiviral antibody produced following natural viral infection is found in the body secretions, so-called secretory IgA antibody (see p. 394). This antibody plays a major role in resistance to infection with virus, as dramatically illustrated by the demonstration that in the absence of secretory antibody and despite the presence of serum antibody, localized gastrointestinal infection with poliovirus may still occur. There is also further suggestive evidence that secretory antibody may play an important role in the prevention of virus-induced hypersensitivity reactions (see below).

The specific role of immune responses to virus-associated proteins in the mechanism of host resistance to viral infection is not known. However it is known that the presence of antibody to the hemagglutinin of rubella virus, hemagglutination-inhibiting (HAI) antibody, signifies immunity to infection with this virus. Because of the sensitivity and simplicity of the HAI test it is used in preference to the viral neutralization test and provides accurate information for use in the clinical setting.

In general, antibody molecules function efficiently and effectively in vivo and in vitro to provide immunity to the offending pathogen. Antibodies which function ineffectively have been recognized and may provide some of the answers to the problem of chronic viral infections. Antibody has been described which combines with virus but fails to neutralize the virus thus giving rise to circulating infectious virus-antibody complexes.[35] Furthermore the infectious complexes are resistant to neutralization by effective neutralizing antibody. These complexes are, however, rendered non-infectious by anti-gamma globulin antibody, an observation which may be of great significance in relation to the occurrence of antiglobulin (rheumatoid) factors in connective tissue disorders as well as in certain chronic infections.

Of great interest in tumour immunology is the occurrence of a serum factor, presumably a 7S antibody, which inhibits the cytotoxic effect of sensitized lymphocytes on tumour cells, so-called blocking or enhancing antibody.[20] A similar blocking effect of serum has been observed on the in vitro killing of target cells chronically infected with mumps virus by mumps-immune lymphoid cells.[47] Further studies of the interaction of humoral and cell-mediated immunity in viral infections are needed because of the importance of this interaction in the pathogenesis of chronic infections.

In the clinical setting, analysis of serum for the type and quantity of antiviral antibody is of immediate practical value. The mere presence of antiviral antibody indicates that the host has been exposed to virus. To determine if infection has been recent, in most instances paired acute and convalescent sera are needed to demonstrate a rise in the actual level of antibody. While exceedingly high values of antibody in a single specimen are more common during the convalescent period of virus infection, the great individual variability of immune responsiveness makes it impossible to draw conclusions from the level of antibody in a single specimen. Because in most primary infections the first antibody formed is of the IgM class and because in most self-limited infections IgM antibody production ceases in the convalescent period, the finding of this class of antibody in a single serum specimen is usually taken as presumptive evidence of recent infection. Unfortunately the identification of IgM antibody requires special procedures, ultracentrifugation or meticulous immunofluorescent tests and therefore is not routinely available. Similarly antibodies with different biologic activity appear in a characteristic temporal sequence. For example, in acquired rubella virus infection, complement-fixing antibody falls during late convalescence while the HAI antibody level is maintained for a prolonged period of time. Thus a high complement-fixing antibody level may be used as an adjunct in the timing of rubella virus infection.

Cell-Mediated Immunity

The prototype cells of cell-mediated immunity (CMI) are lymphocytes and macrophages. While both cell types are involved in CMI and in resistance to virus infection, their functions are probably separate, although in some instances complementary.

It has been shown experimentally that macrophages or the phagocytic cells of the reticuloendothelial system may play a role in host resistance to viral infection by preventing the dissemination of virus.[45] In some systems this is an age-dependent function in that macrophages from neonatal animals are unable to inactivate viruses. Whether macrophages from an immune host are intrinsically more efficient in virus neutralization or whether this increased efficiency is a function of antibody in the cell suspension or on the macrophage surface is not clear. As mentioned below, macrophages from immune animals, on re-exposure to the virus in vitro, produce more interferon than non-immune macrophages. This may be a function of immune lymphocytes present in the macrophage preparations as it is known that stimulation of lymphocytes by antigen or mitogens in vitro induces interferon production.[18]

Lymphocytes do not normally interact with viruses in such a way as to cause virus neutralization. Small lymphocytes are not susceptible to virus infection unless they are transformed into large blast-like cells by antigen or mitogen.[54] Latency of viruses within lymphoid cells may be a common phenomenon, though not easily demonstrable. Viruses which have been recovered from cultured "normal" lymphoid cells include the Epstein-Barr virus, rubella, and rubeola.

In their capacity as mediators of cellular immunity through the elaboration of soluble factors, lymphocytes may play a large role in host resistance to viral infection. Since CMI is directed preferentially against cell-associated antigens, i.e., as on tissue grafts and tumours, and since virus-infected cells carry new antigens, making them similar to foreign tissue grafts, it becomes apparent that CMI might play a role in eliminating or destroying such cells.

Because CMI to viral antigens is still not completely understood, little use has been made clinically of its demonstration. In vivo skin tests with viral antigen have been used for a number of years, but because of the impurity of the antigens false positive responses are common. In vitro correlates of CMI to viral antigens have been developed using the blast transformation response,[34] macrophage migration inhibition,[52] and target cell lysis techniques.[47] These procedures are as yet useful only for investigative purposes, while for routine purposes they provide no information not readily available from serologic tests.

Interferon

Interferons are a class of protein produced or released by cells following stimulation by viruses and certain other microbial and nonmicrobial agents. Interferon acts on host cells to inhibit both RNA and DNA viruses; indirect evidence suggests that interferon itself is not antiviral, but acts in turn upon other host cells to induce the formation of another intracellular substance (presumed to be protein) which mediates antiviral activity. The exact mechanism by which viral replication is inhibited in interferon-treated cells remains somewhat controversial, but the end result seems to be an inhibition of viral protein synthesis.[46] There is frequently a rough correlation between the ability of a virus to induce interferon production and its sensitivity to the antiviral action of interferon. In general, these determinants are related to an overall consideration of the "virulence" of a virus. Polioviruses, for example, may be virulent because of limited adsorption to host cells most active in interferon production or because they rapidly and effectively shut off protein synthesis (including interferon) once they have entered susceptible host cells.[21]

Interferon is relatively species-specific in that it induces maximal antiviral activity in other cells of the same species in which it was produced and gives little or no antiviral protection to cells of other species. This has important implications for any future usefulness of exogenous interferon in the control of human viral infections since the interferon would have to be produced in human cells. Because of this limitation, recent efforts have been directed toward inducing endogenous interferon in humans with polyribonucleotides such as polyinosinic-polycytidylic acid (polyI:C).[14] The mechanism of action of these complexed double-stranded polyribonucleotides in the induction of interferon is presumed to be similar to that of double-stranded viral RNA.

Although the interferon system is generally regarded as a component of the host's non-immune rather than immune defence mechanisms, a discussion of interferon is pertinent to this review. Since the precise role of interferon in human viral infections cannot be studied wholly in isolation from other host defence mechanisms, evidence that interferon contributes significantly to the recovery process under natural conditions of viral infection remains somewhat circumstantial. However, since interferon has virus-inhibitory properties and has been detected during the course of naturally-acquired and experimentally-produced viral infections of man, it appears probable that it plays an active role in suppressing the infection. Present evidence suggests that interferon reduces the dissemination of virus in the host by protecting normal cells from subsequent viral attack. Thus, interferon may prove beneficial in the treatment of chronic diseases where the illness may be perpetuated by continuing viral infection of normal cells.[53]

The contribution of interferon to recovery from disease may thus be related to its ability to reduce the dissemination of viruses, thereby permitting the host to activate a humoral or cell-mediated immune response, or both, suggesting an interesting relationship between the interferon system and the immune response. Clinical evidence of this possible relationship has been demonstrated recently in patients with Hodgkin's disease where there is evidence of depressed lymphocyte function. Patients with malignant disease who had depressed lymphocyte function or lymphopenia (or both) produced ten-fold less interferon in the vesicle fluid of varicella and vaccinia lesions and had a poorer clinical response to viral infection in comparison to normal individuals or cancer patients without leukopenia.[1]

Glasgow[18] has reviewed the experimental evidence that immune lymphocytes or macrophages may have an altered capacity to react to a virus on re-exposure to that agent and that enhanced interferon production may be one feature of this altered reactivity. The recent demonstration by Epstein et al.[13] of interaction between human macrophages and lymphocytes in the production of interferon raises the question of its relationship to macrophage-lymphocyte interactions in cellular immunity and antibody production. These authors speculated that if interferon production associated with blastogenic transformation of lymphocytes is an important mechanism of host defence, then an explanation might be provided for the unusual severity and increased frequency of viral infections in patients with impairment of lymphocyte transformation and delayed hypersensitivity.

CONDITIONS ASSOCIATED WITH UNDUE SUSCEPTIBILITY TO VIRAL INFECTION

Immaturity of the Host

In experimental animals and in natural infections of man it has been shown that the immature host is more susceptible to certain viral infections. In some models this can be correlated with the inability of the macrophages from immature animals to prevent dissemination of virus.[45] As vigorous interferon production has been demonstrated in fetal tissues it is unlikely that increased susceptibility of the immature host to viral infection is related to a deficiency in the interferon system.[6, 40] Specific immune competence is not fully developed in some animals at birth, although in man both CMI and antibody synthesis appear at the end of the first trimester.[49] Thus the reason for this increased susceptibility may be multifactorial and is still not well understood.

Congenital infection with rubella virus has been studied as a model of chronic viral infection in man.[12] Maternal infection in the first trimester may result in chronic viral excretion by the infant for prolonged periods after birth despite evidence of effective circulating antibody in the serum of such infants. Studies of interferon responses, CMI, and antibody production have failed to demonstrate any consistent defect to explain this puzzling immunologic phenomenon. Further studies may reveal qualitative defects of antibody function such as ability to fix complement, presence of secretory antibody, presence of blocking antibody, or abnormalities of specific CMI to rubella virus antigens. Such studies are of considerable importance, as they will lead to a better understanding of the mechanism of chronic viral persistence in other infections as well.

Primary Immune Deficiency States

Studies in experimental animals have indicated that compromise of immune competence by various methods increases their susceptibility to viral infection as judged by increased virus dissemination and lethality.[2, 18] In general, impairment of CMI has a more profound effect but in many instances nonspecific factors as well as humoral immunity may have also been compromised so that the relative importance of the different parameters of host defence in resistance to viral disease is not yet known. The primary immunodeficiency diseases, while still incompletely understood, have provided some insight into this question. The lethal effects of vaccinia virus in patients with the combined immune deficiency states (both cellular and humoral) as well as in some patients with isolated cellular immune deficits and normal humoral immunity suggest a vital role for CMI in recovery from vaccinial infection.[16] Measles virus has also been reported to cause lethal infections in these patients in the absence of the usual dermal manifestations. The giant cell pneumonia associated with this type of lethal infection may reflect the widespread dissemination resulting from a deficient immune response.

Isolated immunoglobulin deficiencies in general do not appear to be associated with an increased susceptibility to viral diseases. Classically, patients with Bruton's congenital agammaglobulinemia do not have increased morbidity or mortality from potentially lethal viral infections such as vaccinia, measles, or chickenpox. An increased incidence of hepatitis has been reported in these patients but this does not appear to be a general phenomenon. The explanations for these observations are (1) that antibody is not important in resistance to this type of infection; (2) that these patients make small but sufficient amounts of antibody; and (3) that most patients receive passive immunity in the form of poly-specific immune globulin as soon as the diagnosis is made and those who do not survive succumb to bacterial rather than viral infections.

Patients with the Wiskott-Aldrich syndrome[9] (eczema, thrombocytopenia, and recurrent infection) display an increased susceptibility to viral infections, particularly herpes simplex virus. The primary immune defect in these patients appears to be an inability to process polysaccharide antigens and to produce IgM antibody. As the disease progresses, a secondary impairment of CMI develops. Whether the increased susceptibility to viral infection is due to this or to the primary IgM-producing defect is not known.

Patients with deficiency of IgA production, as in ataxia telangiectasia or isolated IgA deficiency, do not show an increased susceptibility to viral infection. The role of viruses with minimal or unrecognized pathogenicity in the intact host in causing disease in patients with various forms of immunodeficiency is not known and deserves further study.

It is of interest that patients with abnormalities of neutrophils and other phagocytic cells, such as in chronic granulomatous disease, do not demonstrate an increased susceptibility to viral infection.

Secondary Immune Deficiency States

IMMUNOSUPPRESSIVE THERAPY. With the increasing use of immunosuppressive drugs in the therapy of a wide variety of diseases, particularly those of so-called autoimmune etiology, an increased incidence of infectious complications might be expected. While the increased hazard of infection, particularly secondary to corticosteroid use, is appreciated, inordinate susceptibility to viral diseases has rarely been reported. This may reflect the fact that in most instances the drugs are not used for prolonged periods of time, nor are they used in doses which are, in fact, immunosuppressive. Furthermore, many such patients possess antiviral antibody prior to the institution of therapy. It is well known that immunosuppression may have little or no effect on an established humoral immune response, which we have indicated is a major factor in protection against viral infections.

The most significant exception to these observations is the renal transplant patient who often is markedly immunosuppressed as a result of therapy with chemicals, irradiation, or antilymphocyte serum. Experimentally all these agents augment viral infection so that it is not surprising that transplant patients display a marked susceptibility to viral infection and other pathogens which do not commonly cause disease in the intact host. Increased susceptibility has been described to herpes zoster, cytomegalovirus, warts virus, Pneumocystis carinii and a number of fungal agents.[33, 48] Quite often, combined infections occur, thereby complicating the clinical picture and therapeutic approach. It is therefore important to be aware of the wide variety of agents which can infect these patients so that those conditions amenable to treatment may be recognized. In so far as viral infections are concerned, because available therapeutic measures are few, untried and potentially toxic, current efforts must be aimed at careful monitoring of immunosuppressive therapy and diligent clinical surveillance coupled with intelligent use of viral diagnostic procedures, assisted where indicated by increased use of lung biopsy for histology and isolation of organisms.

MALIGNANCY. Patients with malignant disease have a twofold problem in terms of their host defence mechanisms (see p. 501). Neoplasia is associated with impaired immunologic competence, often aggravated by therapy which is itself immunosuppressive. Patients with malignancies of the lymphoreticular system are at even greater risk because they have more profound defects in immunologic competence. In general, individuals with neoplastic disease are subject to the same spectrum of viral, protozoal, and fungal infections as are renal transplant patients, although the frequency of infection is less.

Malignancies of the lymphoreticular system have been of major interest in the study of host resistance because of the selective nature of the immune deficiency in various disorders. Hodgkin's disease is characterized by impaired CMI, and the severity of this impairment parallels the severity of the disease. These patients are inordinately susceptible to herpes zoster infection. While rarely fatal, the dissemination of zoster carries a poor prognosis in terms of life expectancy. This susceptibility to infection and particularly to the dissemination of infection is thought to be due to decreased CMI. It has recently been shown that patients with Hodgkin's disease and other lymphoreticular malignancies who develop disseminated varicella-zoster infections have an impaired local interferon response.[1] As discussed above this observation has been interpreted to indicate that the interferon response may play a major role as a mediator of CMI with respect to viral infection.

Patients with other forms of lymphoreticular malignancy have an increased incidence of viral infection; however, no specific pattern has emerged from which definitive conclusions could be drawn with respect to the type of viral infection and the nature of immunologic impairment present. For example, patients with chronic lymphocytic leukemia have an increased susceptibility to both herpes zoster and progressive vaccinia infection. These patients may have defects in lymphocyte function, in isolation or in combination with impaired immunoglobulin production. In acute lymphocytic leukemia of childhood, decreased host resistance appears to be due solely to decreased neutrophil levels. No significant cellular or humoral immunologic deficit intrinsic to the malignant process itself has been reported. However, these patients show a marked susceptibility to dissemination of measles infection and possibly to chickenpox.

Herpes zoster occurs with increased frequency and many patients are found at autopsy to have disseminated cytomegalovirus infection. It is not known to what degree this is due to chemotherapy, nor is it known which parameters of host defence are lacking to account for this susceptibility. As a practical note it is recommended that serologic evidence of immunity to measles virus be documented in patients with malignancy so that gamma globulin prophylaxis may be given when measles is known to be prevalent in the community. Disseminated measles infection has occurred following administration of live measles vaccine, thus precluding this form of prophylaxis. In this regard it is felt that no live virus vaccines should be given to any patients on immunosuppressive therapy or any patients with malignant disease.

ALTERED REACTIVITY TO VIRUSES

Measles Virus

An atypical response to measles virus has been observed in children previously immunized with an inactivated alum-precipitated measles virus vaccine.[15] The presenting complaint is usually fever accompanied by abdominal pain, headache, or myalgia. A feature common to all of the cases has been clinical or radiographic evidence of pneumonitis, often accompanied by some degree of pleural effusion.[56] The rash, which does not develop in all cases, usually begins 2 or 3 days after the onset of fever and is strikingly different from the rash of "normal" measles both in its appearance and distribution; although usually maculopapular, some patients have a distinctly vesicular eruption not unlike that of varicella, or the rash may have a hemorrhagic or urticarial appearance. It has a strikingly centrifugal distribution, frequently with complete sparing of the face and trunk.

Laboratory studies show very low or absent titers of measles antibody (hemagglutination-inhibiting and complement fixing) in the serum at the onset of disease but the titers of antibody (particularly complement fixing antibody) rise to very high levels within a matter of a few days. Studies on recipients of killed measles virus vaccine have shown almost 100 per cent skin reactivity to the intradermal inoculation of measles antigens. Fulginiti and Arthur[17] have postulated that delayed hypersensitivity to measles virus in the absence of serum antibody results in susceptibility to atypical measles.

An alternative hypothesis has been proposed by Bellanti et al.[3] who have shown that immunization with live measles virus vaccine regularly induced the production of secretory IgA antibody in nasal secretions, whereas inactivated measles vaccine induced nasal antibody in less than 50 per cent of cases. Serum antibody reached comparable peak titers in recipients of either killed or live virus vaccine. It was speculated that upon exposure of recipients of killed measles vaccine to natural measles, viral replication in the respiratory tract and an anamnestic antibody response occurred. The presence of antigen and antibody together provides the conditions for the formation of immune complexes in the lung with subsequent tissue injury. Skin biopsies from children immunized previously with inactivated measles virus vaccine who developed a local reaction at the site of a subsequent live measles virus vaccination showed the presence of IgG, measles antigen, and complement within blood vessel walls, suggesting that an Arthus-type reaction is the basis of the altered reactivity of these children to measles virus.

Respiratory Syncytial Virus (RSV)

This virus is the most important respiratory tract pathogen of early life, with the most serious cases often occurring in those infants who possess the highest levels of passively transferred serum neutralizing antibody. Particularly serious cases of RSV infection have also been observed in infants with high titers of serum neutralizing antibody induced following parenteral administration of an inactivated alum-precipitated vaccine. These serious clinical responses are probably the result of interaction between serum antibody and RSV antigen in the lungs of children who lack respiratory tract secretory antibody or who possess a level of this antibody which is insufficient to confer protection.[8] These situations of qualitative abnormalities of immune responses have drawn attention to the importance of the local immune reaction in providing safe and effective protection against viral infection.

CHRONIC, PERSISTENT OR LATENT VIRAL INFECTIONS

Subacute Sclerosing Panencephalitis (SSPE)

SSPE is a progressive, fatal degenerative disease of the central nervous system, considered to be caused by measles virus, which can be isolated from brain tissue of these patients.[41] Particles resembling Papova viruses have been observed by electron microscopy in association with the measles-like viruses in brain tissue removed from cases of SSPE, suggesting that the disease may involve an interaction between the two viruses.[25] Titers of measles antibody are markedly elevated in the serum and cerebrospinal fluid of these patients, a point which is of some diagnostic value.[23] However, the pathogenesis of SSPE may be related to an abnormality of cellular rather than humoral immunity.[5] In addition to defective host factors, the aberrant adaptation of measles or a measles-like virus to neural tissue must be considered as a possible mechanism in the pathogenesis of SSPE.[27]

Arthritis Associated with Rubella

Persistent viral infection in the congenital rubella syndrome has been discussed above. Recent studies have suggested that a prolonged viral infection may occasionally occur in persons vaccinated with live attenuated rubella virus vaccines. Both children and adults have developed a recurrent form of arthritis beginning several weeks after the vaccination, and occasionally have symptoms persisting for upwards of a year.[28] Ogra[37] has reported the isolation of vaccine strains of the virus from the joint fluid of children with arthritis as long as 4 months after vaccination. The association of viruses and connective tissue diseases will be discussed below.

Herpes Simplex

Recurrent cold sores and recurrent keratitis caused by herpes simplex virus are often considered as examples of reactivation of a latent viral infection in man. More recent evidence[24, 29] has suggested that there may be continuous excretion of virus from persistently infected tissues but that the manifestations of disease, i.e., cold sores or keratitis, are held in check by normal host defence mechanisms. It is only when these defence mechanisms break down through the effect of hormonal inbalance during menstruation, exposure to ultraviolet light, fever, emotional distress, etc., that the so-called latent infection becomes apparent. The role of various host defence mechanisms such as interferon production and secretory antibody in persistent herpesvirus infections remains unclear. Infectious virus-antibody complexes have been demonstrated in experimental herpes keratitis, indicating that ineffective, non-neutralizing antibody may be a contributing factor to the pathogenesis of chronic herpesvirus infections.[7]

Herpes Zoster

The varicella-zoster virus causes both chickenpox and herpes zoster infection but the pathogenesis of the two diseases is quite different. Whereas chickenpox is primarily a disease of early childhood, herpes zoster infection is uncommon before the age of 50. The question remains whether herpes zoster represents a reactivation of a virus which has remained latent in the dorsal root ganglion or perhaps even respiratory tissues in the body or whether reinfection with the virus occurs in people with waning immunity to the primary chickenpox infection.[30] Epidemiological studies have shown that chickenpox in children rarely leads to herpes zoster in close family contacts, nor do patients with zoster give rise to secondary cases of zoster in contacts. However, when cases of chickenpox do give rise to cases of zoster in contacts, the incubation period in the latter is believed to be much shortened, that is, only 3 to 7 days as opposed to the 2 to 3 week incubation period of chickenpox. The fact that antibody titers reach higher levels and develop earlier in zoster than in varicella does not clearly differentiate between exogenous reinfection and activation of latent virus. The predilection for zoster to occur in patients with malignant disease is discussed above.

HUMAN ONCOGENIC VIRUSES

That viruses cause a wide variety of cancers in animals is now clearly appreciated, and current efforts are being directed toward determining the role of viral agents in the etiology of human malignancy. In this section we will review briefly some recent developments in this area.

Burkitt's Lymphoma

The isolation of the Epstein-Barr virus (EBV) from tumour cells of patients with Burkitt's lymphoma along with the demonstration of very high antibody levels to EBV in the serum of such patients indicated an etiologic link of the virus with this malignancy.[36] During the course of an investigation attempting to clarify this link, it was strongly implicated that EBV is the cause of infectious mononucleosis. It has further been demonstrated that patients who have had EBV infection either clinically or subclinically, diagnosed on the basis of circulating anti-EBV antibody, may harbour this virus in their peripheral lymphocytes. It has been proposed that Burkitt's lymphoma probably develops in patients previously infected with EBV who undergo hyperstimulation of the reticuloendothelial system, in Africa most commonly as a result of chronic plasmodial infection. The role of EBV in the etiology of malignancies in non-African settings is under continued study.

Human Breast Cancer

While a role for viruses in the etiology of murine mammary adenocarcinoma has been accepted for many years, it is only recently that evidence is accumulating for a similar role in human breast cancer.[31] Viral particles have been isolated in high frequency from the milk of women who have a family history of breast cancer. These particles are morphologically and physicochemically identical to the RNA B-type particles which induce breast cancer in susceptible mouse strains. Reverse transcriptase activity has been demonstrated in viral particles purified from human milk.

Sarcoma

A number of human tumours have now been shown to have tumour-specific antigens which in many cases are common to all tumours of the same histologic type. In experimental animals, tumours caused by a single strain of oncogenic virus have been shown to share common tumour-specific antigens, thus the observations in human tumours are compatible with a postulated viral etiology. Human connective tissue sarcomas have been shown to possess a common antigen to which most patients have high levels of antibody, as has been found in other types of human tumours. However, the recent isolation[32] of an agent from cultures of these tumours which causes in vitro transformation of normal human fibroblasts and induces in these cultures the appearance of tumour-specific antigens and the demonstration of viral particles with a morphology identical to animal sarcoma viruses, represent an exciting advance toward the demonstration and possible isolation of a human oncogenic virus.

Carcinoma of the Cervix

The demonstration of a high frequency of antibody to the genital strain (type 2) of herpes simplex virus in patients with cancer of the cervix and in women with a high risk of developing this malignancy as compared to appropriate controls indicated that this virus might have an etiologic relationship to cancer of the cervix.[43] No conclusive evidence is yet available to clarify the nature of this association.

In summary, while the evidence continues to accumulate that viruses play a role in the causation of human malignancy, it must be repeatedly emphasized that oncogenesis is a multifactorial process. It depends not only on a specific inciting agent but in many cases promoting factors as well as inherent genetic susceptibility and other host factors. Notwithstanding, it is clear from animal studies that pre-existing immunity to a specific oncogenic virus protects the animal from developing cancer following exposure to this virus. This fact is ample justification for the current hot pursuit of human cancer viruses.

VIRUSES AND CONNECTIVE TISSUE DISEASE

The clinical picture and evidence from numerous experimental models of autoimmune disease make it highly probable that these disorders are caused by infectious agents. Among the best investigated animal models are the so-called slow virus infections in which a persistent virus infection occurs with chronic progressive tissue damage, such as in lymphocytic choriomeningitis virus infection in mice and Aleutian disease of mink.[42] In these situations the pathogenesis of the lesions involves the deposition of immune complexes of virus, antibody and complement in various tissues such as kidney, liver, erythrocytes, and vascular endothelium. The clinical picture so resembles disseminated lupus erythematosus that a viral etiology has been avidly sought in this disease; however, despite the most assiduous efforts, little progress has been made. Elevated levels of humoral antibody to certain common viruses, particularly the myxoviruses and paramyxoviruses have been found in lupus, however, this probably reflects the generalized immunological hyperreactivity of these patients.[22]

A similar search for an infectious etiology of rheumatoid arthritis has failed to bear fruit, although some interesting observations have been made which give impetus for continued studies.[11] The striking similarity of infectious mycoplasma arthritis of swine to human rheumatoid arthritis has prompted numerous studies on the relationship of mycoplasmas to this disease in man, but to date no etiologic link has been demonstrated. A high frequency of antibody to one strain of mycoplasma, M. fermentans, has been reported in patients with rheumatoid arthritis and a majority of such patients have in vitro evidence of CMI to this organism.

Synovial cell cultures from patients with rheumatoid arthritis demonstrate altered growth patterns and biochemical behaviour in vitro. Furthermore these cultures are resistant to superinfection with rubella virus and Newcastle disease virus. These observations suggest that synovial cells in rheumatoid arthritis may be chronically infected with an interfering agent, presumably a virus. While preliminary, these findings provide the most compelling evidence for the presence of an infectious agent in human rheumatoid arthritis. Although the above studies do not implicate rubella virus as the cause of rheumatoid arthritis, this virus seems to have a peculiar tropism for joint tissues. Arthritis in association with natural or vaccine-induced infection is a common phenomenon (see above) and congenital infection in rabbits with rubella virus results in chronic persistance of viral antigen in articular tissues.

Rheumatoid arthritis may be a manifestation of chronic infection with a variety of agents which have a tropism for joint tissues causing primary or secondary (immunologic) tissue destruction. On the other hand the joint may, like the kidney in lupus erythematosus, be damaged as an innocent bystander by ongoing immune complex deposition. With our increasing sophistication in virus identification and isolation it is certain that we shall soon see the ultimate solution of some of these problems.

ACKNOWLEDGMENT

The excellent assistance of Mrs. Linda Roberts in the preparation of this manuscript is gratefully acknowledged.

REFERENCES

1. Armstrong, R. W., Gurwith, M. J., Waddell, D., and Merigan, T. C.: Cutaneous interferon production in patients with Hodgkin's disease and other cancers infected with varicella or vaccinia. New Eng. J. Med., 283:1182, 1970.
2. Baron, S.: The biological significance of the interferon system. Arch. Intern. Med., 126:84, 1970.
3. Bellanti, J. A., Sanga, R. L., Klutinis, B., Brandt, B., and Artenstein, M. S.: Antibody responses in serum and nasal secretions of children immunized with inactivated and attenuated measles-virus vaccines. New Eng. J. Med., 280:628, 1969.
4. Berry, D. M., and Almedia, J. B.: The morphological and histological effects of various antisera on avian infectious bronchitis virus. J. Gen. Virol., 3:97, 1968.
5. Burnet, F. M.: Measles as an index of immunological function. Lancet, 2:610, 1968.
6. Carter, W. A., Hande, K. R., Essien, B., Prochownik, E., and Kaback, M. M.: Comparative production of interferon by human fetal, neonatal, and maternal cells. Infect. Immunol., 3:671, 1971.
7. Centifanto, Y. M., and Kaufman, H. E.: Secretory immunoglobulin A and herpes keratitis. Infec. Immun., 2:778, 1970.
8. Chanock, R. M., Kapikian, A. Z., Mills, J., Kim, H. W., and Parrott, R. H.: Influence of immunological factors in respiratory syncytial virus disease. Arch. Environ. Health, 21:347, 1970.
9. Cooper, M. D., Chase, H. P., Lowman, J. T., Krivit, W., and Good, R. A.: Immunologic defects in patients with Wiskott-Aldrich syndrome. Birth Defects Original Article Series, 4:378, 1968.
10. Craddock, C. G., Longmire, R., and McMillan, R.: Lymphocytes and the immune response. New Eng. J. Med., 285:324, 378, 1971.
11. Dent, P. B., and Avila, L.: Experimental models of rubella virus infection. Proceedings of the Fourth Canadian Conference on Research in the Rheumatic Diseases, Toronto, October 1970 (in press).
12. Dent, P. B., and Rawls, W. E.: Human congenital rubella: The relationship of immunologic aberrations to viral persistence. Ann. N.Y. Acad. Sci., 181:209, 1971.
13. Epstein, L. B., Cline, M. J., and Merigan, T. C.: The interaction of human macrophages and lymphocytes in the phytohemagglutinin-stimulated production of interferon. J. Clin. Invest., 50:744, 1971.
14. Field, A. K., Young, W., Krakoff, I. H., Tytell, A. A., Lampson, G. P., Nemes, M. M., and Hilleman, M. R.: Induction of interferon in human subjects by PolyI:C. Proc. Soc. Exper. Biol. Med., 136:1180, 1971.
15. Fulginiti, V. A., Eller, J. J., Downie, A. W., and Kempe, C. H.: Altered reactivity to measles virus. Atypical measles in children previously immunized with inactivated measles virus vaccines. J.A.M.A., 202:1075, 1967.

16. Fulginiti, V. A., Kempe, C. H., Hathaway, W. E., Pearlman, D. S., Sieber, O. F., Eller, J. J., Joyner, J. J., and Robinson, A.: Progressive vaccinia in immunologically deficient individuals. Birth Defects Original Article Series, 4:129, 1968.

17. Fulginiti, V. A., and Arthur, J. H.: Altered reactivity to measles virus. Skin test reactivity and antibody response to measles virus antigens in recipients of killed measles virus vaccine. J. Pediat., 75:609, 1969.

18. Glasgow, L. A.: Cellular immunity in host resistance to viral infections. Arch. Intern. Med., 126:125, 1970.

19. Green, M.: Oncogenic viruses. Ann. Rev. Biochem., 39:701, 1970.

20. Hellstrom, K. E., and Hellstrom, I.: Immunological enhancement as studied by cell culture techniques. Ann. Rev. Microbiol., 24:373, 1970.

21. Ho, M.: Factors influencing the interferon response. Arch. Intern. Med., 126:135, 1970.

22. Hollinger, F. B., Sharp, J. T., Lidsky, M. D., and Rawls, W. E.: Antibodies to viral antigens in systemic lupus erythematosus. Arthritis Rheum., 14:1, 1971.

23. Jabbour, J. T., Garcia, J. H., Lemmi, H., Ragland, J., Duenas, D. A., and Sever, J. L.: Subacute sclerosing panencephalitis. A multidisciplinary study of eight cases. J.A.M.A., 207:2248, 1969.

24. Kaufman, H. E., Brown, D. C., and Ellison, E. M.: Recurrent herpes in the rabbit and man. Science, 156:1628, 1967.

25. Koprowski, H., Barbanti-Brodano, G., and Katz, M.: Interaction between Papova-like virus and paramyxovirus in human brain cells: A hypothesis. Nature, 225:1045, 1970.

26. Larke, R. P. B.: The effects of therapeutic measures in diseases caused by viruses. Canad. Med. Assoc. J., 95:961, 1966.

27. Lehrich, J. R., Katz, M., Rorke, L. B., Barbanti-Brodano, G., and Koprowski, H.: Subacute sclerosing panencephalitis. Encephalitis in hamsters produced by viral agents isolated from human brain cells. Arch. Neurol., 23:97, 1970.

28. Lerman, S. J., Nankervis, G. A., Heggie, A. D., and Gold, E.: Immunologic response, virus excretion, and joint reactions with rubella vaccine. A Study of adolescent girls and young women given live attenuated virus vaccine (HPV-77:DE-5). Ann. Intern. Med., 74:67, 1971.

29. Lindgren, K. M., Douglas, R. G., Jr., and Couch, R. B.: Significance of herpes virus hominis in respiratory secretions of man. New Eng. J. Med., 278:517, 1968.

30. Miller, L. H., and Brunell, P. A.: Zoster, reinfection or activation of latent virus? Observations on the antibody response. Amer. J. Med., 49:480, 1970.

31. Moore, D. H., Charney, J., Kramarsky, B., Lasforgues, E. Y., Sarkar, N. H., Brennan, M. S., Burrows, J. H., Sirsat, S. M., Paymaster, J. C., and Vaidya, A. B.: Search for a human breast cancer virus. Nature, 229:611, 1971.

32. Morton, D. L., Malmgren, R. A., Gall, W. I., and Schidlovsky, G.: Immunologic and virus studies with human sarcomas. Surgery, 66:152, 1969.

33. Murray, J. F., Haegelin, H. F., Hewitt, W. L., Latta, H., McVickar, D., Rasmussen, A. F., Jr., and Rigler, L. G.: Opportunistic pulmonary infections. Ann. Intern. Med., 65:566, 1966.

34. Naspitz, C. K., and Richter, M.: The action of phytohemagglutinin in vivo and in vitro, a review. Progr. Allergy, 12:1, 1968.

35. Notkins, A. L., Mahar, S., Scheele, C., and Goffman, J.: Infectious virus-antibody complex in the blood of chronically infected mice. J. Exper. Med., 124:81, 1966.

36. O'Conor, G. T.: Persistent immunologic stimulation as a factor in oncogenesis, with special reference to Burkitt's tumor. Amer. J. Med., 48:279, 1970.

37. Ogra, P. L., and Herd, J. K.: Arthritis associated with induced rubella infection. J. Immunol., 107:810, 1971.

38. Oldstone, M. B. A., and Dixon, F. J.: Pathogenesis of chronic disease associated with persistent lymphocytic choriomeningitis viral infection. II. Relationship of the anti-lymphocytic choriomeningitis immune response to tissue injury in chronic lymphocytic choriomeningitis disease. J. Exper. Med., 131:1, 1970.

39. Oroszlan, S., and Gilden, R. V.: Immune virolysis: effect of antibody and complement on C-type RNA virus. Science, 168:1478, 1970.

40. Overall, J. C., and Glasgow, L. A.: Fetal response to viral infection: Interferon production in sheep. Science, 167:1139, 1970.

41. Payne, F. E., Baublis, J. V., and Itabashi, H. H.: Isolation of measles virus from cell cultures of brain from a patient with subacute sclerosing panencephalitis. New Eng. J. Med., 281:585, 1969.

42. Porter, D. D.: A quantitative view of the slow virus landscape. Progr. Med. Virol., 13:339, 1971.

43. Rawls, W. E., and Kaufman, R. H.: Herpesvirus and other factors related to the genesis of cervical cancer. Clin. Obstet. Gynecol., 13:857, 1970.

44. Roizman, B., and Spring, S. B.: Alteration in immunologic specificity of cells infected with cytolytic viruses. Proceedings of the Conference on Cross-Reacting Antigens and Neoantigens. (Edited by J. J. Trentin.) Baltimore, Williams and Wilkins, 1967, p. 85.

45. Silverstein, S.: Macrophages and viral immunity. Seminars Hematol., 7:185, 1970.

46. Sonnabend, J. A., Kerr, I. M., and Martin, E. M.: Development of the antiviral state in response to interferon. J. Gen. Physiol., No. 1, Part 2, 172s, 1970.
47. Speel, L. F., Osborn, J. E., and Walker, D. L.: An immuno-cytopathogenic interaction between sensitized leukocytes and epithelial cells carrying a persistent noncytocidal myxovirus infection. J. Immunol., 101:409, 1968.
48. Spencer, E. S., and Andersen, H. K.: Clinically evident, non-terminal infections with herpesviruses and the wart virus in immunosuppressed renal allograft recipients. Brit. Med. J., 3:251, 1970.
49. Sterzl, J., and Silverstein, A.: Developmental aspects of immunity. Adv. Immunol., 6:337, 1967.
50. Summers, D. F.: Biochemistry of animal virus replication. New Eng. J. Med., 276:1016, 1076, 1967.
51. Temin, H. W.: Malignant transformation of cells by viruses. Perspect. Biol. Med., 14:11, 1970.
52. Tompkins, W. A. F., Adams, C., and Rawls, W. E.: An in vitro measure of cellular immunity to fibroma virus. J. Immunol., 104:502, 1970.
53. Wheelock, E. F., Larke, R. P. B., and Caroline, N. L.: Interference in human viral infections: Present status and prospects for the future. Progr. Med. Virol., 10:286, 1968.
54. Wheelock, E. F., and Edelman, R.: Specific role of each human leukocyte type in viral infections. III. 17D yellow fever virus replication and interferon production in homogeneous-leukocyte cultures treated with phytohemagglutinin. J. Immunol., 103:429, 1969.
55. Wiktor, T. J., Kuwert, E., and Koprowski, H.: Immune lysis of rabies virus-infected cells. J. Immunol., 101:1271, 1968.
56. Young, L. W., Smith, D. I., and Glasgow, L. A.: Pneumonia of atypical measles. Residual nodular lesions. Amer. J. Roentgen., 110:439, 1970.

Department of Pediatrics
McMaster University
Hamilton, Ontario
Canada

The Changing Pattern of Diseases Associated with M Components

W. Pruzanski, M.D., F.R.C.P.(C). F.A.C.P., and
M. A. Ogryzlo, M.D., F.R.C.P.(C)***

Changes in disease patterns are invariably the direct consequence of an ever expanding knowledge resulting from new discoveries. An example of this is the considerable progress which has been made in the last decade, relating to a better understanding of the clinical, pathologic and immunologic aspects of diseases associated with dysproteinemia and dysproteinuria. The recognition of γ, α and μ heavy chain diseases[13, 16, 60] and the discovery of IgD and IgE globulins[31, 57] are illustrative of this rapidly expanding field. At a somewhat slower yet detectable pace, changes have also occurred in the management of the dysproteinemias. The use of combined therapy for multiple myeloma and more effective control of its various complications herald a more promising future in the management of this disease. Moreover, the early detection of M components, resulting from a greater awareness of these diseases and the widespread use of sensitive immunochemical techniques, make it possible to institute treatment measures at an earlier stage.

M COMPONENTS

Definition and Classification

Under physiologic conditions, the heterogeneous population of immunoglobulin-producing cells in the body, i.e., plasmacytes and lymphocytes, are capable of producing and secreting a large variety of immunoglobulins. Thus far five main classes of immunoglobulins have been identified, IgG, IgA, IgD, IgE, and IgM, depending on their distinctive heavy chain component (γ, α, δ, ϵ, μ). Each may be divided into those having either kappa (κ) or lambda (λ) types of light chains, and further

From the Immunoproteins Research Laboratory of the University of Toronto Rheumatic Disease Unit, The Wellesley Hospital, Toronto, Ontario, Canada

*Assistant Professor of Medicine; Director, Immunoproteins Research Laboratory

**Professor of Medicine; Director, University of Toronto Rheumatic Disease Unit

Supported in part by a grant-in-aid from the Ontario Cancer Treatment and Research Foundation (220).

subdivided according to the subclass of heavy or subtype of light chains, genetic factors, and other differences. For a detailed discussion of the immunoglobulins, the interested reader is referred to the review by Deutsch and Fudenberg.[11]

In pathologic circumstances, the uncontrolled replication of a single precursor results in a homogeneous population of immunoglobulin-producing cells. The immunoglobulin synthesized by these cells is invariably homogeneous (monoclonal); i.e., all of its molecules have a single and identical class of heavy chains and a single type of light chains. When formed in excess, this homogeneous immunoglobulin constitutes what has been called an M component. However, not infrequently such proliferating cells may produce and secrete incomplete molecules of immunoglobulins, rather than the usual whole molecules. These may constitute light chains only, half molecules, molecules with partial deletion of the heavy or of the light chain, as well as Fc-related fragments which have almost complete deletion of the Fd piece and complete absence of light chains. All of these may be included in the family of proteins which may give rise to the appearance of M components.

The standard definition of an M component as a sharp peak or narrow band of protein on electrophoresis, or a precipitation line of greater density and sharper convexity toward the antibody reservoir on immunoelectrophoresis, is still valid in the majority of instances (Fig. 1). However, important exceptions to this definition may be encountered. Examples include the broad band of globulin frequently observed in gamma heavy chain disease, the absence of a narrow band of protein on electrophoresis in many patients with alpha heavy chain disease, which may appear as an extended line of precipitation in immunoelectrophoresis, and Bence Jones proteins recognized in the serum by immunoelectrophoresis but not by electrophoresis (Fig. 2).

Frequency

Hallen[23] has reported that about 0.9 per cent of the adult population in a community have M components detectable by electrophoresis. This incidence rises to 3 per cent when a population over 65 years of age is screened. Similar results have been reported by Hobbs,[24, 27] who found that 0.8 per cent of 7200 patients in a hospital population on whom electrophoresis was performed, had M components, and also by Takatsuki[68] who recorded 0.8 per cent with M components among 5327 hospitalized patients.

Although M components have been observed more frequently in adults and especially in elderly people, children and also infants with M components have occasionally been observed. Illustrative examples include a 3 month old infant with an IgG cryoglobulin[67] and a 12 year old child with Wiskott-Aldrich syndrome and a serum M component.[55]

Kinetics

Since an M component usually represents an overproduction of a single protein, resulting from an uncontrolled neoplastic proliferation of immunoglobulin-producing cells, it would be expected to be progressive

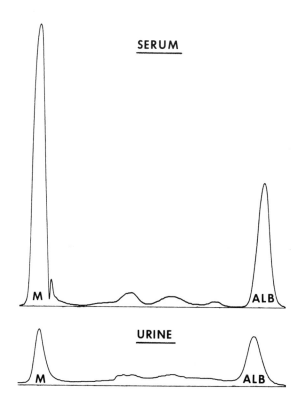

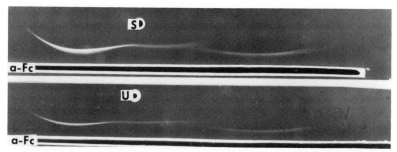

Figure 1.   Sharp peak of an M component in serum and urine, identified immunoelectro-phoretically as an IgG. Partial spontaneous split into Fc and Fc′ fragments is observed. (Modified from Pruzanski, W., and Ogryzlo, M. A.: Adv. Clin. Chem., 13:335–382, 1970, by permission.)

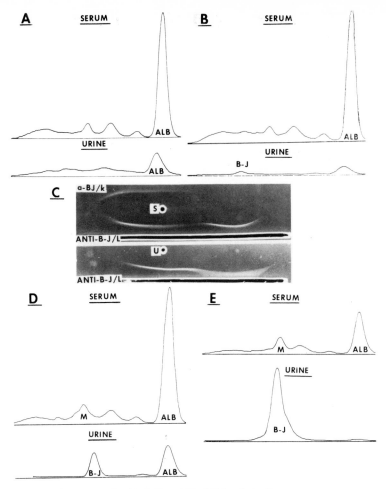

Figure 2.   Four examples (*A, B, D* and *E*) of light-chain disease.
A, No spikes of M components detectable in serum or urine electrophoresis. Immunoelectrophoresis (C) identifies fast moving Bence Jones types lambda globulin in both fluids. B, Minor abnormality of electrophoretic curve only. Diagnosis by immunoelectrophoretic analysis. *D* and *E*, Spikes of M component in serum and urine were identified immunoelectrophoretically as Bence Jones globulin. (Modified from Pruzanski, W., and Ogryzlo, M. A.: Adv. Clin. Chem., *13*:335–382, 1970, by permission.)

and not self limited. Also, the concentration of the M component in the serum would depend on the relationship between the rate of production on the one hand and the rates of catabolism and excretion of the globulin on the other. However, recent observations would suggest that the problem is more complicated than this.

Krause[35] has shown that rabbits hyperimmunized with streptococcal polysaccharides exhibit narrow, M-like bands of protein, detectable on serum electrophoresis, which subsequently disappear after the immunization has been discontinued. Similar M-like bands have been induced in rabbits by prolonged immunization with bacterial vaccines prepared from pneumococci, meningococci, Salmonella typhi and Proteus vulgaris.[21, 33, 35] Furthermore, some of the rabbits which produced large amounts of homogeneous antibody also exhibited features of a myeloma-like disease. These included anemia, extensive rouleaux formation, hyperviscosity, high sedimentation rate, and extensive infiltration of the bone marrow with globulin-containing cells. The manifestations persisted in one rabbit until death, but disappeared in another when the antibody concentration dropped spontaneously.[33]

Counterparts to this experimental model have also been described in human beings. Hobbs[24] observed a patient with chronic lymphocytic leukemia and hypogammaglobulinemia who suffered an episode of pneumococcal pneumonia. In the course of the illness, serum electrophoresis showed an M component identified immunoelectrophoretically as an IgG (λ). The concentration of this protein increased up to the third week of the illness and then gradually disappeared.

Osserman[44] reported a patient who developed an IgG (κ) M component and Bence Jones proteinuria during a hypersensitivity reaction to Gantrisin. After the drug was discontinued and the patient coincidentally developed serum hepatitis, the M component disappeared and was not observed to recur during 3½ years of follow-up.

Similar "transient" M components have been noted by others,[22, 26, 27, 61] suggesting that the production of M components is not always progressive and uncontrolled in a malignant sense. Furthermore, in patients with nonmalignant disorders associated with M components, the monoclonal protein is usually present in low concentration and remains fairly constant over many years. For example, out of 304 patients with M components in one series, 68 showed this benign course for at least 3 years.[27]

As a consequence of these observations, a new concept of a "benign"

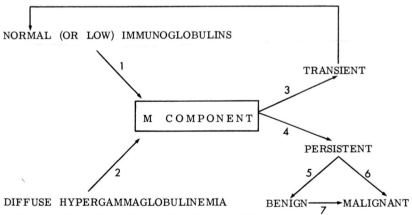

Figure 3. Alternative pathways of development of M components.

$1 \rightarrow 4 \rightarrow 6$ – Multiple myeloma, macroglobulinemia

$\left.\begin{array}{l} 1 \rightarrow 3 \\ 2 \rightarrow 3 \end{array}\right\}$ – Infectious diseases, hypersensitivity, hyperimmunization, and others[21, 22, 24, 26, 27, 33, 35, 44, 59, 61]

$\left.\begin{array}{l} 2 \rightarrow 4 \rightarrow 5 \\ 2 \rightarrow 4 \rightarrow 6 \end{array}\right\}$ – Chronic liver diseases and others[56, 71]

$1 \rightarrow 4 \rightarrow 5 \rightarrow 7$ – Transformation of "benign gammopathy" into multiple myeloma.[36, 59]

versus "malignant" M components has emerged. The "benign" form defines those cases in which there is no malignant disease and the concentration of the serum M components remains lower than 2 gm. per 100 ml. without increasing substantially over the years. Frequently there is no concomitant hypogammaglobulinemia or Bence Jones proteinuria. The "malignant" form, on the other hand, is usually associated with a neoplastic behaviour and a progressive increase in the concentration of the serum M component, usually accompanied by Bence Jones proteinuria. However, there are exceptions in both groups.

Classical multiple myeloma may sometimes have a slow, insidious course, without Bence Jones protein in the urine and only a very gradual increase in the concentration of the M component in the serum. Similarly, the usual stable course of "benign" monoclonal gammopathy may occasionally develop into a progressive, malignant disease.[36, 66] Along a similar line, the rare transformation of a nonspecific, diffuse hypergammaglobulinemia into a monoclonal gammopathy may herald either the development of a malignant transformation[56, 71] or may remain essentially benign[71] (Fig. 3).

Distribution

Diseases with M components are classified as to whether they are neoplastic in Table 1.

Multiple myeloma and macroglobulinemia constitute the most common forms of monoclonal gammopathy, but comprise only a portion of all M components reported. Among a series of 809 patients with M components, these two diseases represented only 46 per cent of the cases.[43] In another series of 691 patients with M components, 74 per cent occurred in malignant diseases (including myeloma, macroglobulinemia, cancer, lymphoma and leukemia) whereas 23 per cent were not associated with

Table 1. *Classification of Diseases with M Components*

NEOPLASTIC*	NON-NEOPLASTIC
Multiple myeloma	Primary generalized amyloidosis
Plasma cell leukemia	Lichen myxedematosus
Macroglobulinemia	Collagen diseases (including rheumatoid arthritis)
γ-Heavy chain disease	Hepatobiliary diseases
α-Heavy chain disease	Chronic cold agglutinin syndrome
μ-Heavy chain disease	Hypergammaglobulinemic purpura
Epithelial neoplasms	Idiopathic cryoglobulinemia
Lymphomas	Benign monoclonal gammopathy**
Leukemias	Others†

*Some other rather ill-defined syndromes have also been described; such as: (a) a syndrome with production of IgG half-molecules; (b) a syndrome with biclonal IgG-IgM gammopathy; (c) a syndrome with production of 7S IgM molecules.

**It is not clear if the term "benign monoclonal gammopathy" should imply an absence of any disease (spike only) or if it denotes a presence of M component in any nonmalignant condition in which there is no clinically recognizable increase in bone marrow plasma cells and no progressive increase in the concentration of the M component.

†A variety of diseases in which M components have been detected, such as Gaucher's disease, polycythemia vera, pyoderma gangrenosum and others.

any malignant condition.[26] The presence of M components in patients with epithelial cancer, sarcoma, lymphoma, and leukemia have been well documented.[26, 43, 46, 56] According to Osserman, adenocarcinoma and adenomatous polyp of the rectosigmoid accounted for 38.4 per cent of 128 patients with tumors associated with M components. Carcinoma of the prostate was responsible for another 18 per cent and carcinoma of the breast for 11 per cent of this group.[43]

Serum and/or urinary M components have also been observed in a great variety of other diseases, including aberrations of lipid metabolism,[32, 56] diabetes mellitus,[56] hepatobiliary diseases,[71] collagen disorders,[56, 70] Gaucher's disease,[50] and lichen myxedematosus,[17] as well as other diseases. Primary generalized amyloidosis, which is frequently associated with serum and urinary M components, is somewhat unique and should be considered separately.[43, 48]

DISEASES WITH M COMPONENTS

Multiple Myeloma

In the United States, myeloproliferative disorders affecting the plasma cells are estimated to account for an annual death rate of 1.7 per 100,000 population.[38] However, the etiology of this apparently neoplastic spectrum of diseases affecting immunoglobulin-producing cells has not yet been elucidated. In addition to the classic search for a viral etiology and physical or chemical irritants, recent attention has been directed towards two additional factors. The first of these concerns the possibility of an hereditary-familial factor. The second concerns the prolonged antigenic stimulation of the reticuloendothelial system resulting in an uncontrolled proliferation of immunoglobulin-producing cells and their precursors.

At least 40 families have now been described in which more than one member has shown an M component.[7, 61, 64] These have included (1) families with two or more cases of multiple myeloma or macroglobulinemia, (2) myeloma or macroglobulinemia in one member of a family and unexplained M components in others, and (3) multiple M components in several members of the same family. Since these disorders have occurred in one or in some cases two generations, including close and distant relatives, it has not been possible to incriminate any common environmental factor. Four sets of spouses with multiple myeloma have recently been reported.[37] Chromosomal aberrations have been noted both in multiple myeloma and in macroglobulinemia,[29] although it is not clear whether these preceded the development of the disease or occurred as a secondary manifestation. On the other hand, there is accumulating evidence that many instances of multiple myeloma are associated with a history of repeated or chronic infection, especially of the biliary or urinary tract. Osserman has reported several instances of a longstanding biliary disease progressing to a monoclonal gammopathy and later terminating in multiple myeloma, macroglobulinemia, or amyloidosis with Bence Jones proteinuria.[44] The demonstration of several M components having antibody activity has stimulated an intensive search for possible antigens in patients with myeloma, which may have been responsible for the production of myeloma proteins. Thus far the search for such antigens has given rather equivocal results.

During its very early stages, the existence of multiple myeloma frequently goes unrecognized, and in most instances the diagnosis is not made until such time as the disease has already become well established. (Table 2). In part, this is because the early phases of the disease may not be associated with any symptoms whatsoever. Moreover, when they do occur, symptoms are often vague, nonspecific, and extremely variable. Since myeloma represents a group of closely related conditions, having in common the neoplastic proliferation of cells capable of producing large quantities of homogeneous immunoglobulin, its early detection is most likely to result from an examination of the protein pattern in the serum and urine by electrophoresis and immunoelectrophoresis. As the disease progresses, the advent of symptoms more directly related to the dysproteinemia, hematologic changes and skeletal involvement, make the diagnosis relatively easier.

The presenting symptoms, clinical findings and natural history of multiple myeloma have been well described in a number of excellent reviews.[6, 46, 47] To a certain extent, the early manifestations, clinical course, type and frequency of complications, therapeutic response, and survival rate may be correlated with the class of M component elaborated by the neoplastic cells.[54] For example, it is possible that the behaviour of the disease may be influenced by differences in the doubling time of the various immunoglobulins (10.1 mos. for IgG, 6.3 mos. for IgA and 3.4 mos. for Bence Jones protein).[25] IgA myeloma, more than any other type, is particularly liable to be associated with bleeding abnormalities and clotting aberrations.[69] Myeloma associated with the exclusive production of Bence Jones type lambda globulin (light chain disease) and IgD

Table 2.   *Clinical Stages of Multiple Myeloma**

Stage 1. Early incipient disease – may be asymptomatic
  An M protein may be discovered during investigation of mild anemia, rouleaux formation, serum anticomplementary activity, elevated erythrocyte sedimentation rate, pneumonia or other infections or unexplained proteinuria. Occasionally, there may be a "solitary" plasmacytoma – skeletal or extraskeletal.

Stage 2. Overt disease – usually symptomatic
  M protein in serum and/or urine, proteinuria, marrow plasmacytosis, osteolytic lesions, osteoporosis, elevated BUN, anemia, hypercalcemia, hyperuricemia, lymphadenopathy, splenomegaly.

Stage 3. Advanced disease
  Renal insufficiency, hypercalcemia, resistant to therapy with prednisone and adequate hydration, inability to maintain a hemoglobin concentration higher than 9.0 gm. per 100 ml. without transfusions, rapidly increasing numbers of plasma cells in peripheral blood. Hyperviscosity syndrome.

Stage 4. Fulminant disease
  Plasma cell leukemia.

---

*Modified from Bergsagel, D. E., and Pruzanski, W.: Postgrad. Med., 43:200–209, 1968.

myeloma are both associated with a more aggressive behaviour, a higher incidence of extra osseous involvement, a greater frequency of renal complications, and a shorter survival time.[5, 25, 54] Only 4 patients have thus far been diagnosed as having an IgE M component, two of whom have had plasma cell leukemia but no osseous lesions on x-ray examination[31, 41, 65] Finally, in a form of multiple myeloma recently described, no M components whatsoever appeared to be formed by the neoplastic cells.[26] The course of the disease was especially malignant. Among 8 such patients, 4 have died within 3 months of diagnosis, and 2 within 6 months. On the other hand, it has become increasingly apparent that the course of the disease cannot readily be related to the morphology of the neoplastic cells, particularly since a great variety of morphologic forms of myeloma cells have been described in each type of myeloma.

Some of the differences observed between the various types of multiple myeloma are summarized in Table 3.

When left untreated, or even despite the application of accepted therapeutic measures, the disease gradually progresses to a more advanced stage. Under these circumstances, the prognosis for survival depends mainly on the ability to correct the existing anemia, to maintain an adequate level of renal function, to prevent the occurrence of excessive hypercalcemia, and to combat infection. In the final stages, the neoplastic process may become widely disseminated, with the appearance of large numbers of plasma cells in the peripheral blood. This terminal leukemic phase however, must be distinguished from that of true plasma cell leukemia.

Patients with multiple myeloma are particularly prone to develop a variety of well recognized complications. Many of these are potentially serious and require the prompt institution of treatment measures before they become irreversible. Infections, especially involving the respiratory or genitourinary tract, are probably related to the inability of the immune mechanism to form normal antibodies in these patients, similar to some of the antibody deficiency syndromes. Hypercalcemia, giving rise to nausea, vomiting, dehydration, loss of muscle tone, and drowsiness, appears to be the direct result of the rapid demineralization of bone.

The risk of renal damage is very real and sometimes difficult to explain. In different patients it may follow the pattern of (a) acute and abrupt renal insufficiency, (b) chronic renal failure, (c) adult Fanconi syndrome with aminoaciduria, glycosuria, and hypophosphatemia, (d) renal tubular acidosis with reduced serum bicarbonate, hyperchloremia, and hypopotassemia, (e) salt-losing nephritis, or (f) nephrotic syndrome. In the investigation of any of these syndromes, the possible existence of multiple myeloma must be seriously considered, since certain diagnostic procedures, such as intravenous pyelography, carry greater risk and may precipitate or induce irreversible, acute renal failure.

Other complications include hyperviscosity syndrome, similar to that occurring in macroglobulinemia, neurological complications such as cord compression from extension of a tumor mass, and amyloidosis with the characteristic distribution of primary amyloid.

The treatment of multiple myeloma must take into consideration

Table 3. *Data on Patients with Multiple Myeloma**

CLASS OF M COMPONENT	TYPE AND FREQUENCY(%) OF LIGHT CHAIN	MEAN AGE YEARS	SEX M/F	AZOTEMIA (BUN >25 mg. per 100 ml.)	HYPER-CALCEMIA (Ca >11 mg. per 100 ml.)	OSTEOLYTIC LESIONS	PLASMA CELL LEUKEMIA	BENCE JONES PROTEINURIA	MEAN SURVIVAL (MONTHS)
IgG	κ−70	62	1/1	8%	33%	55%	2%	61%	35
	λ−30			8%				60%	25
IgA	κ−70	65	1/1	15%	59%	65%	2%	71%	22
	λ−30			11%				67%	19
Bence Jones globulin	κ−50	56	1/1	30%	62%	78%	?**	100%	28
	λ−50			58%					11
	κ−10								
IgD‡	λ−90	56.9	2.7/1	77%	45%	73%	9%	89%	16.6†

*Data compiled from references 2, 25, 52, 54.

**Unknown, but seems to be more frequent than in IgG or IgA myeloma.

†Mean survival from the beginning of symptoms; in other groups from the commencement of therapy.

‡Data on 83 reported patients summarized by the authors.

therapeutic measures directed toward the disease itself and the prevention or treatment of its complications. Although there are a number of well documented reviews on the therapeutic effectiveness of various chemotherapeutic agents, there is a lack of agreement as to which drug or combination of drugs is the most effective. This uncertainty is in part due to the marked variability in the clinical picture, the differing frequency of complications, and also the lack of a uniform standard in evaluating the therapeutic response by various groups of investigators.

In general, however, patients with multiple myeloma can roughly be divided into two groups, so-called responders and non-responders. Responders are those who, during the course of treatment, show improvement in one or more of the following parameters: (1) a decrease of 50 per cent in the concentration of the serum M component; (2) a decrease of 50 per cent in the daily excretion of Bence Jones protein in the urine, and (3) shrinkage of plasmacytomas to 50 per cent of their initial size.[5] It is of interest that slow responders often survive longer than fast responders, who have a greater tendency to relapse.[25]

It has also been reported that use of steroids in conjunction with chemotherapeutic agents, may convert some non-responders into responders.[2, 58] In one series, treatment with cyclophosphamide was shown to prolong a median survival time to 32 months as compared to 9.5 months in an ancillary group.[34] In another, maintenance therapy with melphalan was accompanied by objective improvement in 78 per cent of the patients and subjective improvement in 65 per cent, although only 58 per cent qualified as responders. About 50 per cent of the patients survived for 23 months or longer, after the administration of melphalan.[28] In a third series, only 19 per cent of patients receiving continuous maintenance therapy with melphalan qualified as responders, as compared to 35 per cent of those receiving an intermittent regime and 70 per cent of those receiving intermittent courses of a combination of melphalan with prednisone.[2]

Preliminary results have shown that patients with light chain disease type lambda, show a poorer response to therapy and survive for a shorter period of time than those with light chain disease type kappa.[5] This difference may be related to the more frequent occurrence of renal disease and azotemia in patients associated with Bence Jones protein type lambda in the urine.[2, 18]

Others have also noted that patients with multiple myeloma who produce whole molecules of immunoglobulins (M components in the serum), show a better response to therapy and survive longer when the type of light chain is kappa as opposed to lambda.[2] It is of some interest that patients with the rare types of myeloma such as light chain disease, IgD and IgE myeloma, are more frequently associated with lambda light chains than are the more common types of myeloma (See Table 3). An aggressive approach to the treatment of myeloma has been advocated by some groups. However, triple therapy including melphalan, corticosteroids, and procarbazine,[1] and total body irradiation[4] have not yet been adequately evaluated.

Infections should be treated promptly with suitable antibiotics.

There is no evidence that the parenteral administration of commercial gammaglobulin is helpful in the prevention of recurrent infections. Azotemia can often be prevented or at least improved by adequate hydration. In severe cases, renal dialysis has been found to be a valuable procedure. The anemia associated with myeloma sometimes responds to the administration of anabolic agents such as testosterone. Others may require blood transfusion. Hyperviscosity and hypervolemia are best treated by plasmapheresis. Finally, severe hypercalcemia sometimes responds to the administration of corticosteroids or other agents and adequate hydration, while hyperuricemia may be controlled by the administration of allopurinol.

Plasma Cell Leukemia

Plasma cell leukemia is one of the rarest forms of plasma cell dyscrasia. Its clinical picture has been well documented and includes many of the features of acute leukemia combined with those of multiple myeloma. Low back pain, pathologic fractures, abnormal bleeding tendency, general malaise, and fever, accompanied by a rapid deterioration in general health, are the main clinical manifestations. Immunoglobulin abnormalities are of the same type and appear with the same frequency in plasma cell leukemia as in multiple myeloma. Bence Jones proteinuria is commonly present. The disease usually runs a fulminant course despite treatment with corticosteroids and chemotherapeutic agents used in various combinations, with an average survival time of 4.8 months from the onset of subjective complaints.[53]

Macroglobulinemia

Macroglobulinemia is usually of insidious onset, most often appearing in late adult life with rather vague symptomatology. Included in the early manifestations are such nonspecific symptoms as weakness, weight loss, fever with excessive perspiration, shortness of breath, headaches, vasomotor manifestations of the Raynaud type, arthralgias, and skin rashes with pruritus. More severe symptoms may include visual disturbances, central nervous system manifestations, congestive heart failure, or evidence of peripheral vascular occlusion. Lymphadenopathy and hepatosplenomegaly are common.

The diagnosis is usually verified by the demonstration of an M component in the serum on electrophoresis and its identification as a macroglobulin immunoelectrophoretically. Ultracentrifugation usually shows an increase in fractions 17 to 32 S, although in a proportion of patients 7S IgM has also been found. The Sia test is usually positive. Cryoprecipitation of the abnormal protein or cryogelification of the serum are not uncommon. Cold agglutinins are also present in some patients producing the so-called chronic cold agglutinin syndrome.

The serum is frequently hyperviscous, giving rise to the hyperviscosity syndrome. Coagulation defects involving fibrinogen, prothrombin, factors V and VII, and a release of factor 3 from the platelets are also encountered.[9] Bence Jones proteinuria is present in 40 per cent of cases.[51] (Fig. 4).

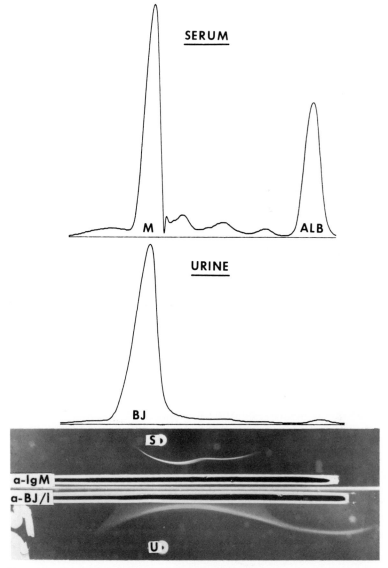

Figure 4.   Macroglobulinemia of Waldenström with IgM(λ) component in the serum and Bence Jones type lambda in the urine. (Modified from Pruzanski, W., and Ogryzlo, M. A.: Adv. Clin. Chem., 13:335–382, 1970, by permission.)

Either the peripheral white blood cells are normal, or there is a lymphocytosis and occasionally an eosinophilia. The platelets are either normal or reduced. Anemia is not uncommon and is often associated with rouleaux formation. The bone marrow may be infiltrated with small lymphocytes and varying numbers of plasma cells or intermediate forms. An increased number of tissue mast cells has been found in some cases.

Complications usually include the hyperviscosity syndrome with various combinations of ocular, cardiovascular, and neurologic manifestations. Congestive heart failure that is resistant to digitalis, acute or chronic encephalopathy, mononeuritis or polyneuritis, or peripheral vascular and cerebrovascular occlusions may also be encountered. Other complications may include chronic hepatitis, Sjögren's or Mikulicz syndromes, renal failure, and amyloidosis.

Macroglobulinemia is usually a chronic disease with a favourable prognosis and an average life expectancy of 38 to 40 months from the first complaints.[9] The better prognosis may be related to the rather long doubling time of the M component. However, several instances have been reported in which the disease has run a more malignant course with a rapidly fatal outcome. Acute renal failure with Bence Jones proteinuria has been described in macroglobulinemia.[3] A leukemic form of macroglobulinemia has been observed in several patients.[53] As in the case of multiple myeloma, one might speculate that macroglobulinemia, also, may not be a single entity but rather a group of closely related but prognostically different conditions.

Macroglobulinemia is most often treated with chlorambucil, sometimes combined with corticosteroids. Splenectomy and radioactive phosphorus have also been tried in several patients. More recently, clinical trials have been conducted with cyclophosphamide[8] and melphalan, but these still require long term evaluation.

HEAVY CHAIN DISEASES

With the demonstration of the basic four-chain structure of the immunoglobulin molecule and the subsequent identification of the different types or classes of light and heavy chains, it was predictable that among the diseases characterized by the presence of abnormal M components, there would be found examples related to the overproduction of each of the different components constituting such molecules. Examples of the exclusive overproduction of each of the two types of light chain (kappa and lambda) were soon recognized and have already been mentioned under the name of so-called, light-chain disease. They most closely resemble multiple myeloma. However, examples of the exclusive overproduction of the known classes of heavy chain fragments, so-called heavy-chain diseases, were not recognized until sometime later. Up to the present time three types of heavy chain disease have been recognized, γ, α and μ heavy chain disease. No cases of heavy-chain disease have yet been identified conforming to Δ or ϵ heavy chains.

GAMMA HEAVY-CHAIN DISEASE. The first 5 examples of gamma heavy chain disease were recognized and described in 1964.[16, 45] Thus far, 21 patients have been identified as having this disorder.[15] The clinical picture includes fever, general malaise, susceptibility to infection, hepatosplenomegaly, and lymphadenopathy. Palatal and uvular swelling has occurred in several patients. Anemia with eosinophilia and the presence of immature plasma cells in the peripheral blood have been noted in many patients. In one patient, atypical lymphocytes constituted 19 per cent of the white blood cells. The microscopic appearance of the bone marrow and lymph nodes resembles a mixed neoplastic proliferation of plasmacytic, lymphocytic and reticular elements. Osseous lesions are not a feature of the disease. Electrophoresis of the serum has shown broad-based spikes of beta mobility. Similar spikes have been detected in the urine, although the protein has not shown the thermoprecipitation properties of Bence Jones protein. Immunochemical studies have shown that the M components are completely devoid of light chains and of part of the Fd fragment. Rather they are closely related to the Fc fragment of the heavy chain of IgG. The sedimentation constant of these components has varied from 2.8 to 4S, with a molecular weight of 52,000 to 56,000. There is no therapy which is particularly effective for this plasmalymphocytic disease.

ALPHA HEAVY-CHAIN DISEASE. The first three patients with alpha heavy chain disease were reported by Seligmann et al. in 1968.[60] Thus far, 25 patients with alpha heavy chain disease have been described.[60, 62, 63] All, except one, had come from the Mediterranean area, North Africa, Far East, or South America. The disease has been documented in one additional patient from the Netherlands.

Clinically, 24 of the patients presented with malabsorption syndrome associated with an abdominal lymphoma. The microscopic picture was that of a diffuse lymphoplasmacytic infiltration of the small intestine and mesenteric lymph nodes. An abnormal protein related to the heavy chain of IgA has been identified in the serum, jejunal fluid, saliva, and urine, as well as in the proliferating malignant cells. The protein, devoid of light chain, is closely related to the Fc fragment of IgA and has invariably been of the alpha-1 subclass. Only half the patients have shown an abnormal band of beta-alpha mobility in the serum on electrophoresis. In all of the patients, an abnormal precipitation line of α-β mobility has been detected in immunoelectrophoresis. The molecular weight has varied from 34,500 to 43,000. Proteinuria ranged from 5 to 180 mg. per 100 ml. The patients have been treated with a variety of chemotherapeutic agents used in lymphomatous disorders.

MU HEAVY-CHAIN DISEASE. Forte et al. reported the first case of μ heavy-chain disease in 1969.[13] Thus far, 3 patients with a picture resembling chronic lymphocytic leukemia have been described with this abnormal protein in the blood. The bone marrow has been infiltrated by a mixture of lymphocytes and peculiar plasma cells with large cytoplasmic vacuoles. Immunochemical studies have shown a low molecular weight protein related to the heavy chain of IgM present in the serum and in the urine. Two of the patients also excreted Bence Jones globulin in the urine.[15]

PRIMARY SYSTEMIC AMYLOIDOSIS

Primary systemic amyloidosis appears to be related to the broad spectrum of plasma cell dyscrasias. Synthesis of M components and marrow plasmacytosis have been well documented in many patients with this disorder.[48] The distribution of the amyloid deposits resembles that occurring in amyloidosis complicating multiple myeloma and may involve the blood vessels and parenchyma of virtually every organ and tissue in the body. The presenting symptoms are quite variable and are frequently associated with a bizarre clinical picture. Nephrotic syndrome has been observed in more than 60 per cent of cases. Congestive heart failure caused by cardiomyopathy, and myopathy involving different striated muscles have often been reported. Macroglossia, carpal tunnel syndrome, hepatosplenomegaly, and involvement of the skin, synovial membranes, or peripheral or central nervous system has been described in this disease.

Similarities between primary amyloidosis and multiple myeloma include the presence of M components in the serum with a diminished level of normal immunoglobulins, the excretion of Bence Jones globulin in the urine, and bone marrow plasmacytosis. These similarities have led Osserman to speculate that there may be a relationship between the gamma globulin-producing system and the formation of amyloid.[42] This presumption has only recently received significant support, with the demonstration that the amino acid sequence of amyloid is similar to that of kappa light chains.[20] Osteolytic lesions resulting from plasma cell proliferation are usually absent in primary amyloidosis, although punched out areas comprised of amyloid deposits have been reported.[19] Among more than 75 patients with primary amyloidosis and M components in the serum, IgG has been found in approximately 50 per cent and Bence Jones globulin in 25 per cent, with the remainder almost equally divided between IgM and IgA classes. Out of 55 typed urinary Bence Jones globulins in primary amyloidosis, only 24 have been of type kappa.[48] This represents a reversal of the ratio of kappa to lambda type, as compared to multiple myeloma. There is no effective treatment for primary amyloidosis, although Missmahl has reported some improvement in several patients treated with chloroquine and methotrexate.[40]

LICHEN MYXEDEMATOSUS (PAPULAR MUCINOSIS, SCLEREMYXEDEMA)

Lichen myxedematosus is primarily a skin disease with the appearance of whitish lichenoid macules which coalesce and form plaques. The lesions are distributed symmetrically in rows and produce a remarkable thickening of the skin. Biopsy usually shows proliferation of fibroblasts in the corium and the presence of an amorphous substance which stains positive for acid mucopolysaccharides. An abnormal M component has been found in the serum in 16 well documented cases, usually appearing as a spike of slow gamma or post gamma mobility on electrophoresis.[12, 14, 17, 26, 30, 39, 49] In all cases in which immunoelectrophoretic identification has been undertaken, the M component has been of the IgG (λ) type. The same immunoglobulin has been demonstrated in the skin in the amorphous substance. In some cases there has been an increase in the plasma cells in the bone marrow, while in others no significant increase in plasma cells have been reported.[30] One patient showed a dramatic response to melphalan therapy with significant improvement in the skin condition and a decrease in the level of abnormal protein in the serum.[12] Two patients treated with methotrexate did not show significant improvement.[49] The disease is benign, with no instances of progression to multiple myeloma over a period of 20 years.[17]

PYODERMA GANGRENOSUM

Pyoderma gangrenosum is another skin disease in which abnormal M components have been reported.[10] These may represent any one of the three major classes of immunoglobulins, namely IgG, IgA, or IgM. However, among 10 patients with this disease, 6 have shown an IgA M component. Some of these have been shown to possess an ability to agglomerate red cells in vitro. Available information is inadequate for an evaluation of the relationship between this skin disorder, the presence of M components, and plasma cell dyscrasia.

REFERENCES

1. Alexanian, R., Bonnet, J., Gehan, E., Hewlett, J., Lane, M., Monto, R., and Wilson, H.: Melphalan-prednisone-procarbazine therapy for multiple myeloma. Abstract Volume, p. 352, XIII International Congress of Hematology, Munich, Aug. 2-8, 1970. J. F. Lehmanns Verlag, München.
2. Alexanian, R., Haut, A., Khan, A. U., Lane, M., McKelvey, E. M., Migliore, P. J., Stuckey, W. J., Jr., and Wilson, H. E.: Treatment for multiple myeloma. Combination chemotherapy with different melphalan dose regimens. J.A.M.A., 208:1680–1685, 1969.
3. Argani, I., and Kipkie, G. F.: Macroglobulinemic nephropathy. Acute renal failure in macroglobulinemia of Waldenström. Amer. J. Med., 36:151–157, 1964.
4. Bergsagel, D. E.: Total body irradiation for myelomatosis. Brit. Med. J., 2:325, 1971.
5. Bergsagel, D. E., Migliore, P. J., and Griffith, K. M.: Myeloma proteins and the clinical response to melphalan therapy. Science, 148:376–377, 1965.
6. Bergsagel, D. E., and Pruzanski, W.: Recognizing and treating plasma cell neoplasia. Postgrad. Med., 43:200–209, 1968.
7. Berlin, S.-O., Odeberg, H., and Weingart, L.: Familial occurrence of M components. Acta Med. Scand., 183:347–350, 1968.
8. Bouroncle, B. A., Datta, P., and Frajola, W. J.: Waldenström's macroglobulinemia. Report of three patients treated with cyclophosphamide. J.A.M.A., 189:729–732, 1964.
9. Cohen, R. J., Bohannon, R. A., and Wallerstein, R. O.: Waldenström's macroglobulinemia. A study of ten cases. Amer. J. Med., 41:274–284, 1966.
10. Cream, J. J.: Pyoderma gangrenosum with a monoclonal IgM red cell agglomerating factor. Brit. J. Derm., 84:223–226, 1971.
11. Deutsch, H. F., and Fudenberg, H. H.: Immunoglobulin structure and function. Adv. Int. Med., 15:377–396, 1969.
12. Feldman, P., Shapiro, L., Pick, A. I., and Slatkin, M. H.: Scleromyxedema. A dramatic response to melphalan. Arch. Derm., 99:51–56, 1969.
13. Forte, F. A., Prelli, F., Yount, W. J., Jerry, L. M., Kochwa, S., Franklin, E. C., and Kunkel, H. G.: Heavy chain disease of the μ (γM) type: report of the first case. Blood, 36:137–144, 1970.
14. Fowlkes, R. W., Blaylock, W. K., and Mullinax, F.: Immunologic studies in lichen myxedematosus. Arch. Derm., 95:370–374, 1967.
15. Franklin, E. C., and Frangione, B.: Heavy chain disease: Defects in protein synthesis and their genetic implications. The New York Academy of Sciences Conference on Immunoglobulins, New York, March 8-10, 1971.
16. Franklin, E. C., Lowenstein, J., Bigelow, B., and Meltzer, M.: Heavy chain disease – a new disorder of serum γ globulins. Amer. J. Med., 37:332–350, 1964.
17. Fudenberg, H. H., Epstein, W. L., Shuster, J., and James, K.: Diagnostic paraprotein in papular mucinosis. Bibl. Haemat., 29:318–321, 1968.
18. Galton, D. A. G.: Treatment of myelomatosis — M. R. C. Trial. Brit. Med. J., 2:323–324, 1971.
19. Gardner, H.: Bone lesions in primary systemic amyloidosis. A report of a case. Brit. J. Radiol., 34:778–783, 1961.

20. Glenner, G. G., Terry, W., Harada, M., Isersky, C., and Page, D.: Amyloid fibril proteins: Proof of homology with immunoglobulin light chains by sequence analyses. Science, 172:1150-1151, 1971.
21. Haber, E.: Antibodies of restricted heterogeneity for structural study. Fed. Proc., 29:66-71, 1970.
22. Hällen, J.: Discrete gammaglobulin (M-) components in serum. Clinical study of 150 subjects without myelomatosis. Acta Med. Scand., Suppl. 462, 1966, pp. 1-127.
23. Hällen, J.: Frequency of "abnormal" serum globulins (M components) in the aged. Acta Med. Scand., 173:737-744, 1963.
24. Hobbs, J. R.: Disturbances of the immunoglobulins. Sci. Basis Med. Ann. Rev., 1966, pp. 106-127.
25. Hobbs, J. R.: Growth rates and responses to treatment in human myelomatosis. Brit. J. Haemat., 16:607-617, 1969.
26. Hobbs, J. R.: Immunocytoma o' Mice an' Men. Brit. Med. J., 2:67-72, 1971.
27. Hobbs, J. R.: Paraproteins, benign or malignant? Brit. Med. J., 3:699-704, 1967.
28. Hoogstraten, B., Sheehe, P. R., Cuttner, J., Cooper, T., Kyle, R. A., Oberfield, R. A.. Townsend, S. R., Harley, J. B., Hayes, D. M., Costa, G., and Holland, J. F.: Melphalan in multiple myeloma. Blood, 30:74-83, 1967.
29. Houston, E. W., Ritzmann, S. E., and Levin, W. C.: Chromosomal aberrations common to three types of monoclonal gammopathies. Blood, 29:214-232, 1967.
30. James, K., Fudenberg, H., Epstein, W. L., and Shuster, J.: Studies on a unique diagnostic serum globulin in papular mucinosis (lichen myxedematosus). Clin. Exper. Immunol., 2:153-166, 1967.
31. Johansson, S. G. O., and Bennich, H.: Immunological studies of an atypical (myeloma) immunoglobulin. Immunology, 13:381-394, 1967.
32. Killander, J.: Immunoglobulin M components with antibody-like activity against lipids. The New York Academy of Sciences Conference on Immunoglobulins, New York, March 8-10, 1971.
33. Kimball, J. W., Pappenheimer, A. M. J., and Jaton, J.-C.: The response in rabbits to prolonged immunization with type III pneumococci, J. Immunol., 106:1177-1184, 1971.
34. Korst, D. R., Clifford, G. O., Fowler, W. M., Louis, J., Will, J., and Wilson, H. E.: Multiple Myeloma. II. Analysis of cyclophosphamide therapy in 165 patients. J.A.M.A., 189:758-762, 1964.
35. Krause, R. M.: Factors controlling the occurrence of antibodies with uniform properties. Fed. Proc., 29:59-65, 1970.
36. Kyle, R. A., and Bayrd, E. D.: "Benign" monoclonal gammopathy: A potentially malignant condition? Amer. J. Med., 40:426-430, 1966.
37. Kyle, R. A., Heath, C. W., Jr., and Carbone, P.: Multiple myeloma in spouses. Arch. Int. Med., 127:944-946, 1971.
38. Lingeman, C. H.: Plasma cell neoplasms of man and animals. National Cancer Institute Monograph, 1969, vol. 32. pp. 303-311.
39. McCarthy, J. T., Osserman, E., Lombardo, P. C., and Takatsuki, K.: An abnormal serum globulin in lichen myxedematosus. Arch. Derm., 89:446-450, 1964.
40. Missmahl, H. P.: Follow-up studies for a 30-year period on patients with amyloidosis; diagnostic methods; treatment. In Mandema, E., Ruinen, L., Scholten, J. H., and Cohen, A. S., eds.: Amyloidosis. Amsterdam, Excerpta Medica Foundation, 1968, pp. 429-437.
41. Ogawa, M., Kochwa, S., Smith, C., Ishizaka, K., and McIntyre, O. R.: Clinical aspects of IgE myeloma. New Eng. J. Med., 281:1217-1220, 1969.
42. Osserman, E. F.: Amyloidosis: Tissue proteinosis: gammaloidosis. Ann. Int. Med., 55:1033-1036, 1961.
43. Osserman, E. F.: Considerations regarding pathogenic mechanisms of plasma cell dyscrasias in man. The New York Academy of Sciences Conference on Immunoglobulins, New York, March 8-10, 1971.
44. Osserman, E. F., and Fahey, J. L.: Plasma cell dyscrasias. Current Clinical and Biochemical Concepts. Amer. J. Med., 44:256-269, 1968.
45. Osserman, E. F., and Takatsuki, K.: Clinical and immunochemical studies of four cases of heavy (H$^{\gamma 2}$) chain disease. Amer. J. Med., 37:351-373, 1964.
46. Osserman, E. F., and Takatsuki, K.: Plasma cell myeloma: gamma globulin synthesis and structure. A review of biochemical and clinical data, with the description of a newly recognized and related syndrome, "H$^{\alpha-2}$-chain (Franklin's) disease." Medicine, 42:357-384, 1963.
47. Owen, D. M.: Multiple myeloma. A review based on 98 cases. Geriatrics, 20:1048-1064, 1965.
48. Parr, D. M., Pruzanski, W., Scott, J. G., and Mills, D. M.: Primary amyloidosis with plasmacytic dyscrasia and a tetramer of Bence Jones type lambda globulin in the serum and urine. Blood, 37:473-484, 1971.
49. Piper, W., Hardmeier, T., and Schafer, E.: Das Skleromyxödem Arndt-Gottron: eine Paraproteinamische Erscheinung. Schweiz. Med. Wschr., 97:829-838, 1967.

50. Pratt, P. W., Estren, S., and Kochwa, S.: Immunoglobulin abnormalities in Gaucher's Disease. Report of 16 cases. Blood, 31:633–640, 1968.
51. Pruzanski, W., and Ogryzlo, M. A.: Abnormal proteinuria in malignant diseasés. Adv. Clin. Chem., 13:335–382, 1970.
52. Pruzanski, W., and Ogryzlo, M. A.: Anomalous urinary proteins in patients with serum M components. Canad. Med. Assoc. J., 104:581–588, 1971.
53. Pruzanski, W., Platts, M. E., and Ogryzlo, M. A.: Leukemic form of immunocytic dyscrasia (plasma cell leukemia). A study of 10 cases and a review of the literature. Amer. J. Med., 47:60–74, 1969.
54. Pruzanski, W., and Rother, I.: IgD plasma cell neoplasia: clinical manifestations and characteristic features. Canad. Med. Assoc. J., 102:1061–1065, 1970.
55. Rádl, J., Masopust, J., Houštěk, J., and Hrodek, O.: Paraproteinemia and unusual Dys-γ-globulinemia in a case of Wiskott-Aldrich syndrome. Arch. Dis. Child, 42:608–614, 1967.
56. Ritzmann, S. E., and Levin, W.: Polyclonal and monoclonal gammopathies. In Laboratory Synopsis. Montreal, Canada, Hoechst Pharmaceutical Co., 1969, 2nd ed., vol. 2, pp. 9–54.
57. Rowe, D. S., and Fahey, J. L.: A new class of human immunoglobulins. I. A unique myeloma protein. J. Exper. Med., 121:171–184, 1965.
58. Schilling, A., Shnider, B. I., Lenhard, R., Jr., and Horton, J.: Intermittent prednisone therapy for myeloma patients no longer responsive to alkylating agents. Abstracts of the Tenth International Cancer Congress, Houston, 1970, pp. 489–490.
59. Seligmann, M., Danon, F., and Clauvel, J. P.: Natural history of monoclonal immunoglobulins. Brit. Med. J., 2:321–322, 1971.
60. Seligmann, M., Danon, F., Hurez, D., Mihaesco, E., and Preud'homme, J.-L.: Alpha-chain disease: A new immunoglobulin abnormality. Science, 162:1396–1397, 1968.
61. Seligmann, M., Danon, F., Mihaesco, C., and Fudenberg, H. H.: Immunoglobulin abnormalities in families of patients with Waldenström's macroglobulinemia. Amer. J. Med., 43:66–83, 1967.
62. Seligmann, M., and Mihaesco, E.: Alpha chain disease. The New York Academy of Sciences Conference on Immunoglobulins, New York, March 8-10, 1971.
63. Seligmann, M., Mihaesco, E., Hurez, D., Mihaesco, C., Preud'homme, J.-L., and Rambaud, J.-C.: Immunochemical studies in four cases of alpha chain disease. J. Clin. Invest., 48:2374–2389, 1969.
64. Spengler, G. A., Bütler, R., Fischer, C., Ryssel, H. J., Schmid, E., and Siebner, M.: On the question of familial occurrence of paraproteinemia. Helv. Med. Acta, 33:208–219, 1966.
65. Spiegelberg, H. L.: Personal communication, 1971.
66. Stevens, A. R., Jr.: Evolution of multiple myeloma. Arch. Int. Med., 115:90–93, 1965.
67. Stoop, J. W., Ballieux, R. E., and Weyers, H. A.: Paraproteinemia with secondary immune globulin deficiency in an infant. Pediatrics, 29:97–104, 1962.
68. Takatsuki, K.: Personal communication, 1971.
69. Vigliano, E. M., and Horowitz, H. I.: Bleeding syndrome in a patient with IgA myeloma: Interaction of protein and connective tissue. Blood, 29:823–836, 1967.
70. Zawadzki, Z. A., and Benedek, T. G.: Rheumatoid Arthritis, dysproteinemic arthropathy, and paraproteinemia. Arthr. Rheum., 12:555–568, 1969.
71. Zawadzki, Z. A., and Edwards, G. A.: Dysimmunoglobulinemia associated with hepato-biliary disorders. Amer. J. Med., 48:196–202, 1970.

Immunoproteins Research Unit
The Wellesley Hospital
Toronto, Ontario
Canada

Immune Mechanisms of Mucosal Resistance

John Bienenstock, M.D.,[*]
and Daniel Y. E. Perey, M.D.[**]

In utero and at birth the normal human infant is germ-free. The fetus has been preserved in this state by protective mechanisms such as the placental barrier and the antibodies supplied through the cord blood from the maternal circulation. From its first breath and first swallow the baby is exposed to a potentially hostile environment. This raises the important question of how pathogenic bacteria and viruses in the external environment are prevented from causing damage to the infant. Since the portals of entry of these agents in the intact infant can only be primarily through the mouth and nostrils, these agents must first pass the initial barrier of the natural mucous membrane defense mechanisms of the upper and lower respiratory and gastrointestinal tracts.

Historically the study of defense mechanisms, in particular the immunologic defense mechanisms, has been primarily related to the responses to injected material, such as that contained in vaccines, or those responses to pathogenic organisms once these have maintained viability long enough to initiate disease. The information as to the normal physiologic mechanisms of maintaining the integrity of the organism at the level of the mucous membranes, though fundamentally important, has only been explored systematically in the last decade.

The present article will deal primarily with the question of immunologic mechanisms of resistance at the mucous membrane level, although it is clear that a number of apparently non-immunologic factors are important in this regard. The latter would for example include the nonspecific effects of various mucopolysaccharides, iron and other metallic ion–binding proteins such as transferrin and lactoferrin, specific for secretions which bathe mucous membranes, enzymes such as lysozyme, and the complement system. It is now clear that in the complement sys-

From the Departments of Medicine and Pathology, McMaster University, Hamilton, Ontario

[*]M. R. C. Scholar
[**]Queen Elizabeth II Scientist

Supported by the Medical Research Council of Canada.

tem, which classically has been associated with specific immunologic activation, activation can occur without mediation by antibody.[21] Specific
factors relating to viral resistance such as interferon are referred to elsewhere in this series by Dent and Larke; however, it is important to point
out that interferon, although classically regarded as a specific antiviral
agent, has now been shown to have the ability to interfere with the
viability of protozoa, rickettsiae, and some bacteria.

The effector mechanisms of the immunologic response can be mediated primarily through two arms; the first being the antibody or immunoglobulin effector arm, and the second being through cells. Immunoglobulins in man are endowed with specificity for a particular antigen and are of 5 major classes IgG, IgA, IgM, IgD, IgE.[22] Only the IgG
and IgM classes have the ability to interact primarily with the complement sequence. This mechanism is important in opsonization of bacteria
for immune phagocytosis by white cells,[37] and is also cytocidal for microorganisms. In addition, factors generated through complement activation
can mediate specific chemotaxis for white cells. In addition to these
biologic properties, some IgG antibodies have the ability to attach to
white cells, endowing the white cells with the specific property of interacting with the antigen against which the antibody is directed. These
antibodies are referred to as cytophilic antibodies.

The cellular immunologic mechanisms which have been referred to
are mainly those relating to the delayed hypersensitivity type of reaction,
which is mediated by lymphocytes.[22] There is evidence now that in
delayed hypersensitivity, interaction between lymphocytes and macrophages may have to occur in a cooperative process. Activated lymphocytes involved in this pathway are able to release cytotoxic factors which
themselves are capable of causing both the specific ingress of certain
types of other cells and the immobilization of others (including macrophages) so as to retain their presence at the appropriate sites. In addition,
upon specific activation, lymphocytes can produce interferon, previously
regarded as a nonspecific antiviral substance, relatively nonspecifically
stimulated. Lymphocytes (delayed hypersensitivity mechanisms) appear to be an important pathway of resistance to viral, fungal, mycobac-
terial, and some other intracellular pathogens.

ANATOMY OF MUCOUS MEMBRANE IMMUNOLOGIC RESPONSES

Mucous membranes differ in their distribution of lymphoid tissue
from those organs classically associated with participation in the immune response such as spleen and peripheral lymph nodes. Generally, in
mucous membranes lymphoid tissue is of two types: the first is a diffuse
scattered population of lymphoid cells in the lamina propria which are
predominantly synthesizing IgA. The concentration of these cells, for example in the gastrointestinal tract lamina propria, is remarkably high,
there being on an average 350,000 such cells per cu. mm. of intestine.[13]
The second type of lymphoid tissue is organized into follicles. The best
example of this would be the Peyer's patches of the gastrointestinal tract.

Real controversy exists as to the nature of these follicles and their relationship to peripheral lymph nodes.[35]

It can be accurately stated that there are several differences between this type of lymphoid tissue and the classical peripheral lymph node. This follicular lymphoid tissue is disseminated throughout the body in mucous membranes and is present in the bronchial tree, the gastrointestinal tract, tonsils, and urinary bladder.

The normal sequence of events leading to antibody production is processing of antigen by macrophages with subsequent production of antibody by activated lymphocytes (plasma-like cells). Specific antibody production clearly occurs in the lamina propria mainly in the IgA class. It also occurs in tonsillar tissue[51] but does not appear to occur in the Peyer's patches[6] or in the bronchial lymphoid aggregates. Thus there is a gradation from the organized lymphoid tissue of the respiratory and gastrointestinal tracts, that in the nasopharynx, and that found in the lymph node. It is possible that one of the functions of the Peyer's patch type of tissue is to provide cells destined for IgA production to the lamina propria of local[14] and other mucous membranes but it also appears to supply other classes of immunoglobulin-producing cells to other peripheral lymphoid tissue.[11, 23] This appears to be a characteristic of the sentinel type of lymphoid tissue found at the potential portals of entry of microorganisms into the body.

MUCOUS SECRETIONS

Mucous secretions, which bathe mucous membranes, contain a number of immunologic resistance factors, which include lymphocytes, macrophages, and antibody. Not all complement components are generally found in secretions, but certain secretions are relatively rich in certain of these components and the biological significance of this aspect of resistance is unknown. The IgA molecule found in secretions differs from its counterpart in serum on the basis of a number of characteristics.[46] First, it is a larger molecule; second, it has unique antigenic characteristics not found in serum IgA; third, it is endowed with resistance to proteolysis as compared to serum IgA. The molecule appears to be synthesized in the lamina propria cells and finds its way across the basement membrane into the lateral intercellular channels between epithelial cells and is then transported through the cells to the surface of the mucous membrane.[47] On its way it becomes coupled to a non-immunoglobulin protein moiety known as secretory component.

This polypeptide is apparently synthesized by the epithelial cells and is not found in lymphocytes or plasma cells. Its function is unknown, but it appears to endow the secretory IgA molecule with many of its unusual characteristics. The secretory IgA molecule is found in the nasal, salivary, mammary, gastrointestinal, bronchial, biliary, lacrimal, cervical, prostatic, and bladder secretions as well as in urine. It does not appear in internal secretions such as synovial fluid or cerebrospinal fluid.

The biologic functions of IgA in general are not known. Secretory IgA appears to play little role in opsonic or cytophilic type of activity. It however does appear to have some involvement, together with complement and lysozyme, in bacteriocidal reactions.[1] It may in addition be able to activate the complement sequence in an unusual way through the terminal acting components, through a by-pass mechanism of the initial complement sequence, since this has been demonstrated to occur in the serum IgA.[41]

IgE, which has been identified as the reaginic or anaphylactic antibody in man, appears to have a similar distribution to IgA insofar as cell localization is concerned in mucous membranes.[27] Thus the largest numbers of IgE-containing cells are found in the nasal, bronchial, and gastrointestinal mucosa. IgE does not contain secretory component or activate the complement sequence, has cytophilic affinity for mast cells, and upon interaction with antigen is capable of degranulation and release of mast cell constituents such as histamine.

CONCEPT OF LOCAL IMMUNITY

Antibodies

It has been apparent from some of the earliest immunologic investigations of this century that successful immunization with subsequent resistance to infection could be accomplished in experimental animals by oral immunization against enteropathogens. Besredka[4] in 1927 published a monograph entitled *Local Immunization.* Except for intermittent pioneering studies which occurred during the following several decades no consistent investigation of these phenomena occurred,[7, 15, 17, 36, 44] and immunization practice was in essence confined to parenteral administration of antigen, so that local vaccination procedures fell into disrepute. It was only in the last decade in which investigation of the types of antibodies found in secretions was undertaken that this whole question was reopened and the concept of local immunization was placed on a sound scientific basis.[16]

There is now a large body of literature pertaining to this subject.[5, 24, 46] It is now true to say that local presentation of antigen to the respiratory tract, gut, eye, and even vagina appears to preferentially induce local antibody which can better be correlated with subsequent resistance to reinfection than parenteral administration of that antigen. It has long been known that oral polio vaccination not only could be correlated with resistance to poliomyelitis and subsequent reinfection, but that this method of immunization would also eradicate the disease carrier state. This was found not to hold true for the inactivated parenteral vaccine which appeared to be able only to prevent the disease. Ogra and co-workers[34] demonstrated that the former local immunization produced local (predominantly secretory IgA) antibody as well as a circulating antibody response, whereas the latter resulted only in a circulating antibody response without secretory antibody. This type of observation has now been made for a number of viruses: rhino, parainfluenza, respiratory syncytial, influenza, measles, and rubella viruses in the upper and lower respiratory tracts. Similar observations have also been made for staphylococci, streptococci, diphtheriae, pneumococci, meningococci, and F. tularensis with regard to the upper respiratory tract.[16] Apart from polio antibodies referred to earlier, similar observations have been made in relation to most of the gut pathogens, including cholera. A local immunoglobulin response can be stimulated by trachoma in the eye, and S. typhi in the female genital tract. Recently Waldman et al.[49] have shown that secretory IgA antibody responses to fungi such as candida albicans occur in the cervical secretions, and sperm-immobilizing substances,[43] probably of an antibody nature, have been demonstrated to occur with increasing frequency among groups of women investigated for infertility.

Cells

Although the emphasis of most of these investigations has been on the antibody content of the secretions bathing the particular mucous membrane investigated, it has been clear for some time that cell-mediated immunity might well be involved in specific resistance at these levels. Indeed it has recently been reported that local delayed hypersensitivity (lymphocyte)-mediated immune mechanisms can occur in the respiratory tract without generalized evidence of this type of immunity.[50] It is interesting to note that in man, mycoplasma infection which is localized to the epithelium of the respiratory tract does not apparently give rise to a predominantly IgA antibody response locally. In fact it has been shown recently that although the local antibody response is predominantly IgM, a major component of resistance in this type of infection in the experimental animal appears to be related to local lymphocyte-mediated immune mechanisms.[18]

One surprising feature of the local immune system is the observation that immunologic memory and recall do not appear to exist on rechallenge.[33]

In summary, several general principles in regard to local immunity may be presented.

1. If the antigen is presented locally, a local immune response may occur.
2. If the antigen is present in sufficient amounts a systemic immune response may also occur.
3. The predominant immunoglobulin response in normal human secretions is of the IgA class.
4. If the antigen is given locally and replicates with persistence of antigen, a prolonged local immune response may be found.
5. A local immune response can occur after administration of parenteral antigen if sufficient quantity of antigen is introduced or if live replicating antigen (virus) is used.
6. The types of local immunity induced may be of at least two kinds, antibody and cell mediated.
7. There is often a dichotomy between the measurement of immunity, as judged by any criteria, in the secretions and the blood.
8. Not all antigens given locally will produce a local IgA immune response, although this is the exception rather than the rule.

Lastly although the levels of antibody demonstrable locally in the secretions may be low, immunity as demonstrated by resistance to infection may be high, indicating the biologic significance of antibody perhaps at relatively high local concentration in the mucous membranes themselves.

Parasites

As has been mentioned earlier the IgE class of immunoglobulins appears to be cytophilic for mast cells as target organs. Upon subsequent interaction with antigen release of vasoactive materials, such as histamine, occurs. This class of antibody is probably not the only class of immunoglobulins responsible for human reaginic activity; however, the contributions from other classes toward this type of activity appear to be relatively minor. The serum IgE levels from groups of patients selected at random among populations with a high degree of parasitic infestation, such as for example among native Ethiopians, are extremely high.[28] Ascaris extracts are well recognized to be among the most potent allergens recorded in man, having an almost uniform ability to excite reaginic antibody upon immunization.

The biologic function of such antibodies in man is not clearly established. However, on the basis of experimental evidence of nematode infestation in animals, peak reaginic activity in the serum can coincide with a massive expulsion of the worms, by the gastrointestinal tract, accompanied by mast cell degranulation and "self-cure." Although it is not clear from an evolutionary point of view why an antibody with otherwise harmful activity should have been retained, this experimental evidence might suggest that IgE antibody is beneficial from the point of view of host-parasite interaction, particularly of the nematode class.

Dietary Proteins

The human gastrointestinal tract is thought to maintain integrity and not transport macromolecules such as proteins across the gut epithelium.[29] However, 70 per cent of normal healthy adults are said to have antibodies to dietary constituents, such as milk antigens.[39] In premature infants Rothberg[38] has clearly shown that antigenically recognizable bovine serum albumin or fragments thereof are present in the circulation after feeding with a formula containing bovine serum albumin. These observations confirm our general ignorance in the area of protein handling by the gut either in health or disease.

The question therefore as to the type of antibody produced or the general immunologic response which may occur after protein feeding[29] must depend on the type of antigen presented, the quantity of antigen absorbed, the amount of antigen digested by the gastrointestinal enzymes and the amount of antigen available locally to lymphoid tissue in the gastrointestinal tract as opposed to that circulating to peripheral lymphoid organs.

Tolerance

Chase reported experiments in which oral feeding of dinitrochlorbenzene or picryl chloride to animals gave rise to immunologic unresponsiveness on subsequent challenge with antigen.[9] The phenomenon which has received the eponym Sulzberger-Chase phenomenon may be pertinent to some of the points already raised in regard to oral feeding of antigen. Several investigators have now clearly demonstrated that the phenomenon which occurs following oral feeding of a potent sensitizing hapten such as quoted above gives rise to complete tolerance: that is, no antibody production or delayed hypersensitivity can be demonstrated on subsequent challenge. We have shown that this tolerance extends not only to the systemic manifestations but also as far as local immunity is concerned in the gut. The exact relationship of this phenomenon to local immunization is unclear, and one can only speculate that unravelling of this problem on an experimental basis may prove to have important implications for better understanding with regard to oral immunization practice. It is interesting to note that North American Indians are said to have chewed poison ivy leaves to prevent poison ivy contact dermatitis.[31] Recently Lowney has clearly demonstrated that tolerance of a similar nature can be produced in man.[30]

Flora

Several types of natural antibodies in the serum, such as isohemagglutinins, may be the result of the flora maintained in the gastrointestinal tract. This information implies that some of this antibody might well be locally produced in the lymphoid tissue of the gastrointestinal tract itself. In fact, Springer and Horton[42] have shown that it is possible to induce high levels of antibody to blood groups not represented in an individual volunteer by feeding a variety of organisms, tissues, and plant substances which contain as the immmunodominant antigenic substance a sugar characteristic for either blood group A or B. The implications of the converse of this experiment are interesting, since, for example, colonization of an individual of blood group B status with organisms bearing mucopolysaccharides cross-reactive to blood group B substance in their cell surface would become symbiotic or parasitic with the host because of the inability of the host to develop antibodies to the somatic antigens. However, antibodies to other constituents of the organisms such as flagellar antigens would not be suppressed. This type of possibility not only exists with bacteria but clearly extends to viruses in which similar cross reactivity between viral antigens and blood group substances has been reported.[26]

Germ-free animals might reasonably be regarded as analogous to the human neonate. Both have almost nonexistent levels of IgA, either in serum or in secretions.[12] Both have very poorly developed lymphoid tissue in respiratory and gastrointestinal tracts. Both groups are particularly susceptible to respiratory tract and gastrointestinal tract infections. Breast feeding in the neonatal period undoubtedly supplies the infant with a major source of passively acquired antibodies. Since colostrum as well as breast milk contains the highest concentration of secretory IgA in any secretion, the suckling infant receives passive immunity in this natural way. This is of course in addition to the maternal IgG antibody which it has received via the cord blood. The secretory IgA antibody does not cross the gastrointestinal tract and remains relatively unaltered in its passage through the tract by virtue of its higher resistance to normal degradative mechanisms which in any case are poorly developed in the neonatal period.

A further example of the value of breast feeding comes from calves which receive most of their immunity passively through colostrum and milk in the early neonatal period.[19] If such animals are deprived of breast feeding, they invariably die of overwhelming infection. The importance of these observations in regard to neonatal infections, particularly early diarrheas in infants not being breast fed, is clear.

Immune Deficiency Syndromes

Immunoglobulin deficiency states can be absolute or relative, congenital or acquired, and they may be associated with defects in cell-mediated immune mechanisms.[20] Regardless of these complicated issues, they are characteristically associated with repeated life-threatening sinopulmonary and gastrointestinal infections.

Absolute deficiencies of all immunoglobulins are a relatively rare event. However deficiencies of IgA, either absolute or relative, occur with surprising frequency in the population at large. The recorded incidence of IgA deficiency is about 1 in 700, and in these patients the IgA is almost invariably deficient in serum and secretions alike.

Although this condition may be totally asymptomatic, not enough experience has been gained to know whether symptoms may not develop relevant to the respiratory and gastrointestinal tracts at some point in the course of such an individual's life.[10] Many such patients have symptoms and disease referable to the respiratory and gastrointestinal tracts.

These individuals also have a tendency to have elevated autoantibodies such as rheumatoid factor, antinuclear factor, antithyroid antibodies, and antibodies to gastric parietal cells.[2] In addition they have been shown to have an increased incidence of and higher than normal levels of antibodies to dietary proteins.[25]

The absolute significance of these observations is not clear. However, if the local secretory IgA and other immunologic immune mechanisms play a protective role in relation to the mucous membranes, it is an attractive possibility that they may prevent the ingress or access to the immunologic machinery of potentially pathogenic organisms such as viruses and self antigens which would otherwise be potent in producing autoantibody formation. The natural role of secretory antibodies may thus be in part to "tie up" loose antigen in the lumen of the respiratory and gastrointestinal tracts and prevent entry into the host. In those patients who have an absolute IgA deficiency, the deficiency of cells normally synthesizing IgA in the mucous membranes is generally replaced by cells synthesizing IgM, and in this case, although the secretory component is still present in the secretions and actively synthesized, it is not found attached to the IgM molecules in the secretions.

Several patients with IgE deficiencies have been reported. It has been suggested that the disease of those patients with IgA deficiencies and sinopulmonary infections might be explained on the basis of superimposed IgE deficiencies.[3] This relationship was first observed in patients with ataxia-telangiectasia. A subsequent investigation in patients without this disease but with IgA deficiency has not supported this explanation for IgA-deficient patients at large.[40]

Transport

The evidence regarding selective transport of IgA from serum into secretions can be summarized by stating that there is no good evidence in healthy man that this transport occurs.[45] Studies with radiolabelled secretory IgA infused into the circulation also support the concept that circulating secretory IgA is not selectively transported into secretions. However some evidence does exist for selective transport of serum type IgA into some secretions, particularly of the nasal and gastrointestinal tracts, but in these cases the IgA appears to be transported as the serum type molecule, and is not found in the mucosal secretions in the characteristic secretory IgA form.

The implication of these data for therapy of such conditions as immune deficiency states is that gammaglobulin, whether parenterally injected or given in the form of plasma infusions, is unlikely to arrive in any appreciable quantity at the appropriate mucosal site. In addition, most gammaglobulin preparations contain less than 5 per cent IgA, and although plasma infusions have been reported to benefit some of these patients, it has never clearly been shown to be due to the presence of IgA. However, in those conditions in which active inflammation has destroyed the integrity of the mucous membranes, it is quite possible for administered gammaglobulin to potentially arrive at the source of inflammation.

From the therapeutic point of view, trials of gammaglobulin preparations with high IgA content are now under way in centers in Europe, and the possibility exists that passive immunization with secretory IgA antibody preparations by mouth or by aerosol might be a practical possibility in the future.

Allergy

The antibody responsible in the main for this type of clinical manifestation has been referred to earlier as IgE. It is well recognized that the efficacy of desensitization procedures is due to the stimulation primarily of IgG (blocking antibodies) in the serum. Clinical allergists have known for a long time, however, that the success of desensitization procedures is not always correlated with serum levels of blocking antibody. More recently it has become clear, since most IgE antibodies are in fact synthesized at local sites in the target organs (such as nasal and respiratory tract mucosae), that local blocking antibodies may indeed be formed locally and thus there may be an explanation for the lack of good correlation between serum antibody and clinical relief.

Turk et al.[49] have shown recently that in fact most of the blocking antibody in nasal secretions is of the secretory IgA class, so that it might be possible to enhance blocking antibody activity locally by suitable manipulation of the allergen and use of the local immune system to produce the blocking antibody. These types of trials are currently under way in several centers and it is not yet clear what the outcome of this speculative approach will be.

GENERAL COMMENTS

From what has been said above, it is clear that those situations in which local immunity is desired at the mucous membrane level, local presentation of antigen is generally the best method of attaining this end. This concept and the scientific basis for it have in fact revolutionized the whole approach to immunization practice. Indeed successful immunization can practically be achieved by nose drops and oral vaccines without the many attendant problems of parenteral immunization. In some instances the application of these principles has out-paced the experimental evidence upon which they are based. In others, such as with the atypical measles presentations which have occurred in great incidence following the use of parenteral killed virus vaccines, and which may in large part have been due to the relative inefficiency of this type of vaccination to produce protective local antibody (see p. 353), forethought and regard for this question of mucosal antibody might well have prevented this type of problem.

That the secretory immunoglobulin system might indeed be regarded as a first line of defence[22] is very strongly suggested by the evidence of Butler et al.[50] who have clearly demonstrated that nasal secretion IgA is high in the incubation period of viral infection, suggesting the release of preformed secretory IgA even before clinical symptoms begin and certainly before stimulation of local IgA antibody production occurs. In fact the latter appeared only to occur as the clinical illness was subsiding. In addition, at the time that rhinorrhea occurred, transudation of antibody from serum, both IgA and IgG, took place. At the time that local IgA synthesis was stimulated, local IgG antibody was blocked. These important observations would tie in the role of local and serum antibodies in their known cooperative action in resistance to viral disease.

Sources of local antibody in the nasopharynx are the tonsils and adenoids. Removal of these lymphoid organs has been known for more than 30 years to be associated with predisposition to poliomyelitis. Only recently has evidence been brought forward that patients in whom tonsils and adenoids have been removed have reduced or absent antibody activity against polio in the nasopharynx following operation.[32]

Lastly, the role of mucosal immunity in resistance to or enhancement of the growth of tumors occurring in the mucous membranes remains to be explored and promises to be at least one more fertile area for future investigation.

REFERENCES

1. Adinolfi, M., Glynn, A. A., Lindsay, M., et al.: Serological properties of IgA antibodies to Escherichia coli present in human colostrum. Immunol., *10*:517, 1966.
2. Ammann, A. J., and Hong, R.: Selective IgA deficiency and autoimmunity. Clin. Exper. Immunol., 7:833, 1970.
3. Ammann, A. J., Cain, W. A., Ishizaka, K., et al.: Immunoglobulin E deficiency in ataxia-telangiectasia. New Eng. J. Med., *281*:469, 1969.
4. Basredka, A.: Local Immunization. Baltimore, Williams and Wilkins Co., 1927.
5. Bienenstock, J.: The significance of secretory immunoglobulins. Canad. Med. Assoc. J., *103*:39, 1970.

6. Bienenstock, J., and Dolezel, J.: Peyer's patches: Lack of specific antibody-containing cells after oral and parenteral immunization. J. Immunol., *106*:938, 1971.
7. Burrows, W., and Havens, I.: Studies of immunity of Asiatic cholera. V. The absorption of immune globulin from the bowel and its excretion in the urine, and feces of experimental animals and human volunteers. J. Infect. Dis., 82:231, 1948.
8. Butler, W. T., Waldmann, T. A., Rossen, R. D., et al.: Changes in IgA and IgG concentrations in nasal secretions prior to the appearance of antibody during viral respiratory infection in man. J. Immunol., *105*:584, 1970.
9. Chase, M. W.: Inhibition of experimental drug allergy by prior feeding of the sensitizing agent. Proc. Soc. Exper. Biol. Med., *61*:257, 1946.
10. Collins-Williams, C., and Bienenstock, J.: Immunoglobulin A. *In* Speer, F., Dockhorn, R. J., and Shira, J. E., eds.: Allergy and Immunology in Children. In Press.
11. Cooper, G. N., Thonard, J. C., Crosby, R. L., et al.: Development of IgM memory in rats after antigenic stimulation of Peyer's patches. J. Reticuloendothel. Soc., 6:419, 1969.
12. Crabbé, P. A., Bazin, H., Eyssen, H., et al.: The normal microbial flora as a major stimulus for proliferation of plasma cells synthesizing IgA in the gut: The germ-free intestinal tract. Int. Arch. Allerg., 34:362, 1968.
13. Crabbé, P. A., Carbonara, A. O., and Heremans, J. F.: The normal human intestinal mucosa as a major source of plasma cells containing gamma-A-immunoglobulin. Lab. Invest., *14*:235, 1965.
14. Craig, S. W., and Cebra, J. J.: Peyer's patches: an enriched source of precursors for IgA-producing immunocytes in the rabbit. J. Exper. Med., *134*:188, 1971.
15. Davies, A.: An investigation into the serological properties of dysentery stools. Lancet, 2:1009, 1922.
16. Dayton, D. H., Small, P. A., Chanock, R. M., et al.: The Secretory Immunologic System. U.S. Department of Health, Education and Welfare Public Health Service and National Institutes of Health, Washington, D.C., 1971.
17. Fazekas de St. Groth, S.: Influenza: A study in mice. Lancet, *1*:1101, 1950.
18. Fernald, G. W., Clyde, W. A., and Bienenstock, J.: Distribution of immunoglobulin-containing cells in lungs of hamsters experimentally infected with Mycoplasma Pneumoniae. Submitted for publication.
19. Fey, H.: Immunology of the newborn calf: Its relationship to colisepticemia. Ann. N.Y. Acad. Sci., *176*:49, 1971.
20. Fudenberg, H., Good, R. A., Goodman, H. C., et al.: Primary immunodeficiencies: Report of a W.H.O. committee. Pediatrics, 47:927, 1971.
21. Gewurz, H., Shin, H.S., and Mergenhagen, S. E.: Interactions of the complement system with endotoxic lipopolysaccharide: Consumption of each of the six terminal components. J. Exper. Med., *128*:1049, 1968.
22. Good, R. A., and Fisher, D. W.: Immunobiology. Stamford, Conn., Sinauer Associates Inc. 1971.
23. Hanaoka, M., Nomoto, K., and Waksman, B. H.: Appendix and γM-antibody formation I. Immune response and tolerance to bovine γ globulin in Irradiated, appendix-shielded rabbits. J. Immunol., *104*:616, 1970.
24. Heremans, J. F.: Immunoglobulin formation and function in different tissues. Curr. Topics Microbiol. Immunol., *45*:131, 1968.
25. Huntley, C. C., Robbins, J. B., Lyerly, A. D., et al.: Antibodies to ruminant serum and milk proteins in humans with IgA deficiency. New Eng. J. Med., *284*:7, 1971.
26. Isacson, P.: Myxoviruses and autoimmunity. Progr. Allergy, *10*:256, 1967.
27. Ishizaka, K.: Human reaginic antibodies. Ann. Rev. Med., *21*:187, 1970.
28. Johansson, S. G. O., Mellbin, T., and Vahlquist, B. Immunological levels in Ethiopian preschool children with special reference to high concentrations of immunoglobulin E (IgND). Lancet, *1*:1118, 1968.
29. Kraft, S. C., and Kirsner, J. B.: Immunological apparatus of the gut and inflammatory bowel disease. Gastroenterology, *60*:922, 1971.
30. Lowney, E. D.: Tolerance of a contact sensitizer in man. Lancet, *1*:1377, 1968.
31. Mitchell, J. C.: Hardening in allergic contact dermatitis and immunologic tolerance. Trans. St. John's Hosp. Dermat. Soc., 55:141, 1969.
32. Ogra, P. L.: Effect of tonsillectomy and adenoidectomy on nasopharyngeal antibody response to poliovirus. New Eng. J. Med., *284*:59, 1971.
33. Ogra, P. L., and Karzon, D. T.: Poliovirus antibody response in serum and nasal secretions following intranasal inoculation with inactivated poliovaccine. J. Immunol., *102*:15, 1969.
34. Ogra, P. L., Karzon, D. T., Righthand, F., et al.: Immunoglobulin response in serum and secretions after immunization with live and inactivated poliovaccine and natural infection. New Eng. J. Med., 279:893, 1968.
35. Perey, D. Y. E., Frommel, D., Hong, R., et al.: The mammalian homologue of the avian bursa of Fabricius. II. Extirpation lethal x-irradiation and reconstitution in rabbits. Lab. Invest., 22:212, 1970.

36. Pierce, A. E.: Specific antibodies at mucous surfaces. Vet. Rev. Annot., 5:17, 1959.
37. Rabinovitch, M.: Phagocytosis: The engulfment stage. Seminars Hematol., 5:134, 1968.
38. Rothberg, R. M.: Immunoglobulin and specific antibody synthesis during the first weeks of life of premature infants. J. Pediat., 75:391, 1969.
39. Rothberg, R. M., and Farr, R. S.: Anti-bovine serum albumin and anti-alpha lactalbumin in the serum of children and adults. Pediatrics, 35:571, 1965.
40. Schwartz, D. P., and Buckley, R. H.: Serum IgE concentrations and skin reactivity to anti-IgE antibody in IgA-deficient patients. New Eng. J. Med., 284:513, 1971.
41. Spiegelberg, H. L., and Müller-Eberhard, H. J.: Proceedings of first International Congress of Immunology, Washington, 1971. Academic Press. To be published.
42. Springer, G. F., and Horton, R. E.: Blood group isoantibody stimulation in man by feeding blood group-active bacteria. J. Clin. Invest., 48:1280, 1969.
43. Straus, E. K.: Sperm immobilization in the human vagina by induced mucoantibody. Fert. Steril., 16:346, 1965.
44. Thomson, D., Thomson, R., and Morrison, J. T.: Oral vaccines and immunization by other unusual routes. Edinburgh, Livingstone Ltd., 1948.
45. Tomasi, T. B.: Structure and function of mucosal antibodies. Ann. Rev. Med., 21:281, 1970.
46. Tomasi, T. B., and Bienenstock, J.: In Kunkel, H. G., and Dixon, F. J., eds: Advances in Immunology. New York, Academic Press, 1968, vol. 9, p. 1.
47. Tourville, D. R., Adler, R. H., Bienenstock, J., and Tomasi, T. B.: The human secretory immunoglobulin system: immunohistological localization of gamma A, secretory "piece," and lactoferrin in normal human tissues. J. Exper. Med., 129:411, 1969.
48. Turk, A., Lichtenstein, L. M., and Norman, P. S.: Nasal secretory antibody to inhalant allergens in allergic and non-allergic patients. Immunol., 19:85, 1970.
49. Waldman, R. H., Cruz, J. M., and Rowe, D. S.: Immunoglobulin levels and antibody to *candida albicans* in human cervicovaginal secretions. Submitted for publication.
50. Waldman, R. H., and Henney, C. S.: Cell-mediated immunity and antibody responses in the respiratory tract after local and systemic immunization. J. Exper. Med., 134:482, 1971.
51. White, R. G.: Functional recognition of immunologically competent cells by means of the fluorescent antibody technique. *In* The immunologically competent cell: Its nature and origin. CIBA Foundation Study Group No. 16 p. 6 (G. E. W. Wolstenholme and J. Knight eds.) Churchill, London, 1963.

Department of Medicine
McMaster University
Hamilton, Ontario
Canada

HL-A Antigens in Clinical Transplantation

J. A. Falk, B.Sc.,* and R. E. Falk, M.D., F.R.C.S.(C)**

Graft rejection, owing to the recognition of foreign transplantation antigens by the recipient, is a major problem in clinical tissue transplantation. An understanding of the mechanisms of graft rejection is required to insure successful organ transplantation. It should be possible, however, to prevent or reduce graft rejection by selecting donor-recipient combinations matched as closely as possible for transplantation antigens.

Two major antigenic systems have been demonstrated to be transplantation antigens in man; the ABO system[17, 22] and the HL-A system[3, 18, 28] (i.e. Human Leukocyte-Locus A). In this review we will discuss the HL-A system of antigens which, while first detected on leukocytes, appear to be represented on the cell membranes of most body tissues.[59, 113]

HL-A ANTIGENS

Definition

Transplantation or histocompatibility antigens are the genetically determined antigens on cell membranes which may, after transplantation, induce an immune response in the host, resulting in rejection of the graft. The magnitude of this response is in part determined by the degree of incompatibility between the donor and the recipient. Since transplantation antigens differ between nonidentical members of the same species, they constitute an alloantigenic system.

The HL-A system is probably the major histocompatibility system in man and is comparable to the H-2 system in the mouse, the Ag B system in the rat, the B system in the chicken, the DL-A system in the dog, the H-I system in the rabbit. Many of our concepts of the HL-A system have been extrapolated from animal studies, in particular the mouse.[91, 92]

From the Department of Surgery and Institute of Immunology, University of Toronto, Toronto, Canada

*Director, Tissue Typing Laboratory, Toronto Western Hospital
**Assistant Professor, Department of Surgery, University of Toronto; Staff Surgeon, Toronto General Hospital

403

History

Antibodies to human leukocytes were first described by Doan[29] in 1928, but the present extensive studies stem from the work of Dausset[20] in 1954 who reported leukoagglutinating antibodies in 90 per cent of patients who had received multiple transfusions. In 1958 Payne and Rolfs[76] and Van Rood et al.[108] reported the presence of antibodies to leukocytes in the sera of multiparous women. The antibodies formed during pregnancy are directed against paternal histocompatibility antigens present in the foetus.

The first description of a leukocyte antigen was made by Dausset[21] in 1958 and was based on a study of sera from polytransfused patients. Seven of the sera showed a similar pattern of agglutination on testing against a panel of leukocyte donors. The sera did not agglutinate the leukocytes of the antibody producer or of the other 6 patients in the group. Dausset concluded that the antibodies were allospecific and the patients lacked the same antigen which he designated "Mac" (now HL-A 2). The identification of an extensive number of antigens of this polymorphic system has proceeded rapidly and is continuing.

The antigens of the HL-A system appear to be divided into two major groups. In 1962 Van Rood[109] described the "4" series, and in 1964, Payne and Bodmer[77] reported a second, the "La" series. The concept of two series of transplantation antigens determined by two closely associated sites on a single chromosome was proposed on the basis of population and family studies[16, 23, 111] and was presented at the Histocompatibility Workshop in Torino in 1967. This hypothesis has since been sustained by studies in several laboratories.[24, 55, 86, 104] Antigens not confined to one of the two segregant series of the mouse H-2 system have recently been reported. Similar "public" or intermediate antigens may also exist within the HL-A system.[93, 106]

The nomenclature of this antigenic system was initially confusing since each laboratory used different designations for similar antisera. A Nomenclature Committee was established in 1967 under the auspices of the World Health Organization. Antigens which the committee agrees to be reproducibly detected are accepted and designated by an "A" number: e.g., A1, A2, A3. Antigens not as yet accepted are assigned a workshop number: e.g., W5, W18 (see Table 1).

Genetic Concept

The HL-A system consists of at least two segregant series of antigens; the First (or "La") Series and the Second (or "4") Series (see Table 1). These HL-A antigens, which are expressed on the cell membranes, are determined by the inherited genetic information stored at a single region of a chromosome, the HL-A region. This is a complex region with at least two sites on each chromosome as shown in Figure 1. The genetic information at one site determines an antigen of the first series and at the other an antigen of the second series. There is codominance in the expression of the genetic information at the sites of both chromosomes. Therefore, an individual will have four antigens, two of the first series and two of the second series.[26, 50, 59]

Table 1. *HL-A Antigens*

FIRST SERIES		SECOND SERIES	
Antigen	Frequency* (%)	Antigen	Frequency (%)
A1	25.4	A5	9.8
A2	45.9	A7	27.0
A3	29.5	A8	16.4
A9	22.9	A12	26.2
A10	11.5	A13	5.7
A11	13.1	W5	20.5
W19	22.1	W10	10.7
W28	5.0	W27	3.3
		W15	7.0

"A" numbers designate acceptance of antigen by WHO nomenclature committee
"W" numbers refer to fourth Histocompatability Workshop
*Antigen frequency in 122 "disease-free" individuals in Toronto area

These four expressed antigens are defined as the antigen profile or phenotype. They are detectable by serologic methods. If fewer than four are detected the individual may have an as yet unidentified antigen or may have the same antigen expressed twice (i.e., an antigen may be homozygous).

The inherited information present on a single chromosome is a haplotype. It consists of two determinants, one of each series. The genotype of an individual represents two haplotypes, one inherited from each parent, and must be deduced from family studies. It is only possible to detect homozygosity of an antigen if the genotype is ascertained.

The inheritance of haplotypes is shown in Figure 2. The genotype of one parent, "AB," consists of the haplotypes "A" and "B." The genotype of the second parent is represented by "CD." The possible offspring combinations (i.e., genotypes) are thus: AC, AD, BC, and BD. Siblings will have a 1:4 or 25 per cent probability of identity with each other.

Identification

Current methods of histocompatibility testing include the serologic identification and matching of donor-recipient transplantation antigens and the reaction between donor and recipient lymphocytes in tissue culture.

The serologic methods rely on identification of HL-A antigens by an-

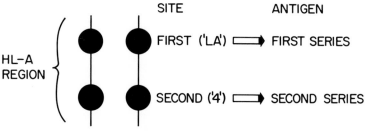

Figure 1.

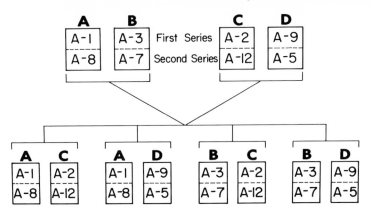

Figure 2.   Mode of inheritance of genetic information determining HL-A antigen.

tisera of known specificity obtained from persons sensitized either during pregnancy or by planned immunization. Antisera must be induced in humans or closely related species, such as chimpanzees, as heteroantisera detecting individual antigenic differences have not yet been produced in other speices. These antisera, selected for "monospecificity", are then utilized to identify antigens on leukocytes purified from peripheral blood or from lymph nodes.

The serologic method routinely used is the microcytotoxicity test first described by Terasaki.[101] When living leukocytes are incubated in the presence of complement with antisera containing known cytotoxic antibodies, those cells which possess the corresponding antigen will be damaged. This antibody-antigen mediated disruption of the cell membrane is indicated by the inability of the membrane to exclude dye. The damaged cells will be stained and are readily identified by inverted miscroscopy.

The microcytotoxicity test has, for routine antigen identification, replaced the agglutination technique, as the former is more reproducible. However, the cytotoxic technique is not a quantitative assay for antigen. Therefore if fewer than four antigens are detected on the cells of an individual, one cannot measure whether one of the antigens is represented twice (i.e., is homozygous). Several investigators are now assessing and standardizing the complement-fixation technique to determine its merits as a quantitative assay capable of detecting homozygous antigens.[19, 98] In this test, the amount of complement fixed by the antigen-antibody reaction is measured using sensitized indicator cells. This method, utilizing platelet fragments as a source of antigen, offers the additional advantage of readily stored antigen for retrospective determinations.

Serologic methods rely on monospecific antibody for identification of leukocyte antigens. However, many sera have been shown to contain cross-reactive components,[24, 59, 97] which complicates interpretation of such data. The cross-reactivity is within each series of HL-A antigens and there are several cross-reactive groups in each series. It might be speculated that these groups of antigens share structural components against which the cross-reacting antibodies are formed,[10] or that there is a quantitative variation in the antigenic determinants.[4] Serologic data might then be explained by variations in the antigen rather than the antibody.

Table 1 lists antigens of this polymorphic system and their frequency in a Caucasian population. Non Caucasian populations have a different distribution of antigen frequency.[13, 56, 59, 88] The number of identified antigens is rapidly increasing as new antigens are detected and as broad antigens are categorized into narrower cross-reactive components.[59] Even so, calculation of the gene frequencies indicates undetected antigens in both series of antigens. The extensive number of possible antigens decreases the likelihood of compatible matching in unrelated donor-recipient transplants. The probability of better matching would be increased if it were demonstrated that antigens which are nonidentical but crossreacting are less immunogenic or even compatible.

A functional method of determining the degree of histoincompatibility between two individuals is the mixed lymphocyte culture (MLC).[8] Lymphocytes, on initial exposure to nonidentical HL-A antigen(s),[6] respond by increased DNA synthesis and transformation into large blastoid cells. Thus, if incompatible cells are mixed in culture under appropriate conditions, the degree of their reactivity may be measured by the uptake of radioisotope. This is a "two-way" MLC, since each cell population may respond to the antigenic stimulus of the other by blastogenesis. To measure the response of the potential recipient's lymphocytes to the potential donor transplantation antigens, the donor cells are usually rendered unresponsive by irradiation or enzyme inhibitors. This is a "one-way" MLC[6] and should represent an in vitro test of the recipient's immunologic reactivity to incompatible donor transplantation antigens. Recent findings suggest that MLC reactivity is elicited by antigens of the second series or a genetic determinant(s) closely linked to this series. This suggests that antigens of the second series are of greater significance in histocompatibility than antigens of the first series.[29a]

Chemical Characteristics

Separation of HL-A antigens from the cell surface membrane and their subsequent purification and characterization may provide essential information which will clarify the genetic concepts and the biological significance of this antigenic system. Furthermore, the induction of specific tolerance or enhancement to donor antigen in clinical transplantation may require purified soluble antigen.

Substances containing HL-A antigenic determinants have been solubilized from crude membrane extracts of spleen cells or lymphoid cell lines by a variety of techniques such as sonication,[51] enzyme degradation (papain),[28, 66, 85] autolysis,[28] and, hypertonic KC1.[53] The released water-soluble antigenic material is purified by centrifugation, chromatography, and electrophoresis. The antigenic activity is determined by the ability of the soluble material (HL-A substance) to inhibit the lymphocytotoxic effect of well defined HL-A antisera.

The properties of the HL-A substance appear to vary depending on the technique used to solubilize. Most studies indicate a molecular weight of soluble HL-A antigen of 40,000 to 50,000, and a second smaller unit in the 14,000 range.[32] The soluble HL-A material is composed primarily of protein with varying carbohydrate content. Autolysis and enzyme digestion release glycoproteins with a carbohydrate content of 5 to

7 per cent but soluble material derived by other methods does not appear to contain carbohydrate. It is not yet established whether or not the antigenic activity is determined by the protein or the carbohydrate moiety. The reported variability of molecular weight and of carbohydrate content may reflect contamination of a small HL-A active unit or may indicate the necessity of a carrier molecule for transplantation antigen activity.

CLINICAL TRANSPLANTATION

Skin Graft Survival

The relevance of the HL-A antigens to transplantation was established by experimental skin transplants between ABO matched individuals. Exchange of first skin grafts between related individuals show an increased graft survival amongst the HL-A identical siblings as compared to non-HL-A identical siblings.[3, 18, 27] In unrelated donor-recipient combinations, skin grafts are rejected rapidly (9 to 13 days), and no correlation between the number of compatible antigens and survival time has been found.[105, 119] Skin grafts in all donor-recipient combinations including HL-A identical siblings, but not monozygotic twins, do reject eventually (usually by 20 to 30 days). One must then assume that minor transplantation antigens exist and have an effect, perhaps an additive one, on graft survival. This would simulate the mouse transplantation system which appears to include many minor antigen systems in addition to a major histocompatibility system.

Kidney Transplantation

DONOR SELECTION. Donors are matched with ABO-compatible recipients in accordance with the HL-A antigens identified. To avoid hyperacute rejection, a direct cross-match should be performed between serum from the recipient and cells from the donor to detect HL-A antibodies in the recipient active against antigen(s) in the donor. If the cross-match is positive, transplants in these high-risk patients are avoided. The presence in the recipient of circulating HL-A antibodies active against the donor antigens may result in an accelerated rejection of the transplanted kidney—usually within a few hours of the re-establishment of circulation.[54, 74] Humoral antibodies may be present in potential recipients as a result of sensitization by pregnancies, previous renal transplants, and transfusions. Recipients with preformed antibodies, even though not reactive with donor antigens, have a significantly poorer transplant outcome than those without detectable antibodies.

Many early failures (the first 6 month period) may be accounted for by grafts into such pre-immunized recipients.[103] As the level of circulating antibody may have fallen below detectable levels at the time of transplant,[75] an assessment of cell-mediated immunity may be required in pre-sensitized individuals.

The match grade is recorded as:

A match: HL-A identity
B match: All the HL-A antigens of the donor are present in the recipient. The recipient has antigens not present in the donor.

C match: The donor has one HL-A antigen not present in the recipient.
D match: The donor has two HL-A antigens not present in the recipient.
E match: The donor has three HL-A antigens not present in the recipient.
F match: The recipient has antibodies active against the donor's HL-A antigen(s).

The determination of the match grade is complicated when less than four antigens can be detected. The calculation of the net histocompatibility ratio (NHR) proposed by Rapaport and Dausset is based on the possibility of undetected antigens constituting an identity or an incompatibility.[80]

The polymorphism of the HL-A system makes it difficult to find closely matched recipients for donor kidneys. The probability of finding an unrelated donor and recipient with identical HL-A phenotypes is less than 1 in 1000 for most individuals, and less for rare phenotypes. The number of recipients available to find a good match for a donor kidney must obviously be large. To create a large pool of recipients, organ-exchange programs have been formed: Eurotransplant,[114] France-Transplant,[81] Scandiatransplant,[57] and the London and Regional Transplant Groups (L.T.G.).[84] These programs have proved successful in improving the proportion of well to poor matched transplants.[38] Collaboration on a wider scale involving exchanges between all the above centres has been established.

Kidney Transplant Survival.   A correlation between the compatibility of the HL-A antigens of donor and recipient and the clinical results of human kidney transplantation was shown as early as 1965 by Terasaki and his co-workers.[115] This was a significant contribution in view of the incomplete information about and the limited identification of transplantation antigens at that time. An early observation, that as the number of matched HL-A antigens increases the chance for a good clinical result also increases, has been confirmed in a number of subsequent reports on the basis of a progressively increasing amount of data.[9, 25, 38, 48, 58, 71, 73, 78, 112] The correlation is better with related than with unrelated (cadaveric) donors. The survival of kidney transplantation in HL-A identical siblings is superior to parental-sibling or non HL-A identical siblings transplants. All are superior to cadaveric transplants.[69] Results from the transplant registry (in 1971) show a one year kidney survival of 52, 77 and 79 per cent in grafts from cadaver, parental, and sibling donors, respectively.[72]

A statistically significant correlation of HL-A typing with the clinical outcome of kidney transplantation in related donors has been documented by many investigators.[25, 48, 78, 87, 102, 110] In a recent report[60] the increased graft survival in the HL-A-matched cases compared to that in the HL-A-mismatched cases of related donor-recipient transplants was highly significant with a $p < 0.0002$. These observations confirm that HL-A antigens are important transplantation antigens. The 1 year survival of kidney transplants was 88.3 per cent in a group of nominally HL-A identical siblings (i.e., identical, with two or more antigens identified) in the North American series typed and reported by Terasaki and co-workers.[69] This series was restricted to the transplants done since January 1, 1967, in which a total of 11 antigens could be identified as compared to 5 or 8 antigens in earlier studies. These results in related kid-

Table 2. *Correlation Between HL-A Typing and Clinical*
Results of Kidney Transplants in Unrelated Donors

CLINICAL RANK	KREISLER ET AL. (1970)		KISSMEYER-NIELSEN ET AL. (1970c)		
	ABC	DF	I+II+III	IV	
Match C	159	87	246	49	9	58
D	110	72	182	13	15	28
	269	159	428	62	24	86

$$x^2 = 0.619 \qquad x^2 = 11.77$$
$$\text{not significant} \qquad p < 0.001$$

ney transplants coincide with the correlation found in skin graft survival between related pairs and confirm the relevance of the HL-A antigen system to transplantation.

Many studies find a significant correlation between HL-A typing and the clinical result of kidney transplants in unrelated (cadaveric) donors. This has been reported in 104 cases by Patel et al.,[73] in 52 cases by Batchelor and Joysey,[9] in 62 cases by Morris and Ting,[71] in 143 cases by Kissmeyer-Nielsen et al.,[58] and in 162 cases by Festenstein et al.[38] In the series reported by Kissmeyer-Nielsen, by Batchelor, and by Morris a significant difference was found in the clinical results between C (one non-identity) and D (two non-identities) matches. Terasaki and co-workers[60, 69] found no significant difference in the clinical outcome between C and D matches. Table 2 shows the clinical significance between C and D matches in the Scandinavian material ($p<0.001$)[58] as contrasted to the lack of significance in the American material.[60] The recently published data of the London and Regional Transplant Groups is shown in Table 3.[38] The cadaveric renal transplants were done in the period March 1969 to December 1970. Recipients and donors were typed with sera defining a total of 21 antigens. In these unrelated donor-recipient transplants 85 per cent having three or four antigens identical were functioning at the time of analysis as compared with 57 per cent of those having two or less antigens identical ($p<0.005$). Thus even in cadaveric kidney transplants, HL-A antigens are clinically important and the results are significantly better when donor and recipient are well-matched.

It must be emphasized, however, that all reports show that many

Table 3. *Transplant Survival (Excluding P.N.F.) in*
Relation to HL-A Matching

GROUPS	NO. OF CASES	FAILED	SURVIVAL
4 and 3 (good match)	41	6	85*
2a and 2b (poor match)	87	37	57

*$p < 0.005$

renal transplants do well despite HL-A incompatibility. The graft survival may be attributed to the effectiveness of immunosuppressive therapy. It could also be explained by variation in the immunologic responsiveness of each recipient, by difference in antigenic strength of incompatible donor-recipient combinations, or by induction of immunologic enhancement or tolerance resulting in graft protection. The delineation of the role of these factors in renal transplantation will be facilitated if the variation in donor-recipient incompatibility is controlled by identification of the HL-A antigens.

ASSESSMENT OF TRANSPLANTATION IMMUNITY

Sensitization to transplantation antigens probably occurs in all transplanted patients, except in a monozygotic twin. Many patients with renal allografts undergo one or more clinical rejection episodes of varying severity even if no HL-A incompatibility is detected. It is necessary to develop a consistent and specific technique for monitoring and characterizing the immune response during allograft rejection. Three in vitro methods utilized to detect sensitization to transplantation antigens will be discussed.

Cytotoxicity of Sensitized Lymphocytes

Sensitized lymphocytes are of fundamental importance in graft rejection. It has been shown in both in vivo and in vitro experimental models that lymphoid cells, in the absence of specific humoral antibody, can destroy target cells, indicating the fundamental importance of sensitized lymphocytes in graft rejection.[2, 46, 68, 90, 118] It is possible to assess by tissue culture techniques the cytotoxic activity of lymphocytes without the interference of humoral antibody and heat labile complement factors. Lymphocytes from specifically immunized animals aggregate to the target cells and kill them within 24 to 48 hours.[14, 40-42, 70, 82, 116, 117] It was recently reported that lymphocytes from persons sensitized to HL-A antigens by skin grafting have a cytotoxic effect on fibroblast monolayers derived from the skin of the sensitizing donors. The killing phenomena was exerted according to HL-A specificity.[64] Studies by the same investigator indicate that measurable cytotoxicity by lymphocytes was observed infrequently in patients with renal allografts.[63] The time period required for the killing phenomena in this system is from 4 to 7 days. This limits the usefulness as related to the clinical transplant situation. A similar cytotoxic effect has been demonstrated with lymphocytes from human beings with autoimmune diseases.[12, 45, 79, 107]

Spontaneous Transformation

This method measures the number of transformed or "blast" cells present in the peripheral blood during a graft rejection crisis. The technique of cell culture is a modification of that described by Bach and Hirschorn.[5] The results suggest that an increased rate of transformation of peripheral blood lymphocytes appears early in the course of rejection. This may reflect the response of the recipient's immunocompetent cells to the presence of the graft tissue.[47, 100] This method has been modified for the use of micro quantities of blood and for a 3 hour culture system.[44] Further studies are required to provide definitive evidence regarding the possibility of false positives due to infection or nonimmunologic tissue injury.

Leukocyte Migration

Several techniques utilizing the migration of human leukocytes derived from peripheral blood have been described. The inhibition of the migration of sensitized cells from capillary tubes in the presence of the specific antigen is considered indicative of a cell-mediated immune response.[34, 36, 83, 94-96] Falk et al. reported that this technique could be utilized to detect immunologically specific reactions to HL-A antigens in individuals sensitized by skin grafting.[35] Other investigators have reported monitoring liver and renal allograft rejection utilizing tissue and leukocyte antigens with a capillary migration technique.[30, 31]

Recently we have modified the technique and utilized the whole leukocyte population derived from the peripheral blood, measuring the degree of reaction to an antigen within 4 hours after initiation of the culture. Good correlation between results obtained at 4 hours plus 20 hours has been observed in response to a variety of different antigens.[37, 65] Subsequently, we have studied 25 patients who have received a renal allograft, prior to transplantation and every third day afterwards. The source of the HL-A antigens utilized has been either lymphocytes obtained from the living donor of the allograft or from a donor who carried HL-A antigens similar to those of the cadaveric donor. More recently we have utilized the spleen of the cadaveric kidney donor harvested at the time of the transplantation. A single cell suspension is prepared from the spleen and maintained at $-70°$ C for subsequent use.

An altered cellular reactivity observed as an inhibition of cell migration has been noted in all cases during a rejection episode. In certain cases the technique was predictive, giving a positive response up to 72 hours prior to elevation of the serum creatinine levels. Following control of the rejection episode, the inhibition of migration to HL-A antigens in pooled human sera was reversed in autologous serum. Inhibition of migration to other antigens, such as tuberculin, to which the transplant patient was sensitized, was maintained in both pooled human sera and autologous serum.

Similar results have been noted by other investigators.[89] While this technique appears to hold promise for detecting cellular immunity in renal allografted patients further studies are required to clearly delineate the phenomena of enhancement and the type of response detectable in patients with chronic rejection.

Biologic Significance of HL-A Antigen

No direct evidence is available at present to define the biologic function of histocompatibility antigens. It is possible that their antigenicity is irrelevant to their function, and this is noted, incidentally, through immunologic methods.

HL-A antigens could be regarded as normal markers to distinguish self from nonself. Thus, if one considers the concept of surveillance, the deletion or alteration of these antigens occurring in abnormal cells would distinguish them from normal cells and allow for their elimination.[46]

Recently, Jerne has advanced a hypothesis[49] which suggests that the function of histocompatibility antigens is the generation of diversity of immunocompetent cells, assuming the clonal selection theory of immunity.[15] In addition, his hypothesis would utilize transplantation antigens as the means of evolving self tolerance. According to Jerne's hypothesis, antibody diversity is the result of somatic mutation during early ontogeny of those cells producing antibodies against the organism's own transplantation antigens. The viable mutants develop into new clones of cells which express antibody molecules of diverse specificities. Nonmutant clones of cells, capable of producing antibodies against histocompatibility antigens which the organism does not possess, will persist.

An association of certain HL-A antigens with neoplastic diseases, e.g., Hodgkin's disease,[1, 33, 39, 121] acute childhood leukemia,[120] and autoimmune diseases, such as disseminated lupus erythematosus,[43] has been reported. In the mouse, the ability to develop humoral[67] and cellular[7] immunity to certain antigens and the resistance or susceptibility to leukemia-inducing viruses are associated with the H-2 system. This association of immune responsiveness with histocompatibility antigens may reflect the range of diversity developed as proposed by Jerne or the presence of a gene influencing immune responsiveness close to or within the histocompatibility chromosomal region.

None of these studies or hypotheses identifies the exact purpose of histocompatibility antigens. This remains to be established through extensive studies involving geneticists, biochemists, immunologists, and clinicians.

REFERENCES

1. Amiel, J. L.: Study of the leukocyte phenotypes in Hodgkin's disease. Histocompatibility Testing, Copenhagen, Munksgaard, 1967. pp. 79–81.
2. Amos, D. B.: The use of simplified systems as an aid to the interpretation of mechanisms of graft rejection. Progr. Allergy, 6:468, 1962.
3. Amos, D. B., Seigler, H. F., Southworth, J. G., and Ward, F. E.: Skin graft rejection between subjects genotyped for HL-A. Transplant. Proc., 1:342–346, 1969.
4. Amos, B., and Yunis, E.: Human leukocyte antigenic specificity HL-A3: frequency of occurrence. Science, 165:300–302, 1969.
5. Bach, F. H., and Hirschhorn, K.: The in vitro response of peripheral blood lymphocytes. Sem. Hematol., 2:68, 1965.
6. Bach, F. H., and Voynow, N. K.: One-way stimulation in mixed leukocyte cultures. Science, 153:545–547, 1966.
7. Bailey, D. W., and Hoste, J.: A gene governing the female immune response to the male antigen in mice. Transplantation, 11:404–407, 1971.
8. Bain, B., Vas, M., and Lowenstein, L.: The development of large immature mononuclear cells in mixed leukocyte cultures. Blood, 23:108, 1964.
9. Batchelor, J. R., and Joysey, V.: Influence of HL-A incompatibility on cadaveric renal transplantation. Lancet, 1:790–793, 1969.
10. Batchelor, J. R., and Sanderson, A. R.: Implications of cross-reactivity in the HL-A system. Transplant. Proc., 2:133–143, 1969.
11. Batchelor, J. R., and Selwood, N. H.: HL-A subloci: are they valid? Histocompatibility Testing, 1970. Copenhagen, Munksgaard.
12. Berg, O., and Källen, B.: Effect of mononuclear blood cells from multiple sclerosis patients on neuroglia in tissue culture. J. Neuropath. Exper. Neurol., 23:550, 1964.
13. Bodmer, J. G., and Bodmer, W. F.: Studies on African Pygmies. IV. A comparative study of the HL-A polymorphism in the Babinga Pygmies and other African and Caucasian populations. Ann. J. Hum. Genet., 22:396–411, 1970.

14. Brondz, B. D.: Interaction of immune lymphocytes in vitro with normal and neoplastic tissue cells. Folia Biol. (Praha), 10:164, 1964.
15. Burnet, F. M.: Clonal Selection Theory of Immunity. Nashville, Tennessee, Vanderbilt and Cambridge University Presses, 1959.
16. Ceppellini, R., Curtoni, E. S., Mattiuz, P. L., Miggiano, V., Scudeller, G., and Serra, A.: Genetics of leukocyte antigens. A family study of segregation of linkage. Histocompatibility Testing, 1967. Copenhagen, Munksgaard, pp. 149–185.
17. Ceppellini, R., Bigliani, S., Curtoni, E. S., and Leigheb, G.: Experimental allotransplantation in man. II. The role of A1, A2 and B antigens. Transplant. Proc., 1:390–394, 1969.
18. Cepellini, R., Mattiuz, P. L., Scudeller, G., and Visetti, M.: Experimental allotransplantation in man. 1. The role of the HL-A system in different genetic combinations. Transplant. Proc., 1:385–389, 1969.
19. D'Amaro, J., Van Leeuwen, A., Van Rood, J. J., and Sevjgaard, A.: The microcomplement-fixation test. II. Serological and comparative studies. Histocompatibility Testing, 1970. Copenhagen, Munksgaard, pp. 539–542.
20. Dausset, J.: Leuco-agglutinins. IV. Leuco-agglutinins and blood transfusion. Vox Sang (Basel), 4:190–198, 1954.
21. Dausset, J.: Iso-leuco-anticorps. Acta Haemat. (Basel), 20:156–166, 1958.
22. Dausset, J., and Rapaport, F.: The role of ABO erythrocyte groups in human histocompatibility reactions. Nature, 209:209–211, 1966.
23. Dausset, J., Ivanyi, P., Colombani, J., Feingold, N., and Legrand, L.: The Hu-1 system. Histocompatibility Testing, 1967. Copenhagen, Munksgaard, pp. 189–201.
24. Dausset, J., Rapapport, F. T., and Legrand, L.: Choice of donors by tissue groups of the Hu-1 system. In Dausset, J., Hamburger, J., and Mathe, G., eds.: Advances in Transplantation. Copenhagen, Munksgaard, 1968, p. 749.
26. Dausset, J., Colombani, J., Legrand, L., and Fellous, M.: Genetics of the HL-A system. Population and family studies. Deduction of 480 haplotypes. Histocompatibility Testing, 1970. Copenhagen, Munksgaard, pp. 53–75.
27. Dausset, J., Rapaport, F. T., Legrand, L., Colombani, J., and Marcelli-Barge, A.: Skin allograft survival in 238 human subjects. Role of specific relationships at the four gene sites of the first and second HL-A loci. Histocompatibility Testing, 1970. Copenhagen, Munksgaard, pp. 381–397.
28. Davies, D. A. L., Manstone, A. J., Viza, D. C., Colombani, J., and Dausset, J.: Human transplantation antigens: the HL-A (Hu-1) system and its homology with the mouse H-2 system. Transplantation, 6:571–586, 1968.
29. Doan, C. A.: The recognition of a biologic differentiation in the white blood cells with a special reference to blood transfusion. J.A.M.A., 86:1593, 1926.
29a. Dupont, B., Staub Nielsen, L., and Svejgaard, A.: Relative importance of Four and LA loci in determining mixed lymphocyte reaction. The Lancet, 2:1336–1340, 1971.
30. Eddleston, A. L., Williams, R., and Calne, R. Y.: Cellular immune response during rejection of a liver transplant in man. Nature, 222:674, 1969.
31. Eddleston, A. L. W. F., Smith, M. G. M., Mitchell, C. G., and Williams, R.: Application of the leukocyte migration test to the diagnosis of rejection after liver transplantation. Transplantation, 12:11–17, 1971.
32. Etheredge, E. E., and Najarian, J. S.: Solubilization of human histocompatibility substances. Transplant. Proc., 3:224–226, 1971.
33. Falk, J. A., and Osaba, D.: HL-A antigens and survival in Hodgkin's disease. Lancet, 2:118, 1971.
34. Falk, R. E., Collste, L., and Möller, G.: In vitro detection of transplantation immunity: The inhibition of migration of immune spleen cells and peripheral blood leukocytes by specific antigens. Immunol., 104:1287, 1970.
35. Falk, R. E., Thorsby, E., Möller, E., and Möller, G.: In vitro assay of cell-mediated immunity: The inhibition of migration of sensitized human lymphocytes by HL-A antigens. Clin. Exper. Immunol., 6:445–455, 1970.
36. Falk, R. E., and Zabriskie, J.: In Vitro Methods in Cell Mediated Immunity. Bloom, B. R., and Glad, P. R., eds., New York, Academic Press, 1971, p. 301.
37. Falk, R. E., Guttmann, R. D., Beaudoin, J. G., Morehouse, D. D., and Oh, J.: Leukocyte migration in vitro and its relationship to human renal allograft rejection and enhancement. In preparation.
38. Festenstein, H., Sachs, J. A., Oliver, R. T. D., Burke, J. M., Adams, E., Divver, W., and Hyams, A., Pegrum, G. D., Blafour, I. C., and Moorhead, J. F.: Multicentre collaboration in 162 tissue-typed renal transplants. Lancet, 2:225–228, 1971.
39. Forbes, J. F., and Morris, P. J.: Leukocyte antigens in Hodgkin's disease. Lancet, 2:849, 1970.
40. Govaerts, A. J.: Cellular antibodies in kidney homotransplantation. J. Immunol., 85:516, 1960.
41. Granger, G. A., and Weiser, R. S.: Homograft target cells. Specific destruction in vitro by contact interaction with immune macrophages. Science, 145:1427, 1964.

42. Granger, G. A., and Weiser, R. S.: Homograft target cells. Contact destruction in vitro by immune macrophages. Science, 151:977, 1966.

43. Grumet, F. C., Coukell, A., Bodmer, J. G., Bodmer, W. F., and McDevitt, H. D.: Histocompatibility (HL-A) antigens associated with systemic lupus erythematosus. New Eng. J. Med., 285:193, 1971.

44. Harris, J. E., Posen, G., and Stewart, T.: Immunologic detection of renal allograft rejection in man: Increased DNA synthesis by peripheral lymphoid cells. Transplantation, in press.

45. Hedberg, H., and Källen, B.: Studies on mononuclear cells obtained from synovial fluid of patients with different types of arthritis. Cytotoxic effect on tissue cultured human fibroblasts. Acta. Path. Microbiol. Scand., 62:177, 1964.

46. Hellström, K. E., and Möller, G.: Immunologic and immunogenetic aspects of tumor transplantation. Prog. Allergy, 9:158, 1965.

47. Hersh, E. M., Butler, W. T., Rossen, R. D., and Morgen, R. O.: Activated lymphocytes (AL): A rapid test to detect allograft rejection. Clin. Res., 18:425, 1970.

48. Hors, J., Feingold, N., Fradelizi, D., and Dausset, J.: Critical evaluation of histocompatibility in 179 renal transplants. Lancet, 1:609, 1971.

49. Jerne, N. K.: The somatic generation of immune recognition. Europ. J. Immunol., 1:71, 1971.

50. Joint report of the Fourth International Histocompatibility Workshop. Histocompatibility Testing, 1970. Copenhagen, Munksgaard, pp. 2–47.

51. Kahan, B. D., Reisfeld, R. A., Pellegrino, M., Curtoni, E. S., Mattiuz, P. L., and Ceppellini, R.: Water soluble human transplantation antigens. Proc. Nat. Acad. Sci., 61:896, 1968.

52. Kahan, B. D., and Reisfeld, R. A.: Transplantation antigens. Solubilized antigens provide chemical markers of biologic individuality. Science, 164:514–521, 1969.

53. Kahan, B. D., Pellegrini, M. A., Papermaster, B. W., and Reisfeld, R. A.: Quantitative serologic parameters of purified HL-A antigens. Transplant. Proc., 3:227–230, 1971.

54. Kissmeyer-Nielsen, F., Olsen, S., Petersen, V. P., and Fjeldborg, O.: Hyperacute rejection of kidney allografts, associated with pre-existing humoral antibodies against donor cells. Lancet, 2:662, 1966.

55. Kissmeyer-Nielsen, F., Svejgaard, A., and Hauge, M.: Genetics of the human HL-A transplantation system. Nature (Lond.), 219:1116–1119, 1969.

56. Kissmeyer-Nielsen, F., Andersen, H., Hauge, M., Kjerbye, K. E., Morgensen, B., and Svejgaard, A.: HL-A types in Danish Eskimos. Tissue Antigens, 3:10, 1971.

57. Kissmeyer-Nielsen, F., and Kjerbye, K. E.: Scandiatransplant. A visual matching system. Histocompatibility Testing, 1970. Copenhagen, Munksgaard, pp. 639–641.

58. Kissmeyer-Nielsen, F., Staub-Nielsen, L., Sandberg, L., Svejgaard, A., and Thorsby, E.: The HL-A system in relation to human transplantation. Histocompatibility Testing, 1970. Copenhagen, Munksgaard, pp. 105–135.

59. Kissmeyer-Nielsen, F., and Thorsby, E.: Human transplantation antigens. Transplantation Review, vol. 4, 1970. ed. Göran Möller, Copenhagen, Munksgaard.

60. Kreisler, M., Singal, D. P., Linscott, S., Mickey, M. R., and Terasaki, P. I.: Relative strength of individual HL-A antigens and haplotypes in 614 kidney transplants. Histocompatibility Testing, 1970. Copenhagen, Munksgaard.

61. Lengerova, A.: Immunogenetics of Tissue Transplantation. Amsterdam, North Holland Publishing Co., 1969.

62. Lilly, F.: The histocompatibility -2 locus and susceptibility to tumor induction. Nat. Cancer Inst. Monogr., 22:631, 1966.

63. Lundgren, G.: Docent thesis; On effector mechanisms in allograft rejection. Stockholm, Tryckeri Balder A. B., 1969.

64. Lundgren, G., Möller, E., and Thorsby, E.: In vitro cytotoxicity by human lymphocytes from individuals immunized against histocompatibility antigens. II. Relation to HL-A incompatibility between effector and target cells. Clin. Immunol., 6:671–680, 1970.

65. Magil, A., Hancock, D. J., Zabriski, J. B., Guttmann, R. D., and Falk, R. E.: A rapid method of assessment of cellular immunity with human blood leukocytes. Canad. Fed. Proc., June 1971.

66. Mann, D. L., Rogentine, G. N., Fahey, J. L., and Nathenson, S. G.: Human lymphocyte membrane (HL-A) alloantigens: Isolation, purification and properties. J. Immunol., 103:282–292, 1969.

67. McDevitt, H. O., and Benacerraf, B.: Genetic control of specific immune responses. Adv. Immunol., 11:31–74, 1969.

68. Medawar, P. B.: The immunology of transplantation. Harvey Lect., 52:144, 1958.

69. Mickey, M. R., Kreisler, M., Albert, E. D., Tanaka, N., Linscott, S., and Terasaki, P. I.: Analysis of HL-A incompatibility in human renal transplants. Tissue Antigens, 1:57, 1971.

70. Möller, E.: Antagonistic effects of humoral isoantibodies on the in vitro cytotoxicity of immune lymphoid cells. J. Exper. Med., 122:11, 1965.

71. Morris, P. J., and Ting, A.: Leukocyte antigens in renal transplantations 9. Matching for the HL-A system and the early course of cadaveric renal grafts. Med. J. Austr., 14:517–519, 1970.

72. Murray, J. E., Barnes, B. A., and Atkinson, J. C.: Eighth report of the human kidney transplant registry. Transplantation, 11:328–337, 1971.
73. Patel, R., Mickey, M. R., and Terasaki, P. I.: Serotyping for homotransplantation. XVI. Analysis of Kidney transplants from unrelated donors. New Eng. J. Med., 279:501, 1968.
74. Patel, R., and Terasaki, P. I.: Significance of the positive cross match test in kidney transplantation. New Eng. J. Med., 280:735, 1969.
75. Patel, R., and Briggs, W. A. Limitation of the lymphocyte cytotoxicity crossmatch test in recipients of kidney transplants having preformed antibodies. New Eng. J. Med., 282:1016, 1971.
76. Payne, R., and Rolfs, M. R.: Fetomaternal leukocyte incompatibility. J. Clin. Invest., 37:1756–1763, 1958.
77. Payne, R., Tripp, M., Weigle, J., Bodmer, W., and Bodmer, J. A new leukocyte isoantigen system in man. Cold Spr. Harb. Symp. Quant. Biol., 29:285–295, 1964.
78. Payne, R., Perkins, H. A., and Najarian, J. S.: The relation between the postoperative course of recipients of renal homografts and compatibility for defined leukocyte antigens. In Dausset, J., Hamburger, J., and Mathe, G., eds.: Advances in Transplantation. Copenhagen, Munksgaard, 1968.
79. Perlmann, P., and Broberger, O.: In vitro studies of ulcerative colitis. II. Cytotoxic action of white blood cells from patients on human fetal colon cells. J. Exper. Med., 117:717, 1963.
80. Rapaport, F. T., and Dausset, J.: Ranks of donor-recipient histocompatibility for human transplantation. Science, 167:1260–1262, 1970.
81. Reveillard, R. J., Leski, M., and Crosnier, J.: Indications et résultats de la transplantation renale. Presse méd., 78:795, 1970.
82. Rosenau, W., and Moon, H. D.: Lysis of homologous cells by sensitized lymphocytes in tissue culture. J. Nat. Cancer Inst., 27:471, 1961.
83. Rosenberg, S. A., and David, J. R.: In Vitro Methods in Cell Mediated Immunity. Bloom, B. R., and Glade, P. R., eds., New York, Academic Press. 1971, p. 297.
84. Sachs, J. A., Festenstein, H., Oliver, R. T., Blandy, J. P., Saloman, J. R., Balfour, I. C., Pegrum, G. D., Williams, G. B., Hopewell, J. P., Moorhead, J. F., Barnes, A. P., and Berwick, M.: International collaboration in renal transplantation. Lancet, 2:228–230, 1971.
85. Sanderson, A. R., and Batchelor, J. R. Transplantation antigens from human spleens. Nature (Lond.), 219:184, 1968.
86. Singal, D. P., Mickey, M. R., Mittal, K. K., and Terasaki, P. I.: Serotyping for homotransplantation. XVII: Preliminary studies of HL-A subunits and alleles. Transplantation, 6:904–912, 1968.
87. Singal, D. P., Mickey, M. R., Terasaki, P. I.: Serotyping for homotransplantation. XXIII. Analysis of kidney transplants from parental versus sibling donors. Transplantation, 7:246–258, 1969.
88. Singal, D. P., Mickey, M. R., and Terasaki, P. I.: Serotyping for homotransplantation, XXIX. Two new HL-A antigens. Transplantation, 8:235–240, 1969.
89. Smith, M. G. M., Eddleston, A. L., Dominiquez, J. A., Evans, D. B., Beweck, M., and Williams, R.: Changes in leukocyte migration after renal transplantation. Brit. Med. J., 4:275, 1969.
90. Snell, G. D.: The immunology of tissue transplantation. In Conceptual Advances in Immunology and Oncology. M. D. Anderson Hospital Symposium, Houston, Texas, 1963.
91. Snell, G. D., and Stimpfling, J. H.: Genetics of tissue transplantation. In Green, E. L., ed.: Biology of the Laboratory Mouse. New York, McGraw-Hill, 2nd ed., 1966, p. 457–491.
92. Snell, G. D.: The H-2 locus of the mouse: observations and speculations concerning its comparative genetics and its polymorphism. Folia Biol. (Praha), 14:335–358, 1968.
93. Snell, G. D., Cherry, M., and Demant, P.: Evidence that the H-2 private specificities can be arranged in two mutually exclusive systems possibly homologous with the two subsystems of HL-A. Transp. Proc., in press.
94. Søborg, M.: In vitro detection of cellular hypersensitivity in man: specific migration inhibition of white blood cells from brucella positive persons. Acta. med. scand., 182:167, 1967.
95. Søborg, M., and Bendixen, G.: Human lymphocyte migration as a parameter of hypersensitivity. Acta. med. scand., 181:247, 1967.
96. Søborg, M.: In vitro migration of peripheral human leukocytes in cellular hypersensitivity. Acta. med. scand., 184:135, 1968.
97. Svejgaard, A., and Kissmeyer-Nielsen, F.: Cross-reactive human HL-A isoantibodies. Nature (Lond.), 219:868–869, 1968.
98. Svejgaard, A., and Kissmeyer-Nielsen, F.: Complement-fixing platelet isoantibodies. Vox Sang (Basel), 14:106–118, 1968.
99. Tennant, J. R., and Snell, G. D.: Some experimental evidence for the influence of genetic factors on viral leukemogenesis. Nat. Cancer Inst. Monogr., 22:61, 1966.

100. Tennebaum, J. I., St. Pierre, R. L., Vasko, J. S., and Cerilli, G. J.: Early detection of allograft rejection: in vitro lymphocyte transformation Vth Leukocyte Culture Conf. Ed. J. Harris, Academic Press, 1971.
101. Teraski, P. I., and McClelland, J. D.: Micro droplet assay of human serum cytoxins. Nature (Lond.), 204:998–1000, 1964.
102. Terasaki, P. I., Vrederoe, D. L., and Mickey, M. R.: Serotyping for homotransplantation. X. Survival of 196 grafted kidneys subsequent to typing. Transplantation, 5:1071, 1967.
103. Terasaki, P. I., Mickey, M. R., and Kreisler, M.: Presensitization and kidney transplant failures. Postgrad. Med. J., 47:89–100, 1971.
104. Thorsby, E.: HL-A antigens and genes. A study of unrelated Norwegians. Vox Sang (Basel), 17:81–92, 1969.
105. Thorsby, E., and Kissmeyer-Nielsen, F.: HL-A antigens and genes. III. Production of HL-A typing sera of desired specificity. Vox Sang (Basel), 17:102–111, 1969.
106. Thorsby, E.: A tentative new model for organization of the mouse H-2 histocompatibility system; two segregant series of antigens. Europ. J. Immunol., 1:1, 1971.
107. Trayanova, T. G., Sura, V. V., and Svet-Moldavsky, G. J.: Destruction of human cells in tissue culture by lymphocytes from patients with systemic lupus erythematosus. Lancet, 1:452, 1966.
108. Van Rood, J. J., Eernisse, J. G., and Van Leeuwen, A.: Leukocyte antibodies in sera from pregnant women. Nature (Lond.), 181:1735–1736, 1958.
109. Van Rood, J. J.: Leukocyte grouping. Thesis, Leiden, 1962.
110. Van Rood, J. J., Van Leeuwen, A., and Bruning, J. W.: The importance of leukocyte antigens in renal transplantation. J. Clin. Pathol., Suppl. 504, 1967.
111. Van Rood, J. J., Van Leeuwen, A., Schippers, A. M. J., Pearce, R., van Blankenstein, M., and Volkers, W.: Immunogenetics of the group four, five and nine systems. Histocompatibility Testing, 1967. Copenhagen, Munksgaard, pp. 203–218.
112. Van Rood, J. J., and Eernisse, J. G.: The detection of transplantation antigens in leukocytes. Seminars Haematol., 5:187–214, 1968.
113. Van Rood, J. J., Van Leeuwen, A., Schippers, A., and Balner, H.: Human histocompatibility antigens in normal and neoplastic tissues. Cancer Research, 28:1415–1421, 1968.
114. Van Rood, J. J., Freudenberg, J., Van Leeuwen, A., Schippers, A., Zweerus, R., and Terpstra, J. L.: Eurotransplant. Transp. Proc., 3:933, 1971.
115. Vredervo, D. L., Terasaki, P. I., Mickey, M. E., Glassock, R., Merrill, J. P., and Murray, J. E.: Serotyping of human lymphocyte antigens. III. Long term kidney homograft survivals. Histocompatibility Testing, 1965. Copenhagen, Munksgaard, pp. 25–35.
116. Wilson, D. B.: The reaction of immunologically activated lymphoid cells against homologous target cells in vitro. J. Cell Comp. Physiol., 62:273, 1963.
117. Wilson, D. B.: Quantitative studies on the behaviour of sensitized lymphocytes in vitro. I. Relationship of the degree of destruction of homologous target cells to the number of lymphocytes and to the time of contact in culture and consideration of the effects of isoimmune serum. J. Exper. Med., 122:143, 1965.
118. Winn, H. J.: The immune response and the homograft reaction. Nat. Cancer Inst. Monograph, 2:113, 1959.
119. Walford, R. L., Colombani, J., and Dausset, J. Retrospective leukocyte typing of unrelated human donor-recipient pairs in relation to skin allograft survival times. Transplantation, 7:188–193, 1969.
120. Walford, R. L., Finkelstein, S., Neerhout, R., Konrad, P., and Shanbrom, E.: Acute childhood leukemia in relation to the HL-A human transplantation genes. Nature, 225:461, 1970.
121. Zervas, J. D., Delamore, I. W., and Israels, M. C. G.: Leukocyte phenotype in Hodgkin's disease. Lancet, 2:634, 1970.

Department of Surgery
University of Toronto
Toronto, Ontario
Canada

The Clinical Application of Antilymphocyte Globulin

*Harold E. Taylor, M.D., F.R.C.P. (Can., Edin.)**

While a great deal is heard about antilymphocyte serum as an effective immunosuppressive agent, the evidence for this depends largely on the observations noted during animal experimentation. Its use in clinical medicine is still experimental, and much further information must be gathered by carefully controlled clinical trials, before its exact use as a therapeutic agent can be defined.

Antilymphocyte serum (ALS) is a cytotoxic heterologous antibody that reacts with and can destroy certain lymphoid cells. The active component of the antiserum is in the gamma globulin fraction. Because of this the crude serum is now fractionated by immunochemical methods to the IgG fraction or antilymphocyte globulin (ALG), before being used for immunosuppressive purposes.

ALS may be raised in a variety of species, e.g. horse, cow, goat, sheep, rabbit, by immunizing them with lymphoid cells from other species. It has been shown that human thymocytes, thoracic duct lymphocytes, and cultured human lymphoblasts are apparently the best antigens to produce the most effective anti-human ALS.

In this essay an attempt will be made to highlight certain facts that are applicable to the clinical use of ALG. The very extensive background of experimentation that has brought ALG to its present status has been well reviewed by Russell and Monaco,[35] James,[17] and more recently by Jeejeebhoy,[20] Sell,[38] and Najarian and Simmons.[31]

Tests for Immunosuppressive Effect of ALG

One of the problems in comparing results in different groups of patients who have been given ALG is the lack of a standard unit. This is due to the lack of a proven, precise method to measure and express the immunosuppressive capacity of different batches of ALG. As yet, there is no single in vitro test that has been proven to correlate directly with the im-

---

*Director, Antilymphocyte Serum Program and Personnel Support Programs, Medical Research Council; Professor, Department of Pathology, University of Ottawa, Ontario, Canada

munosuppressive action of a given antiserum in humans; e.g., the fact that an ALG has a high titer of lymphocytotoxic antibodies and will cause a significant lymphopenia when given in vivo does not necessarily prove that this ALG will be clinically immunosuppressive.

A number of different tests have been devised and investigated for this purpose. Of these, the best correlation at present exists between the effect of ALG in prolonging the survival of skin grafts in higher primates (certain species of monkeys and chimpanzees) and its likely immunosuppressive activity in humans.[5, 6] However, as yet one cannot be positive that evidence of immunosuppression in a monkey necessarily proves that the substance will be immunosuppressive in humans; the accumulating evidence suggests that this is likely true, but more cases are still needed to prove it beyond doubt.

Certain in vitro tests such as the Bach rosette inhibition,[4] lymphocyte transformation inhibition,[14] and opsonization tests[43] may eventually prove to be useful. The effect of an "active" ALG in inhibiting a graft vs. host reaction under the renal capsule of a rat also looks promising as an indication of its immunosuppressive activity in clinical conditions.[36] It has been shown that foreign lymphoid cells, when injected under the kidney capsule of a rat made immunodeficient by prior treatment with cyclophosphamide so that the foreign cells will not be rejected, will cause an intense local graft vs. host reaction in the cortex of the kidney, causing it to increase in weight. Prior treatment of the lymphoid cells to be injected, with an appropriate (as to species) ALS or ALG, will abrogate this graft vs. host reaction if the ALG is "active". There appears to be a significant correlation between this test and the immunosuppressive capacity of the same ALG to prolong the survival of skin grafts.

The effect of ALG in reversing a positive delayed type skin test in humans, e.g. against tuberculin, is also direct evidence of its capacity to abrogate a cell-mediated immune response.[48] We have seen a strongly positive tuberculin skin test become and stay negative for 4 months following the administration of 20 mg. ALG per kg. of body weight, daily, for 2 weeks.

Najarian et al.[32] have reported the prolonged survival of human skin allografts in patients with multiple sclerosis who were treated with anti-human lymphoblast ALG. They also showed a significant dose response: the median survival time of grafts in patients with three Terasaki histoincompatibilities was 15.8 days in patients given 4 mg. ALG per kg.; 17.0 days in those given 10 mg. per kg. and 20.8 days in those given 20 mg. per kg. We have also seen a skin graft survive for 28 days in a patient given 10 mg. ALG per kg. intravenously, daily for 7 days, as compared to the usual rejection at about 9 days.

All this is evidence that certain ALGs are indeed immunosuppressive in man. However, until a satisfactory standard is devised that can be applied to all ALGs, then it is difficult to decide on a satisfactory dose schedule. In fact, in many published papers it is quite impossible to know what dosage was used. For instance, it is meaningless for an author to state that he gave 1 or 5 ml. of ALS daily. One should at least state that so many mg. of immunoglobulin (ALG) were given per kg. of body weight.

The ALS to be used in the Canadian trial of ALG in renal allografts has been fractionated to IgG and then concentrated to 5 gm. protein per 100 ml., so that 1 ml. contains the equivalent of 50 mg. of ALG. It is intended to use as a trial dose, 10 or 20 mg. ALG per kg. of body weight given intravenously daily for 14 days after kidney transplantation.

Mode of Action of ALG

There is plenty of evidence that ALG can interfere with cell-mediated immune responses[26] which are important in the pathogenesis of allograft rejections, in the graft vs. host reaction, and in some forms of autoimmune disease. There is also evidence that it can interfere with the primary response in humoral antibody production. A variety of ideas concerned with the mechanism of action of ALS have been investigated over the past few years.[22] The evidence today which is most generally accepted supports the conclusion that ALS acts by selectively destroying lymphocytes of the recirculating pool, or as Mitchison[28] so aptly describes it: "it is simply the soldiers who stick their heads above the parapet who get shot."

Since ALS acts against those cells which play such a prominent part in graft rejection[45] and are incriminated in the pathogenesis of certain autoimmune disorders, it is logical to wish to try the effect of ALG therapy in these situations in clinical medicine. It must be remembered however, that there are certain important and potentially serious hazards associated with the administration of ALS or ALG, and it is thus most important to weigh the balance between these hazards and an expected beneficial therapeutic effect before giving ALG to any patient or group of patients.

Potential Hazards of ALG Therapy

The intramuscular administration of ALS or ALG usually causes severe pain and oedema at the site of injection; patients also frequently have pyrexia. In addition to these common reactions, there are certain potential hazards that must be recognized when administering ALG. These can be divided into two main groups: (1) complications directly related to ALG (presence of contaminating antibodies, sequelae to administration of a foreign protein); and (2) complications related to the state of immune depression (unusual infections, particularly viral and fungi, and oncogenesis).

CONTAMINATING ANTIBODIES. The antigen used to raise an ALS may be contaminated with erythrocytes, platelets or serum proteins, any of which may stimulate the formation of specific antibodies against them. Thus an ALS may contain antihuman hemolysins or hemagglutinins which could cause an anemia in the patient given such an ALS. Antibodies against human serum proteins could react with the serum proteins of the patient and form immune complexes that could cause serum sickness or anaphylactic reactions; while antibodies against platelets may cause a thrombocytopenia. Two of these contaminating antibodies can be absorbed with human erythrocytes and serum proteins during the production of an ALG,[44] however, sufficient antiplatelet antibodies may be present even after purification to cause a severe thrombocytopenia. Platelet counts may precipitously drop to 40,000 to 50,000 after 2 or 3 days of ALG therapy. In spite of this we have not as yet noted any bleeding in these patients. The platelet counts often show a return towards normal even while the ALG treatment is continued, and a rebound thrombocytosis is sometimes encountered when the treatment is stopped.

Another hazard we encountered in producing a large (100 liter) common pool of equine antihuman thymocyte ALG was the occurrence of an antibody in the ALG that had the capacity to react with a monkey's glomerular basement membranes, causing a fatal nephrotoxic nephritis. It was postulated that this glomerular basement membrane (GBM)-reactive antibody might have developed against contaminating basement membrane antigens (capillary basement membranes, reticulin, etc.) in the thymus homogenate used as antigen in the first phase of immunizing the horses.

This particular ALG was studied further by Wilson et al.[52] who showed that it could cause both immediate and delayed glomerular injury in monkeys following intravenous injection. In other studies, they demonstrated GBM-reactive antibodies in ALGs from 13 of 20 individual horses, and in 7 of 10 serum (ALS) pools from horses immunized with lymphocytes derived from solid lymphoid organs, e.g. spleen, thymus, lymph node, tonsils. They found no such antibodies in ALS prepared against thoracic duct lymphocytes or cultured lymphoblasts.

Recently a similar GBM-reactive antibody has been reported that bound to the glomeruli of human kidneys when given intravenously.[47] However, in only 1 of 11 patients did a glomerulonephritis develop and that was in the only patient who developed an autologous phase to the glomerular-bound equine globulin. On the other hand, 5 Rhesus monkeys given the same ALG showed immunohistochemical evidence of both the heterologous and autologous phases, and they all developed glomerulonephritis. It is possible that the concomitant use of other immunosuppressive drugs in humans may have masked or prevented the development of an active glomerulonephritis. In any case, it is felt that any ALG contaminated with GBM-reactive antibodies should not be used for clinical purposes.

Since the above experience, we have been able to produce an ALG free of such GBM-reactive antibodies, by using as antigen the membrane fraction of thymocytes[23] rather than homogenate of thymus gland and suspensions of whole thymocytes.

One of the important problems still to be mastered in the production of ALGs for clinical use, is to raise and purify one that contains only the (still to be identified) immunosuppressive antibody fraction. Considerable research time is now being expended on studying the use of various fractions of cellular antigens and methods of immuno-absorption, in the hope of developing such an ALG with precise immunosuppressive properties.

REACTIONS TO FOREIGN PROTEINS. The patient who is given ALG is in fact receiving horse or other heterologous species protein, and there is some evidence to suggest that ALG is more immunogenic than its normal IgG counterpart.[18] Antibodies may therefore develop against these proteins, and the well known reactions of serum sickness or anaphylaxis may occur during or subsequent to treatment. A not uncommon manifestation of serum sickness is the occurrence of giant urticaria. Sometimes severe anaphylactic reactions with hypotension and respiratory distress may be seen. Since many patients given ALG also receive steroids and other immunodepressants, e.g. azathioprine, these reactions are not as common as one might expect, and the occurrence of serum sickness nephritis in these patients is rarely encountered.

TOLERANCE TO ALG. Attempts have been made to induce tolerance to horse proteins in patients prior to giving them ALG.[30, 51] Some success has been claimed, particularly in animal experiments; however, there is as yet no assured method for use in man. This is of some importance since antibodies formed against the ALG (horse protein) can hasten its elimination and theoretically interfere with its immunosuppressive capacity.[11] For instance, Simmons et al.[40] have reported that the prolongation of skin grafts in patients given ALG is inversely related to the titer of antihorse globulin (antibodies to ALG) that develop in the recipient.

The induction of tolerance is possibly of greater importance if it is intended to use ALG for prolonged periods. It is in this situation that one is more liable to produce the amount of anti-ALG antibodies needed to form immune complexes, rather than in the short term administration of ALG for 10 to 14 days. Admittedly, even in the latter situation the patient is liable to become sensitized to the ALG, thus precluding its subsequent use.

INFECTIONS. The patient who has received immunosuppressive therapy, with or without ALG, is a candidate for infections, especially those caused by fungi and viruses. Thus unusual infections have to be considered as possible causes of various complications such as pneumonitis, in which Pneumocystis carinii or cytomegalovirus may be the etiologic agent, while more common infections, e.g. herpes simplex or herpes zoster, may be very troublesome.

Of particular importance is the occurrence of Australian antigen and serum hepatitis in immunosuppressed transplant patients who require multiple transfusions. Aronoff et al.[3] reported that 17 of 125 renal transplant patients at the Royal Victoria Hospital, Montreal, developed hepatitis. Immunologic tests for Australian antigen were positive in 11 of 14 patients with clinical evidence of liver disease and in 2 of 37 patients tested with no evident liver disorder. Huang[16] examined liver tissue from 6 of these patients with clinical hepatitis and Australian antigenemia. In 4 surgical biopsies and 1 necropsy,[1] characteristic virus-like particles were found in the nuclei and occasionally in the cytoplasm of hepatocytes.

While the positive identification of hepatitis-associated antigen (HAA) to these virus-like particles must still be established, the evidence is highly presumptive that this is so. Three of these 5 positive cases showed aggressive active chronic hepatitis, and two showed posthepatitic cirrhosis.

ONCOGENESIS. There is considerable evidence that ALS treatment has a tumour-enhancing effect. Thus methylcholanthrene-induced skin cancers occur earlier and have a greater lethal effect in ALG-treated mice. Similarly, certain virus induced tumours are potentiated by ALS.[24] This is particularly so with neoplasms of lymphoreticular tissues, e.g. certain strains of mice that normally resist the leukemogenic effects of the murine leukemia virus (MLV) may be made leukemic at a high frequency and short latent period, following only two injections of ALS. In other cases ALS administration induces the occurrence of reticulum cell sarcomas in the subcutaneous tissues of MLV infected mice. It has also been noted that the growth of transplantable tumours and some spontaneous tumours is enhanced by ALS treatment.

Penn et al.[33] have observed the occurrence of an unusual number of malignant tumours in organ transplant recipients. From their own experience they report the development of 11 de novo malignancies in 236 renal homograft recipients followed for 1½ to 8 years. An additional 29 examples have been collected from other institutions. In these 40 cases 23 of the tumours were of epithelial origin and 17 were mesenchymal; the majority of the latter were reticulum cell sarcomas. No single immunosuppressve agent can be specifically incriminated in this series, and it should be noted that only 8 of the patients who developed tumours received ALS or ALG.

The fact that tumor growth is enhanced in both immunosuppressed experimental animals and apparently in man, suggests that this effect of ALG may be through interference with the postulated immune surveillance that may be concerned with the "control" of some types of neoplastic disease. On the other hand, ALG may have some antibody-enhancing effect; or it may enhance the growth of oncogenic viruses yet to be identified as the cause of the human neoplasms. In any case it seems that ALS and ALG are important tools in neoplasia research and their extended use in that field may prove to be valuable.

THE USE OF ALG IN ORGAN TRANSPLANTS IN MAN

Kidney Transplantation

ALS and ALG have been used in many cases of kidney transplants during the past few years. However, it is very difficult to evaluate the results on any objective basis, since there are so many variables involved. These include different dose schedules, different routes of administration, different methods of producing and "standardizing" the ALS or ALG that has been used in different centers, and indeed the use of different lots of sera in treating a single patient.

It is for this reason that a large controlled clinical trial, with patients being allotted at random to the treatment and control groups, is being undertaken in some 10 Canadian University centers under the auspices of the Medical Research Council.[44] An anti-human equine ALG for this trial has been prepared at the Connaught Medical Research Laboratories, Toronto, using the membrane fraction of human thymocytes as antigen. A common pool of ALS was prepared by immunizing 9 horses. Sufficient absorbed ALG has been prepared from the common pool to treat some 100 recipients of cadaver kidney transplants. The logistics involved in handling and purifying the large quantities of sera involved were considerable and have taken some 2 years of concentrated experimentation to solve.

Starzl et al.[41] were one of the first groups to use ALG extensively in human transplantation. In 1970, they reported that about 140 recipients of kidneys, livers, or hearts had been given intramuscular ALG in combination with azathioprine and prednisone. In their experience the adjunct use of ALG was considered to be beneficial, and it was noted that the 1 year graft survival after intrafamilial renal transplantation rose to more than 90 per cent and after cadaveric renal transplantation to 83 per cent. At the recent First International Congress of Immunology, Penn stated that the 2 year survival figure for the former group was still 90 per cent and for the latter group, 75 per cent.

Monaco et al.[29] also noted a significant decrease in the number of observed acute rejection reactions in a preliminary report of 21 recipients of cadaveric renal allografts which were mis-matched at one or more HLA antigens. These patients were given equine anti-human lymph node ALG, (5 mg. per kg.) for either 21 days after transplantation or for 42 consecutive days, followed by a maintenance dose for 180 days. The preliminary analysis of this small group did not allow definite conclusions, but they were encouraged with the use of ALG and the extremely low incidence of rejection episodes. On the debit side they reported a high incidence of troublesome viral, protozoan, and fungal infections, with two patients dying of overwhelming fungal infection and one of a herpes-like viral infection.

Birtch et al.[8] report on a clinical trial in which 58 renal transplant patients were given an equine ALG prepared against human thoracic duct lymphocytes. Another 37 patients receiving transplants concomitantly were not given ALG. It is difficult to evaluate this series since different doses of ALG and different regimens were used in two groups, one of which received kidneys from relations, the other group from cadavers. However, it was concluded that a short early course of potent ALG reduced the number and severity of early rejection crises, without materially affecting the 1 year survival.

Traeger[48] and his group at Lyons have had experience with equine ALG prepared against human thymocytes or thoracic duct lymphocytes since 1966. They advocate the intravenous route, with a dose of 10 to 20 mg. per kg. daily. They believe it has been effective in lowering the number of rejection crises and also they have found it useful in treating acute and subacute rejection episodes. As yet they are unsure of the long-term effectiveness of ALG in prolonging the survival of kidney grafts.

Najarian and Simmons[31] are enthusiastic with the results they are obtaining with their ALG prepared in horses against cultured human lymphoblasts. They treat their patients intravenously for 2 weeks post transplantation, using a daily dose of 10, 20, or 30 mg. of ALG per kg. of body weight. On the basis of their results in 30 consecutive mismatched cadaver transplants, they now recommend the 30 mg. dose schedule. Table 1 summarizes their results in these 30 patients.

Table 1. *Effect of ALG in Cadaver Kidney Transplants*

	No ALG	4 mg. ALG	10–20 mg. ALG	30 mg. ALG
No. of patients	5	6	11	8
Graft rejection in:	4	4	1	0

The patients given 10 to 20 mg. have been observed 8 to 13 months, and those given 30 mg., 7 to 11 months.

At the Congress of Immunology, Najarian stated that he is convinced that treatment with antilymphoblast ALG is effective in markedly reducing rejection crises, and that his present experience with patients given 30 mg. of ALG per kg. shows an 18 month survival of cadaveric kidney grafts in excess of 90 per cent, which is about double the survival rate noted in his experience prior to the use of ALG. In this connection it is interesting to note that ALG did not apparently improve the 90 per cent 2 year functional survival that pertains to patients given kidneys from related donors.

One of the first controlled clinical trials has recently been reported by Sheil et al.[39] from Australia. They treated 54 cadaver kidney recipients with equine or goat ALG prepared against human thymic and lymph node lymphocytes; another 46 patients received no ALG. Both groups were given uniform treatment with standard immunosuppressive drugs. For the first 3 months of the trial, alternate patients were placed in one or other of the groups, but thereafter ALG-treated patients were selected in an attempt to restore balance to the trial with respect to a number of factors, such as degree of tissue compatibility between donors and recipients. Thus it is neither a double-blind nor a randomized trial in the true sense. Furthermore, the first 34 patients in the "treated" group were given intramuscularly, 0.75 mg. of equine ALG per kg. daily for the first 4 post transplant days and then on alternate days for an average of 7 weeks (the average total dose being 600 mg. IgG); the last 20 patients were given 3 mg. of goat ALG per kg. intravenously daily for 7 days and then on alternate days, until between 1.5 and 15 gm. of a 1.5 gm. per 100 ml. ALG solution had been administered. Thus in this trial there is a marked variation in dosage, route of administration, and type of ALG administered.

In spite of these variables, they report that ALG therapy was effective as judged by the following results. Graft function continues in 83 per cent of the ALG group and in 65 per cent of the controls at a mean time of 13 months for both groups. Graft failure for a variety of reasons occurred in 19 per cent of the ALG group and 41 per cent of controls; 9 per cent of the failures due to rejection were in the "treated" group, and 30 per cent in the control. Prolonged good function was achieved in 72 per cent of the ALG treated patients and in 52 per cent of the controls.

With regard to the low dose schedule adopted, they found it necessary to increase the ALG dose for treatment of the rejection episodes, and they state "if rejection episodes are to be avoided, increased routine dosage is required." They also noted that the goat ALG was largely free of side-effects, compared to their equine product which was thrombolytic and caused a thrombocytopenia in about half the patients on routine therapy, and in almost all when increased treatment was required for rejection.

The foregoing clinical experiences with kidney transplants from a number of centers certainly support the experimental evidence that ALG is actively immunosuppressive and seems to be effective as a therapeutic adjunct in cadaver kidney transplants. The evidence indicates that its use diminishes the number of acute and subacute rejection episodes in the early crucial 30 to 60 days after transplantation. Its effect on long-time survival of functioning grafts must await the future assessment of these groups of treated patients and the results of more carefully controlled and randomized clinical trials. One of the expected benefits will be a reduction in the steroid dosage needed to handle rejection crises as they occur.

A great deal has yet to be learned about the most effective dosage and mode of administration of ALG. The dose will of course depend upon the immunosuppressive characteristics of a given ALG, but with present day methods of production and fractionation a dose level of about 20 mg. IgG (ALG) per kg. of body weight, daily, is indicated. The evidence accumulating also suggests that about 14 days of post transplant treatment will probably produce as good a result as will a long-term maintenance dose schedule. Physicians are now using the intravenous rather than the intramuscular route. The latter almost invariably causes severe and extremely painful local reactions. The intravenous route (central catheter and continuous drip over a period of hours) is less immunogenic, it does not limit the amount of ALG that can be given at anytime, and it can be stopped immediately if allergic reactions occur.[31]

Heart Transplantation

There is less concrete information on the use of ALG in cardiac transplantation than that discussed above. At the Second World Symposium on Heart Transplantation in 1969, Barnard[7] reported the use of antilymphocyte globulin in 5 patients using doses of 5 to 10 ml. intravenously (mg. dose not given) every 12 hours for the first month, then once daily for the second month, and 3 times weekly during the third. However, he did not comment on its specific effectiveness, if any.

Stinson et al.[42] in describing their experiences with 14 heart transplant patients, noted that in 12 ALG was included in the immunosuppressive regimen. In all of these 14 patients, acute rejection episodes were treated one or more times, suggesting that the ALG was not effective in preventing them. Cooley,[12] reporting on 20 transplants, stated that ALG used in conjunction with azathioprine and corticosteroids had provided better control of rejection while allowing smaller doses of the other drugs; Grondin[15] also used ALG in his 9 patients but made no comment regarding its effect. Brendel[10] emphasized the use of high doses of high grade ALG, i.e., 20 ml. per day (again no mg. dose is given), and believed that the survival rate of patients so treated was higher. Lamoureux,[21] however, in attempting to analyze the effectiveness of ALS or ALG in 56 cases of heart transplantation, could reach no conclusion, because of the many variable factors involved.

The eventual outcome of these various cases is now well known and I believe that one can conclude that the use of the then available ALS or ALG did not have any significant effect on the eventual clinical outcome of a patient with a transplanted heart.

Bone Marrow Transplantation

There is accumulating evidence that ALG may be an important therapeutic adjunct in the immunologic manipulations required to abrogate or minimize the host vs. graft and potential graft vs. host reactions that are involved in marrow transplants. In spite of these immunological problems, there seems to be a resurgence of clinical interest in marrow transplantation as a means to correct immune deficient states, and possibly to treat certain hemopoietic disorders, such as aplastic anemia and acute leukemias.[50]

Theoretically it is possible to circumvent the immunologic problems of marrow transplantation by using donor recipients that are highly and mutually compatible, and it has been reported recently that antilymphocyte serum may be useful in conditioning man for a marrow graft.[27] Also, the use of cell separation methods may allow the selection of stem cells for the transplant, that are free from cells that cause the graft vs. host disease.[2]

ALG IN AUTOIMMUNE DISORDERS

Although the pathogenesis of most of the so-called autoimmune diseases is not completely understood, it is very probable that cell-mediated immune reactions are involved, if not in the initiation of these disorders, then possibly in their propagation to chronicity. Based on this assumption, it was natural that the effect of ALG on the pathogenesis of experimental models of autoimmune diseases would be investigated.

It has now been reported that ALG can suppress or modify the natural history and clinical manifestations of a number of such examples including adjuvant arthritis, allergic encephalomyelitis, thyroiditis and Coombs-positive hemolytic anemia in N.Z.B. mice. This evidence has been reviewed in detail by Denman,[13] who emphasizes that this effect of ALG is noted when it was administered before or soon after the disease was induced experimentally – a condition that would not be enjoyed by clinicians contemplating its use in human autoimmune diseases. Jasin and Ziff[19] also note that if experimental results in animals are to be considered in the light of possible use of ALS in human autoimmune disease, the pertinent results are those obtained with treatment at the time when the experimental disease was already established. The report of Leibowitz et al.[25] that ALS prolonged the survival of paralysed animals with allergic encephalomyelitis, and that the treatment was effective even after the onset of paralysis, has led to an interest in treating certain types of multiple sclerosis with ALG.

Multiple Sclerosis

Although the role of immune injury remains to be proven, the similarity (in some respects) of this incurable chronic human disorder to experimental allergic encephalomyelitis has led to the treatment of rapidly progressive acute relapsing cases with ALG. I am indebted to McPherson et al.[37] for preliminary results from a clinical trial that is being conducted at the University of Alberta, Edmonton. To date, they have treated 14 patients with ACTH and ALG and 12 controls with ACTH alone. They are giving ACTH, 40 I.U. per day, and equine anti-human thymocyte ALG, 20 mg. per kg. per day, intravenously for 14 days. The follow-up period is too short to allow an assessment of the effectiveness of ALG to induce a sustained remission; however, their preliminary objective data show fewer exacerbations in the test group than in those given ACTH alone. Based on their experience to date, they believe that it is worthwhile to use ALG as adjunct therapy in acute relapses of multiple sclerosis which do not respond to adequate doses of ACTH.

These results are similar to those reported by Brendel[9] of Munich, at the International Congress of Immunology. He has now treated 14 neurological conditions, of which 10 were cases of acute relapsing multiple sclerosis. Eleven of these patients have shown evidence of remissions. His regimen consists of an effort to induce tolerance by thoracic duct drainage and 10 mg. per kg. of de-aggregated normal IgG given intravenously, daily for 3 days, increased to 30 mg. per kg. daily for another 3 days and then 500 mg. of ALG per patient per day, using equine anti-human-thoracic-duct-lymphocyte ALG for varying periods of time, depending on the clinical results.

Miscellaneous Conditions

Brendel[9] also reported using ALG in 3 cases of dermatomyositis, 3 disseminated lupus erythematosus, 2 of temporal arteritis, and 2 of sympathetic ophthalmia. In some of these cases remissions occurred, and Brendel was convinced that the use of ALG was the turning point. Trepel et al.[49] also report improvement of symptoms in 2 patients with dermatomyositis and one with temporal arteritis when they were given 16 to 38 days' treatment with equine anti-human ALS.

Pirofsky et al.[34] have reported the use of goat anti-human, antilymphocyte and antithymocyte ALG to treat 2 patients with progressive lupus nephropathy and 1 patient with Goodpasture's syndrome, all of whom had been refractory to steroid and azathioprine therapy. Prompt remissions occurred in the latter and one of the former cases.

I believe that one must be very conservative when contemplating the use of ALG in human autoimmune diseases. One must not only consider the potential hazards of administering ALG for long periods of time, but one must also select cases in which it is probable that immune injury plays a significant pathogenetic role, and in which the patient is refractory to presently accepted therapeutic regimens. It does not seem reasonable, for instance, to use ALG to treat chronic rheumatoid arthritis or autoimmune thyroiditis at the present time. A great deal more must be learned about the possible beneficial effects of ALG in a disease already established to warrant its use for that purpose.

CONCLUSIONS

The evidence to date suggests that a potent anti-human ALG can be produced that is immunosuppressive in man. Such an ALG, when used as a therapeutic adjunct in cadaver kidney transplants, may diminish the number of acute and subacute rejection episodes in the immediate crucial weeks following transplantation, and it may allow a decrease in steroid therapy, which in itself would be important. Further follow-up studies and, in particular, carefully planned clinical trials are essential to define its exact role in such cases and to prove its effectiveness in the long-term survival of organ grafts. Since its administration poses a number of hazards, one must balance these against the anticipated results when making the decision to use ALG in a given clinical situation. As yet its use in autoimmune disease is very much in the experimental phase, and here again clinical trials are indicated.

A satisfactory method of isolating the precise immunosuppressive fraction, and that alone, from crude ALS must be found, as well as a proven method of standardizing the resulting ALG. Only then will it be possible to develop exact dose schedules for clinical use.

REFERENCES

1. Ahmed, M. N., Huang, S.-N., and Spence, L.: Australia antigen and hepatitis. An electron microscopic study. Arch. Path., 92:66, 1971.
2. Amato, D., Bergsagel, D. E., Clarysse, A. M., Cowan, D. H., Iscover, N. N., McCulloch, E. A., Miller, R. G., Phillips, R. A., Ragab, A. H., and Senn, J. S.: Review of bone marrow transplants at the Ontario Cancer Institute. Transplant. Proc., 3:397, 1971.
3. Aronoff, A., Huang, S.-N., Lal, S., Wu, K. T., Moinuddin, S. L., Spence, L., MacLean, L. D., and Gault, M. H.: Progressive hepatitis with Australia antigen following renal transplantation. To be published.
4. Bach, J.-F.: In vitro assay for antilymphocyte serum. Fed. Proc., 29:120, 1970.
5. Balner, H., Dersjant, H., Betel, I., and van Bekkum, D. W.: Current state of evaluating anti-human lymphocyte sera by "in vivo" testing. International Symposium on Antilymphocyte Serum. Symposia Series in Immunobiological Standardization, 16:179, 1970 (S. Karger, Basel).
6. Balner, H.: In vivo evaluation of antihuman lymphocyte sera. Fed. Proc., 29:117, 1970.
7. Barnard, C. N.: Experience at Cape Town with human to human heart transplantation. Heart Transplantation Second World Symposium. Les Presses de L'Université Laval, Quebec, Canada, 1969, p. 13.
8. Birtch, A. G., Carpenter, C. B., Tilney, N. L., Hampers, C. L., Hager, F. B., Levine, L., Wilson, R. E., and Murray, J. E.: Controlled clinical trial of antilymphocyte globulin in human renal allografts. Transplant. Proc., 3:762, 1971.
9. Brendel, W.: Communication at ALS Workshop. First International Congress of Immunology, Washington, D.C., August 1971.
10. Brendel, W.: Intravenous use of high dosage of ALG. Heart Transplantation Second World Symposium. Les Presses de L'Université Laval, Quebec, Canada, 1969, p. 149.
11. Butler, W. T., and Rossen, R. D.: Increasing effectiveness of antilymphocytic globulin by prevention of antibody formation to horse IgG. Transplant. Proc., 3:733, 1971.
12. Cooley, D. A., and Hallman, G. L.: Results of cardiac transplantation. Heart Transplantation Second World Symposium. Les Presses de L'Université Laval, Quebec, Canada, 1969, p. 24.
13. Denman, A. M.: Anti-lymphocytic antibody and autoimmune disease: A Review. Clin. Exper. Immunol., 5:217, 1969.
14. Eijsvoogel, V. P., van der Hart, M., du Bois, M. J. G. J., and van Loghem, J. J.: The specificity of antilymphocyte serum "in vitro" and its possible implications "in vivo." International Symposium on Antilymphocyte Serum. Symposia Series in Immunobiological Standardization, 16:291, 1970 (S. Karger, Basel).

15. Grondin, P., and Lepage, G.: Experience of the Montreal Heart Institute. Heart Transplantation Second World Symposium. Les Presses de L'Université Laval, Quebec, Canada, 1969, p. 39.
16. Huang, S.-N.: Hepatitis-associated antigen hepatitis. An electron microscopic study of virus-like particles in liver cell. Amer. J. Path., 64:483, 1971.
17. James, K.: Anti-lymphocytic antibody – A review. Clin. Exper. Immunol., 2:615, 1967.
18. James, K.: Effect of antilymphocytic antibody on humoral antibody formation. Fed. Proc., 29:160, 1970.
19. Jasin, H. E., and Ziff, M.: Influence of antilymphocyte serum on autoimmune processes. Fed. Proc., 29:177, 1970.
20. Jeejeebhoy, H. F.: Heterologous antilymphocyte serum: A Review. Canad. J. Surg., 14:5, 1971.
21. Lamoureux, G.: The use of ALG in 56 cases of heart transplantation. Heart Transplantation Second World Symposium. Les Presses de L'Université Laval, Quebec, Canada, 1969, p. 133.
22. Lance, E. M.: The nature and scope of action of ALS. University of London, Ph.D. thesis. 1968.
23. Lance, E. M., Ford, P., and Ruszkiewicz, M.: Use of subcellular lymphocyte fractions to raise antilymphocyte serum. Fed. Proc., 29:106, 1970.
24. Law, L. W.: Effects of antilymphocyte serum on the induction of neoplasms of lymphoreticular tissues. Fed. Proc., 29:171, 1970.
25. Leibowitz, S., Kennedy, L. A., and Lessof, M. H.: Antilymphocyte serum in the later stages of experimental allergic encephalomyelitis. Lancet, 1:569, 1968.
26. Levey, R. H.: Influences of antilymphocyte serum on cell-mediated and antibody-mediated responses. Fed. Proc., 29:156, 1970.
27. Mathé, G., Amiel, J. L., Schwarzenberg, L., Choay, J., Trolard, P., Schneider, M., Hayat, M., Schlumberger, J. R., and Jasmin, C.: Bone marrow graft in man after conditioning by antilymphocyte serum. Transplant. Proc., 3:325, 1971.
28. Mitchison, N. A.: Mechanism of action of antilymphocyte serum. Fed. Proc., 29:222, 1970.
29. Monaco, A. P., Lewis, E. J., Latzina, A., Hardy, M., Quint, J., Schlesinger, R., McDonough, E., Latham, W., Madoff, M., and Edsall, G.: Clinical use of equine anti-human lymph node lymphocyte serum: Preliminary results in twenty-one mis-matched cadaveric renal transplants. International Symposium on Antilymphocyte Serum. Symposia Series in Immunobiological Standardization 16:355, 1970 (S. Karger, Basel).
30. Najarian, J. S., Simmons, R. L., Gewurz, H., Moberg, A., Merkel, F., and Moore, G. E.: Antiserum to cultured human lymphoblasts: Preparation, purification and immunosuppressive properties in man. Ann. Surg., 170:617, 1969.
31. Najarian, J. S., and Simmons, R. L.: The clinical use of antilymphocyte globulin. New Eng. J. Med., 285:158, 1971.
32. Najarian, J. S., Simmons, R. L., Moberg, A. W., Gewurz, H., Soll, R., and Tallent, B.: Immunosuppressive assay of anti-lymphoblast globulin in man: Effect of dose, histocompatibility and serologic response to horse gammaglobulin. International Symposium on Antilymphocyte Serum. Symposia Series in Immunobiological Standardization, 16:199, 1970 (S. Karger, Basel).
33. Penn, I., Halgrimson, C. G., and Starzl, T. E.: De novo malignant tumors in organ transplant recipients. Transplant. Proc., 3:773, 1971.
34. Pirofsky, B., Bardana, E. J., Jr., Bayracki, C., and Porter, G. A.: Antilymphocyte Antisera in Immunologically Mediated Renal Disease. J.A.M.A., 210:1059, 1969.
35. Russell, P. S., and Monaco, A. P.: Heterologous antilymphocyte sera and some of their effects. Transplantation, 5:1086, 1967.
36. Saleh, W. S., Gordon, J., Lamoureux, G., and MacLean, L. D.: Test to measure immunosuppressive potency of antilymphocyte sera. Transplantation, 8:524, 1969.
37. Seland, T. P., McPherson, T. A., Blain, J. G., and Lamoureux, G.: Multiple sclerosis: Evaluation of anti-thymocyte globulin in acute relapses. A preliminary report. American Academy of Neurologists, New York, February 1971 (abstract).
38. Sell, S.: Antilymphocytic antibody: Effects in experimental animals and problems in human use. Ann. Intern. Med., 71:177, 1969.
39. Sheil, A. G. R., Kelly, G. E., Storey, B. G., May, J., Kalowski, S., Mears, D., Rogers, J. H., Johnson, J. R., Charlesworth, J., and Stewart, J. H.: Controlled clinical trial of antilymphocyte globulin in patients with renal allografts from cadaver donors. Lancet, 1:359, 1971.
40. Simmons, R. L., Moberg, A. W., Gewurz, H., Soll, R., Tallent, M. B., and Najarian, J. S.: Immunosuppressive assay of antilymphoblast globulin in man: Effect of dose, histocompatibility, and serologic response to horse gamma globulin. Surgery, 68:62, 1970.
41. Starzl, T. E., Penn, I., Brettschneider, L., Ono, K., and Kashiwagi, N.: Selected topics on antilymphocyte serum. Fed. Proc., 29:186, 1970.
42. Stinson, E. B., Schroeder, J. S., Harrison, D. C., Dong, E., Jr., Popp, R. L., and Shumway, N.

E.: Experience with cardiac transplantation in fourteen patients. Heart Transplantation Second World Symposium. Les Presses de L'Université Laval, Quebec, Canada, 1969, p. 19.

43. Svehag, S.-E., Manhem, L.: An "in vitro" opsonization test for evaluation of A fG preparations. International Symposium on Antilymphocyte Serum. Symposia Series in Immunobiological Standardization, *16*:307, 1970 (S. Karger, Basel).

44. Taylor, H. E.: Clinical trial of antilymphocyte serum. International Symposium on Antilymphocyte Serum. Symposia Series in Immunobiological Standardization, *16*:343, 1970 (S. Karger, Basel).

45. Taylor, H. E.: Pathology of Organ Transplantation in Man. Pathology Annual, Ed. Sheldon Sommers 1972 (in press) Appleton-Century-Crofts, New York.

46. Taylor, H. E.: The occurrence of glomerular basement membrane-reactive antibodies in antihuman antithymocyte globulin. Transplant Proc., 2:413, 1970.

47. Thiel, G., Moppert, J., Mahlich, J., Buhler, F., Vischer, T., Enderlin, F., Weber, H., and Zollinger, H. U.: Glomerular damage after intravenous administration of antilymphocyte globulin (ALG) in man and rhesus monkeys. Transplant. Proc., 3:741, 1971.

48. Traeger, J., Touraine, J. L., Fries, D., and Berthous, F.: Evaluation of intravenous route for administration of antilymphocyte globulins in humans. Transplant. Proc., 3:749, 1971.

49. Trepel, F., Pichlmayr, R., Kimura, J., Brendel, W., and Begemann, H.: Therapieversuche mit Antilymphocytenserum bei Autoaggressionskrankheiten des Menschen. Klin. Wschr., *15*:856, 1968.

50. van Bekkum, D. W.: Bone marrow transplantation. Transplantation Proc., 3:53, 1971.

51. Weksler, M. E., Bull, G., Schwartz, G. H., Stenzel, K. H., and Rubin, A. L.: Induction of tolerance to antilymphocyte globulin in man. Transplant. Proc., 3:754, 1971.

52. Wilson, C. B., Dixon, F. J., Fortner, J. G., and Cerilli, G. J.: Glomerular basement membrane reactive antibody in anti-lymphocyte globulin. J. Clin. Invest., *50*:1525, 1971.

Medical Research Council
Natural Research Bldg. M-58
Ottawa (KIA OR6) Canada

Human Bone Marrow Transplantation

R. A. Phillips, Ph.D., and D. H. Cowan, M.D., F.R.C.P.(C)***

Since the demonstration that transplanted bone marrow cells can repopulate the hemopoietic system of lethally irradiated animals,[32, 50, 64] there has been interest in applying the technique to the management of human bone marrow failure. Because early clinical attempts were unsuccessful,[15, 66] enthusiasm about transplantation of human bone marrow diminished. However, a number of recent major advances have led to a revival of interest. We shall review some of these advances and discuss the current status of bone marrow transplantation in man. We have limited our discussion to the three areas in which most of the recent work has occurred: aplastic anemias, acute leukemias, and congenital immunologic deficiencies. Rather than including all case reports, we have referred to those recent cases which demonstrate new approaches and advances. The clinical results were last reviewed in the *Medical Clinics* by Miller and Diamond in 1961.[66] Since then, there have been several reviews,[15, 20, 23, 77] the most comprehensive by Bortin[15] in 1969. To avoid repetition and to emphasize the recent procedural and conceptual advances, we have concentrated primarily on the work done since 1969.

PROBLEMS AND APPROACHES

The objective of bone marrow transplantation is to replace defective or missing host hemopoietic cells with functioning cells from a normal donor. In this cell renewal system, only the pluripotent stem cells in bone marrow have sufficient capacities for self-renewal, differentiation, and proliferation to reconstitute permanently the myeloid and lymphoid tissues of the recipient. In cellular terms, then, a bone marrow transplant is simply an attempt to graft stem cells.

The actual transplantation of bone marrow is a simple procedure.[93] The desired quantity of marrow is aspirated from a number (up to 150) of

*Associate Professor, Department of Medical Biophysics, University of Toronto; Division of Biological Research, Ontario Cancer Institute, Canada

**Assistant Professor, Department of Medicine, University of Toronto; Physician, Princess Margaret Hospital in The Ontario Cancer Institute, Canada

Research on bone marrow transplantation at the Ontario Cancer Institutes was supported by a grant from the Ontario Cancer Treatment and Research Foundation.

different sites in the sternum and iliac crest. The whole marrow or some fraction of it (see below) is given to the recipient by intravenous transfusion. A proportion of the stem cells in the graft then migrate to the bone marrow where they begin to produce differentiated progeny. As with transplantation of other tissues, the major problems come after the actual grafting. Three categories of problems are discussed: (1) immunologic problems, (2) maintenance of graft function, and (3) clinical problems of the recipient. For additional information the reader is referred to several extensive reviews.[51, 65, 77, 101]

Immunological Problems

With all allografts, a major barrier to success is the immunological response of the host lymphoid cells resulting in the graft rejection. In addition, when dealing with hemopoietic grafts, there is a unique problem. Suspensions of bone marrow cells, obtained from normal donors, contain large numbers of immunologically competent cells. Upon transplantation, these cells recognize the foreign transplantation antigens of the recipient and mount an immunological reaction against them.[35] This reaction results in a syndrome characterized by wasting, dermatitis, diarrhoea, liver dysfunction, susceptibility to certain infections and, paradoxically, failure of engrafted bone marrow.[101] The syndrome has been called secondary disease or graft-versus-host disease (GVHD). Although both rejection and GVHD are basically immunological problems, there are different approaches for dealing with each.

FACTORS INFLUENCING REJECTION.   Several factors affect the potential rejection of the graft by the recipient. The most important factor is the selection of the donor. The second factor is the type of immunosuppressive treatment given to the recipient. Finally, the degree to which the recipient has been presensitized to the donor's tissues will influence the risk of rejection.

Donor Selection.   The early experience with bone marrow grafts was similar to that with the transplantation of kidneys. Kidney grafts from identical twins functioned without difficulty, but the function of grafts from non-identical, sibling donors were unpredictable.[10] Some grafts survived for long periods, while others were rapidly rejected. With the advent of sophisticated methods of tissue typing, it became apparent in kidney transplantation that siblings whose transplantation and major blood group antigens were identical to those of the recipients made better donors than did siblings who were not identical.[84] Clearly, in animal systems, the degree of histoincompatibility between donor and recipient influences the rate of rejection.[36] Although extensive tests in bone marrow transplantation have not been carried out, the available data indicate that similar matching is important in the transplantation of this tissue. The longest survivors of marrow grafts have been in cases where histocompatibility typing showed identical transplantation antigens and identical major blood group antigens.[20]

Therefore, it is essential in any proposed transplantation of marrow to attempt to select a donor with a suitable tissue match, preferably a sibling. Two methods are commonly used to assess the compatibility of donor and recipient cells.[7] Using specific antisera, it is possible to identify approximately 90 per cent of the transplantation antigens (or human leukocyte antigens, HL-A) in the North American population (see page 337). With these sera, it is usually possible within a single family to determine which of the siblings have identical HL-A antigens. Since these antigens appear to be determined by a single genetic locus in man, there is a one-in-four chance that siblings will have identical HL-A antigens.

The other method commonly used in histocompatibility typing is the mixed leukocyte reaction.[1, 9] When peripheral blood lymphocytes from different individuals are placed in culture, they stimulate each other to proliferate. However, if cells from individuals with identical transplantation antigens are placed in culture no stimulation occurs. Thus, one can determine whether or not two individuals have identical tissue type by observing whether or not their cells stimulate the other's cells in culture.

Immunosuppression of the Recipient. Except in the case of truly identical twins, the presence of identical HL-A antigens on the donor and recipient cells does not prevent the rejection of the graft. For this reason, it is necessary to use immunosuppressive agents to prevent rejection of bone marrow allografts. The only exception, of course, is in immunologically deficient recipients who have lost the capacity to reject foreign tissue grafts.

Three agents are commonly used to suppress graft rejection: radiation, cyclophosphamide, and antilymphocyte globulin (ALG). Because radiation and cyclophosphamide also suppress bone marrow function, they must be given prior to transplantation. Total body irradiation is the oldest method of preparing recipients for marrow grafts. Doses in the range of 800 to 1000 rads provide sufficient immunosuppression to prevent rejection of the grafted bone marrow cells.[90] Doses in excess of 1500 rads cause severe gastrointestinal side-effects and must be avoided.[90]

A number of drugs are known to be powerful immunosuppressive agents. Of these, cyclophosphamide has been the most widely used agent in the preparation of recipients for bone marrow transplantation. Because Santos et al. have shown that cyclophosphamide is most effective as an immunosuppressive agent if given after an antigenic stimulus,[78] a unit of donor blood is usually given to the recipient one day before the drug to initiate a reaction of the recipient cells against those of the donor. Cyclophosphamide is then administered in a high dose (45 to 60 mg. per kg. of body weight) daily for 4 days.[77, 79] The half-life of this drug in the circulation is very short,[37] and the transplant is given 24 hours after the last dose. Successful engraftment has been obtained by several groups following this protocol.[2, 8, 38, 79] Because both x-rays and cyclophosphamide also kill leukemic cells,[19] these methods of immunosuppression have been most commonly applied in leukemic patients.

Another method of immunosuppression is the pretreatment of the recipient with ALG.[54] ALG has no antileukemic effect and is thus ineffective in controlling leukemia,[54] but because of its low toxicity, ALG is the agent of choice in conditions such as aplastic anemia. To achieve adequate immunosuppression, ALG is administered daily for 5 to 10 days before the transplant. Following this protocol, Mathé et al. have achieved several grafts in patients with aplastic anemia.[54]

Presensitization of Recipients. Patients who are potential recipients of bone marrow grafts have usually received multiple transfusions in the management of their disease. It has been suggested that immunization against transplantation antigens on leukocytes and platelets in the transfused blood may explain the subsequent failure of bone marrow grafts in some patients.[88] Certainly, in kidney transplantation, the presence of circulating antibodies against the donor antigens leads to immediate, acute rejection of the kidney.[46] In dogs, transfusion of the recipient with donor blood prior to transplantation increases the chance of rejection.[88] However, it is important to note that the presensitized dogs did not necessarily show cytotoxic antibodies in their serum. As a general rule, patients who are prospective transplant recipients should not receive blood transfusions from potential donors. In addition, prior to transplantation, the recipient's serum should be tested for the presence of antibodies cytotoxic to the cells of the donor. The presence of such antibodies will generally rule out possibility of a transplant.

FACTORS INFLUENCING THE DEVELOPMENT OF GRAFT-VERSUS-HOST DISEASE (GVHD). Factors that influence rejection of the marrow graft also tend to influence the development of GVHD. One of the most important factors in attempting to minimize the severity of GVHD is the selection of a suitably matched donor. In mice, GVHD is clearly determined by the degree of histoincompatibility between the donor and recipient.[99] In both animals and humans, the rapidity of skin graft rejection is markedly reduced in closely matched donors and recipients.[4, 36] It is reasonable to assume that the severity of other cellular immune reactions, such as GVHD, will be similarly influenced by the degree of histoincompatibility. However, lethal GVHD can occur in recipients of HL-A identical bone marrow,[2, 38, 79, 89] and other precautions must be used in conjunction with careful selection of the donor to prevent this complication. Three other methods are commonly used to decrease the severity of GVHD: drugs, specific antisera, and cell separation.

Drugs. Two cytotoxic drugs, methotrexate and cyclophosphamide, are useful in minimizing the complications of GVHD. The timing of the administration of these drugs is crucial; they must be given after the transplant but before the onset of the symptoms of GVHD, i.e., within the first 10 days after grafting. Once the symptoms of GVHD occur, therapy is ineffective.[68] Santos usually gives cyclophosphamide, 7.5 mg. per kg. of body weight, on days 1, 3, 5, 7, and 9 after transplantation,[77-79] while Thomas and his colleagues administer methotrexate in doses of 10 mg. per sq. meter of body surface area on days 1, 3, 6, and 11, and then weekly thereafter.[89, 91] Both of these procedures markedly reduce the severity of GVHD and, in some cases with HL-A identical donors and recipients, eliminate it entirely. When HL-A differences exist between the donor and recipient, drug therapy is less effective.[38, 79, 89]

Antisera. With experimental animals, pretreatment of donors with ALG reduces the incidence of GVHD.[102] Mathé has shown that the procedure is also effective in humans.[54] In 11 cases where both the donor and the recipient were pretreated with ALG before the bone marrow graft, he observed no GVHD. Surprisingly, in the same series, 5 recipients who were pretreated with ALG but received marrow from untreated donors also had no overt signs of GVHD. This latter result suggested that pretreatment of the recipient alone was sufficient to prevent the onset of GVHD.

In numerous model systems with animals, it has been demonstrated that cellular immune reactions, such as those responsible for GVHD, can be suppressed with specific antibody.[67, 87, 103] The enhancement of tumor growth by specific antitumor antibody[42, 67] is an example of this phenomenon. The administration of specific antisera to animals prevents immunologically competent cells from reacting against the tumor and allows the tumor to grow and kill the host. An obvious extension of this observation is to use enhancing antisera to prevent other cell-mediated immune responses, such as graft rejection and GVHD. In fact, Batchelor et al. have reported the successful use of antisera to enhance a human kidney graft.[11] In addition, Hellström et al. have observed enhancing factors in the serum of dogs given bone marrow grafts;[43] these factors suppress cell-mediated immune responses in tissue culture. More recently, similar serum blocking factors have been observed in immunologically deficient children successfully reconstituted with bone marrow transplants.[48] At present, the planned use of such factors offers perhaps the most promising approach for overcoming the problems of GVHD. The major attraction of this application of enhancing factors is their specificity; they prevent GVHD without suppressing other immune reactions.

Buckley and her colleagues have attempted to use specific antisera to prevent GVHD in recipients of HL-A incompatible bone marrow grafts. In three attempts, they report one partially successful reconstitution of a child with combined immunologic deficiency disease.[20, 21] In this instance, the mother had naturally occurring enhancing factors, presumably resulting from multiple pregnancies, and her serum was used to prevent the development of GVHD. Except for an eosinophilia, the child had no overt signs of GVHD. Unfortunately, attempts with other recipient-donor pairs to produce enhancing factors by planned immunizations have been unsuccessful.[20, 34] Hopefully, work currently in progress in several laboratories will lead to reliable methods for the production and use of enhancing factors in tissue transplantation.

Cell Separation. The objective in the transplantation of bone marrow is to graft stem cells. The problems associated with acute onset of GVHD are caused by the mature lymphocytes present in the aspirate of bone marrow.[29, 35, 72] It is obvious that the component of GVHD caused by the mature lymphoid cells could be eliminated if it were possible to separate the stem cells from the lymphocytes.

Experiments in animals and in humans have shown that the stem cells are larger[3, 72, 104] and less dense[29, 104] than the mature lymphoid cells that cause GVHD. Thus, physical procedures that separate cells either on the basis of size or density should yield suspensions of stem cells that are

relatively free of lymphoid contamination. Both types of separation procedures have been tested in animal systems and shown to be effective in
preventing GVHD.[29, 72] In humans the physical separation techniques are
still being tested. Dicke et al. have used the method of density separation
to prepare stem cells for transfusion into children with immune deficiency diseases.[26, 27] We have obtained stem cells by velocity sedimentation fractionation and transfused the large, rapidly sedimenting stem cell
fractions into both leukemic patients and children with immune deficiency diseases.[2] Both types of separation procedures appear to reduce
the severity of acute GVHD which is generally manifest within 2 weeks
after transplantation. However, delayed indications of GVHD, as indicated by moderate to severe skin rashes, have been observed in patients
that have received stem cells prepared by either method.[2, 26, 27, 34, 49]

There are two disadvantages to the use of cell separation techniques
in the prevention of GVHD. First, the techniques currently available are
cumbersome and difficult to use, especially when large numbers of bone
marrow cells are required. Second, even though it is possible to prepare
fractions of stem cells depleted of lymphocytes, after transplantation the
stem cells probably proliferate and differentiate to give additional lymphocytes, that are capable of reacting against the recipient's tissues.[48]
Thus, while separation is able to prevent the acute GVHD, it may have to
be combined with other methods of therapy to prevent the delayed type of
GVHD presumably associated with differentiation of stem cells.

Maintenance of Graft Function

The assessment and maintenance of graft function is a problem in
the transplantation of any organ or tissue. In bone marrow transplantation there are three discrete problems associated with the function of the
grafted tissue.

SIZE OF THE GRAFT.   Transplantation of bone marrow is unlike the
transplantation of whole organs in that the size of the graft can be variable. The required number of cells varies according to the type of patient
being grafted and the route by which the grafted bone marrow is given.
Children with some immune deficiency diseases cannot reject allografts
and do not require immunosuppressive treatments. In addition, their
need for a graft, at least in terms of myeloid function, is not as acute as in
other patients. For these reasons, small grafts, utilizing as few as 5×10^7
nucleated cells per kg. are commonly given to such recipients;[34, 49, 100] if
the donor cells are subjected to a separation procedure, even smaller
numbers of cells can be used.[29] The small graft has the added advantage
of minimizing the severity of GVHD.[34, 49] The situation is different in patients with bone marrow aplasia and leukemia. In addition to the pancytopenia induced by the x-ray or chemotherapy given in preparation for
the graft, these patients usually have severe deficiencies in normal
peripheral blood elements as a result of their disease. For these reasons
they have an acute need for rapid restoration of their myeloid and
lymphoid systems and require a large tissue graft, generally in excess of
4×10^8 nucleated cells per kg.[101] However, despite the administration of
these relatively large numbers of bone marrow cells, the peripheral

leukocyte and platelet counts do not increase until 13 to 21 days after transplantation (e.g., 52).

The route of administration of the bone marrow graft also affects the number of cells required for transplantation. More cells are required for engraftment by the intraperitoneal route than by the intravenous route, but the magnitude of the decreased efficiency of intraperitoneal injection is unclear. In mice, 50 times more cells are required if the cells are given intraperitoneally.[94] In monkeys the difference in efficiency of the intraperitoneal and intravenous routes is much less,[27] perhaps differing by only a factor of 2. However, because in adult patients one is usually working with relatively small numbers of cells, the most efficient method of administration should be used.

IDENTIFICATION OF THE GRAFTED TISSUE. Because the grafted cells become disseminated to many parts of the body, and are mixed with those of the recipient, it is often difficult to determine whether or not the cells observed in the peripheral blood or bone marrow belong to the donor or the recipient. Several kinds of markers are useful in attempting to distinguish between donor and recipient cells. If the donor and recipient are of different sex, karyotypic analysis of the dividing cells is a useful method for identifying donor cells. In cases where the donor and recipient are the same sex, minor antigenic differences between the donor and recipient are often used to distinguish the origin of cells. Minor blood group antigens are particularly good markers for the myeloid system (e.g., 55) while immunoglobulin allotypes can distinguish between donor and recipient lymphoid systems (e.g., 55). The disadvantage to using antigens to search for the presence of donor cells is the long time required before such cells are present in sufficient number to be detected by current techniques. Donor antigens are difficult to detect in the circulation prior to one month after transplantation. Donor karyotypes, however, can be detected in the bone marrow as early as 2 weeks after transplantation.[8]

MAINTENANCE OF GRAFT FUNCTION. With any tissue graft, a major problem is to maintain the function of the graft until it becomes permanently established. Bone marrow is not unique in this regard. A common experience is for the graft to function well for short periods of time and then to fail. The reasons for the graft failure are unclear. The high degree of immunosuppression used in conjunction with marrow grafts makes it unlikely that rejection is the cause of this failure, but this possibility has not been ruled out. It is also possible that unknown factors in the foreign environment have adverse effects on the function of the transplanted cells. There is evidence from studies on hemopoietic stem cells in animals that the environment in which the cells are growing can have marked effects on the function of the grafted cells, especially when there are histocompatibility differences between the donor and recipient.[25, 61] These host effects on the growth of transplanted stem cells are probably not related to immunologic reactions against the transplanted cells.[25, 61] As mentioned above, significant advances in bone marrow transplantation can be expected when it becomes possible to study quantitatively and precisely the influence of these environmental factors. At present, one can only hope that the graft is functioning well in its new environment.

Problems Associated with Maintenance of the Patient

Although the actual infusion of the bone marrow cells is a relatively simple procedure, the "postoperative" supportive care is no less complicated than that of the most major surgical or medical illness. A highly skilled team of medical, nursing, and paramedical personnel is mandatory. Aside from the general deterioration of metabolic, renal, pulmonary, cardiac, and hepatic functions that may be expected in severely ill patients, there are the specific problems associated with deficient hemopoietic functions that require special attention. All the complications of anemia, granulocytopenia, thrombocytopenia, and suppression of the immune system must be expected.

Anemia and thrombocytopenia can be managed with transfusions of red blood cells and platelets, respectively. Infection remains the most life-threatening complication.[85] Either as a result of the underlying disease or the use of immunosuppressive drugs, these patients suffer from the effects of profound granulocytopenia and immunologic depression. In addition, the occurrence of GVHD can further increase the risk of infection since one consequence of GVHD is lymphoid aplasia.[101] Therefore, the patients are at risk for both common bacterial pathogens and the less common, opportunistic bacterial, viral, fungal, and protozoal infections. Most transplantation groups utilize some form of protected environment in an attempt to reduce the occurrence of infection. Prompt diagnosis and treatment of infection with appropriate agents is of course mandatory. Transfusion of granulocytes may also be helpful.

It must be appreciated that transfusions of red cells, platelets or leukocytes all contain lymphoid cells in sufficient quantities to induce GVHD,[52] especially in patients with defective immune responses. Therefore, all transfusions given in the early post-transplantation period must be pretreated in some way to prevent the initiation of GVHD, which can be lethal.[39, 52] Irradiation of the transfused blood is probably the simplest procedure for inactivating potentially reactive lymphocytes. The exact dose required is not clear; doses from 1500 to 5000 rads have been recommended.[24, 39] Preliminary tests indicate doses much higher than these have little effect on the survival of platelets[40] or on the phagocytic function of macrophages.[70] Other pretreatments of transfused blood elements, such as incubating at 37°C. or freezing and thawing,[34, 49, 52] have been reported to destroy GVHD activity.

CLINICAL RESULTS

Bone marrow transplantation has potential applications in many diseases. For example, the problem of rejection of any organ graft could be eliminated if the recipient's lymphoid tissue were replaced with that of the donor by a concomitant bone marrow graft. Many genetic defects, such as sickle cell anemia and thalassemia, might be cured by transplantation of bone marrow from normal donors. More intensive therapy of disseminated malignant disease would be feasible if bone marrow transplantation could reliably protect patients from drug-induced bone marrow aplasia. However, at present, bone marrow transplantation is a high-risk, experimental procedure that is being tested in only a limited number of diseases. The three areas in which there is most information are discussed in detail below.

Acute Leukemia

Two aspects of bone marrow transplantation may be useful in the treatment of acute leukemia. First, therapists could give potentially curative doses of chemotherapeutic agents if the transplant could prevent the lethal complication of aplasia induced by the drugs.[18, 77] Second, transplanted bone marrow may react immunologically against the leukemic cells, thus providing another mechanism for elimination of the malignant cells. Although such immunologic reactions can cure leukemia in mice,[14] it has proven difficult in humans to manipulate graft-versus-host reactions to the benefit of the patients.[55] In fact, GVHD appears to be especially severe in leukemic recipients[45] and remains a major problem in the application of bone marrow transplantation to this disease.

It is obvious, therefore, that leukemic recipients must be pretreated with agents that have both immunosuppressive and antileukemic properties. As mentioned above, ALG has no antileukemic effect;[54] the two most commonly used agents are whole body irradiation and cyclophosphamide. Early experiments by Thomas using total body irradiation showed that doses between 800 and 1500 rads gave sufficient immunosuppression to prevent rejection of the grafted bone marrow tissue.[90] However, in the majority of recipients the disease was not eliminated and the patients died of recurrent leukemia. Although there has been one reported case where the patient survived for more than 1 year after this procedure,[53] it is unlikely that radiation alone will be a suitable treatment for leukemia. Measurement of the radiation sensitivity of leukemic cells indicates that the doses of radiation in the allowable range (<1500 rads) are insufficient to kill all of the leukemic cells.[44]

Santos has pioneered the use of cyclophosphamide in the pretreatment of leukemic patients.[77-79] This agent is a powerful immunosuppressive agent, and it is clear that engraftment and temporary control of leukemia is possible after this treatment.[2, 8, 38, 79] However, among the recently reported cases, only 1 patient has survived for more than 6 months with maintenance of the graft and absence of leukemia.

Thomas and his colleagues have used whole body irradiation in conjunction with either cyclophosphamide[89] or immunotherapy.[92] There is 1 long-term, approximately 1 year, survivor in each series. These apparent successes using combinations of therapy suggest that transplantation may be an effective treatment for leukemia if the problems associated with transplantation can be overcome.

However, a recent report from the group in Seattle calls into question the rationale for carrying out bone marrow transplants in leukemic patients.[31] They reported a case in which a female patient with acute leukemia was irradiated and then given marrow from her HL-A identical brother. The leukemia recurred 62 days after transplantation. At that time, 100 per cent of the bone marrow karyotypes were XY, indicating that the leukemia had recurred in the donor cells! The possible implica-

Table 1. *Summary of Recent Bone Marrow Transplants*

	LEUKEMIA[*]	APLASTIC[†] ANEMIA	IMMUNE[‡] DEFICIENCY DISEASES
HL-A compatible donors§			
Total attempts	28	7	12
No. of takes	17	3	10
No. with GVHD	16	1	8
Longest surviving	>14 mos.	>8 mos.	>3 yrs.
Per cent surviving >6 mos.			
with functional graft	11% (3/28)	14% (1/7)	50% (6/12)
HL-A incompatible donors:			
Total attempts	12	1	17
No. of takes	9	1	11
No. with GVHD	4	0	9
Longest surviving	6 mos.	–	14 mos.
Per cent surviving >6 mos.			
with functional graft	8% (1/12)	–	6% (1/17)

[*]Data from references 2, 39, 54, 62, 79, 86, 89
[†]Data from references 54, 62, 75, 86
[‡]Data from references 2, 20, 27, 34, 49, 62
§These data exclude identical twin donors

tions of this finding are enormous and bear not only on the future of bone marrow transplantation in leukemic patients but also on the underlying mechanism of the induction of leukemia.

In summary, the results of bone marrow transplantation in patients with acute leukemia have been disappointing. Table 1 gives a summary of recent transplant attempts and shows that only about 10 per cent of the leukemic recipients have survived for more than 6 months with a functioning graft. In the cases we reviewed, the median survival of those treated by bone marrow transplantation is 77 days for acute lymphoblastic leukemia and 42 days for acute myeloblastic leukemia. It must be appreciated that many of these patients received a transplant at a time when conventional therapy was no longer effective and would have had a short life expectancy with any treatment. Because of these discouraging results and because of improved results in the chemotherapy of acute leukemia,[41] the wisdom of attempting transplants in the early stages of this disease must be seriously questioned.

These considerations create a dilemma for the clinical scientist. Because at the present time bone marrow transplantation cannot be considered as an alternative to conventional therapy, only patients at advanced stages of disease are usually candidates. These patients are generally poor risks and many deaths occur before it is possible to assess graft function or remission of the leukemia. Certainly there remain many unanswered questions concerning the feasibility of transplantation in leukemic patients. More experiments are required to devise procedures for eradicating the underlying disease and for minimizing the severity of GVHD. In addition, it is essential that the possibility of leukemia recurring in the donor cells be carefully evaluated.

Bone Marrow Aplasia

The transplantation of normal bone marrow is the obvious treatment for severe bone marrow aplasia, and many attempts have been made to use this form of therapy. Among the early attempts, most successes occurred in recipients whose donor was an identical twin. Although it is impossible to prove the existence of a graft from an identical twin because of the absence of markers on the donor cells, the timing of the hemopoietic recovery in these recipients made it likely that the new cells came from the grafted tissue. Thomas has recently reported the long-term follow-up on 4 such cases;[92] these patients remain alive and well 3 to 10 years after transplantation.

In contrast, nearly all the earlier attempts of the transplantation of allogeneic bone marrow were unsuccessful.[15] These grafts were performed without HL-A typing, and in the majority of instances marrow was obtained from donors likely to be histoincompatible (e.g., from parents or unrelated donors). Little or no immunosuppression was used and, in most cases, only small numbers of bone marrow cells were infused. In light of our present knowledge, it is not surprising that the aplasia failed to respond to transplantation. However, among these early attempts there were several apparent exceptions.

In 1959, Mathé reported transplantation in 5 patients involved in a radiation accident.[56] Five of the 6 accident victims received ABO-compatible marrow from unrelated, volunteer donors. A transient graft, indicated by the presence of donor erythrocytes, was observed in some recipients. Four of the 5 recipients survived. A proven bone marrow graft was also obtained in a patient with drug-induced aplasia following chemotherapy for Hodgkin's disease.[12] In this case the donor was an ABO-compatible sister. Tissue typing was, of course, not available at that time, but it is important to note that there is at least a 25 per cent chance that the donor and recipient were HL-A identical.

Despite the use of immunosuppressive agents and a selection of HL-A identical donors, the recent results (Table 1) are still discouraging in that there are few long-term survivors. The most promising approach appears to be the use of ALG for immunosuppression. Using this procedure, Mathé has reported two successful grafts in four cases attempted;[54] Rogentine et al. have also used ALG to obtain a successful graft in a patient with aplastic anemia.[75] Although the complications of GVHD were avoided by the use of ALG, the potential of this treatment must await the long-term follow-up of the survivors.

Immune Deficiency Disorders

The most promising application of bone marrow transplantation at present is in the treatment of children with immune deficiency disorders. Both the improved methods of tissue typing and the rapid increase in our understanding of the differentiation of the immune system have played large parts in the improved therapy of these patients. A discussion of the differentiation of this system is found elsewhere in this issue (see p. 319).

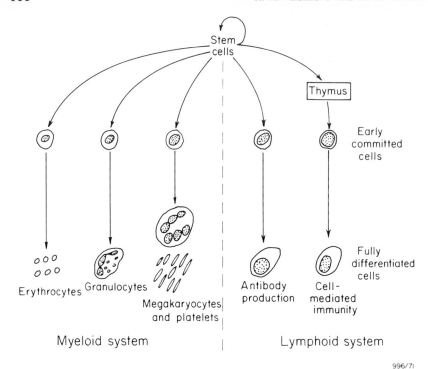

996/71

Figure 1.   Pathways of differentiation for stem cells in bone marrow.

As shown in Figure 1, there are basically two types of lymphoid cells in the immune system. A thymus-dependent lymphoid cell is responsible for cell-mediated immune responses such as graft rejection, graft-versus-host disease, and delayed hypersensitivity reactions; a thymus-independent lymphoid cell differentiates into progeny that synthesize specific antibody, i.e., the humoral immune response.

In a recent review, Gatti and Good[33] showed that genetic defects may occur at any stage in differentiation. Genetic defects in the stem cells would be expected to affect both cellular immune responses and antibody production. Combined immunologic deficiency or Swiss-type agammaglobulinemia is probably an example of such a stem cell defect.

Genetic lesions could also occur in either of the two lymphoid pathways leading to defects in humoral or cellular immune responses, but not both. Bruton-type agammaglobulinemia in which children have defective antibody production but normal cellular immune responses is probably an example of a defect in the thymus-independent lymphoid cells. On the other hand, children with the Wiskott-Aldrich syndrome have defective cell-mediated responses, but near-normal immunoglobulin levels; such children may represent defects in the thymus-dependent lymphoid cells. Cellular immune responses can also be altered if there is a defect in the thymic environment. Children with the diGeorge syndrome have an apparent congenital lack of the thymus and defective cellular immune responses.

On the basis of the knowledge of the differentiation of the immune system and a knowledge of the cellular basis for these immunologic defects, one would predict that children with combined immunologic deficiency disease, the Bruton-type agammaglobulinemia, and the Wiskott-Aldrich syndrome would respond to bone marrow transplantation, but children with the diGeorge syndrome would require a thymus graft.

Recent clinical results tend to confirm the above predictions. Several children with combined immunologic deficiency disorders have been immunologically reconstituted with bone marrow grafts from HL-A identical sibling donors.[20, 26, 27, 34, 49, 62] There has also been one successful reconstitution of a child with Wiskott-Aldrich syndrome treated by bone marrow transplantation.[8] However, there have been no successful bone marrow grafts reported for the treatment of Bruton-type agammaglobulinemia. Since cellular immune reactions are normal in such children, immunosuppressive drugs should probably be used in conjunction with transplantation, but in a recently reported attempt[62] no immunosuppression was used. With combined immunologic deficiency diseases no immunosuppression is required. In the Wiskott-Aldrich syndrome, the situation is less clear. The proposed cellular basis for the defect suggests that immunosuppression should not be required. However, Bach et al. found that a graft was achieved only after the child had been pretreated with cyclophosphamide.[8] Finally, there have been two reports of the successful immunologic reconstitution of children with diGeorge syndrome following the transplantation of fetal thymus.[5, 22]

Table 1 gives a summary of the recent attempts to reconstitute children with immune deficiency diseases. Although all diseases, with the exception of the diGeorge syndrome, have been combined for presentation in this table, the majority of the attempts have been for combined immunologic deficiency. The striking fact from this table is the difference between HL-A compatible and incompatible donors. With compatible sibling donors, 80 per cent of the grafts resulted in successful takes, and 50 per cent of the children are alive more than 6 months after transplantation with a functional graft. In contrast, only 30 per cent of the grafts with incompatible donors functioned even transiently. Only one recipient survived for more than 6 months with a functional graft; this child had only minimal immunologic reconstitution and died of pneumonia 14 months after the first of two bone marrow grafts.[21] The data with regard to GVHD are somewhat misleading. The apparent high proportion of recipients with GVHD in the compatible series is a reflection of the greater number of takes compared to the incompatible series. What is not indicated in the table is that GVHD in recipients of compatible marrow is mild and, in general, not life-threatening. In contrast, the GVHD observed in recipients of HL-A incompatible bone marrow is usually severe and results in the death of the recipient.

In future transplants with an HL-A identical sibling donor, GVHD will probably not be a major problem. Although the group in the Netherlands has used cell separation to prevent this complication in such cases,[26, 27] more recent data from the group in Boston indicates that, simply, transplantation with small numbers (5×10^7 cells per kg.) of bone marrow cells is sufficient to prevent the occurrence of severe GVHD.[34, 49] Recipients of small numbers of unfractionated, HL-A identical bone marrow develop a mild skin rash that spontaneously disappears about 3 weeks after transplantation.

When an HL-A identical donor is not available, as is the case in most instances, other measures are required to prevent GVHD. The two most encouraging results with HL-A incompatible donors involve the use of cell separation techniques and antisera to prevent GVHD. In one case, a child in Copenhagen was given bone marrow from its father.[27] Prior to transplantation, the recipient was given ALG and the cells were separated on density gradients to prepare a stem cell fraction depleted of GVHD activity. There was a partial immunologic reconstitution within 5 weeks after transplantation, and donor lymphocytes were observed in the peripheral blood. However, despite the separation procedure and ALG treatment, the child developed a severe skin rash and died of sepsis 70 days after transplantation.

In a second case, donor bone marrow from the mother was also separated on a density gradient. In addition, since the mother's serum contained factors with some of the properties of enhancing antibody, the child was given a single infusion of maternal plasma prior to transplantation and several other plasma infusions after grafting.[21] The child showed some reconstitution of its immunologic responses and had no signs of GVHD except for an eosinophilia that began shortly after transplantation. Unfortunately, there were no markers available to prove the existence of a graft. The child maintained some immune responses as indicated by positive skin tests to candida and low antibody titers but eventually died of pneumonia 14 months after the initial graft. Although no patients have been permanently reconstituted immunologically with HL-A incompatible bone marrow, these two indications of partial reconstitution lead to the hope that a combination of methods will soon allow the successful treatment of these recipients of HL-A incompatible bone marrow.

CONCLUSION

In only two situations can bone marrow transplantation be considered as the treatment of choice. Both situations are rare: patients with aplastic anemia whose donor is a normal identical twin, and infants with combined immunologic deficiency disease whose donor is a normal, HL-A identical sibling. In these combinations, there is a high success rate and the complications following transplantation are minimal. With all other combinations of donors and recipients, bone marrow transplants should not be attempted except as an experimental procedure.

However, there are indications that bone marrow transplantation may soon become a reliable procedure in some other situations. The use of cell separation techniques and specific antisera has shown limited success in grafts of HL-A incompatible marrow in patients with combined immunologic deficiency. Pretreatment with ALG shows promise of overcoming problems associated with allogeneic grafts in patients with aplastic anemia. The results with leukemic recipients are most discouraging.

Whether or not these improvements in technique will also help eradicate disease in patients with acute leukemia must await further evaluation, but the few long remissions obtained recently indicate that transplantation may be an effective form of therapy in some patients.

Although theoretically many patients could benefit from a bone marrow transplant, it is perhaps best to end this review on a note of caution. The few successes in recent years should not be interpreted as a signal for the routine application of bone marrow transplantation. Except for the two situations mentioned above, it remains a high-risk, experimental procedure that should be attempted only in selected patients where the outcome will contribute to our understanding of the problems associated with the transplantation of this tissue. The indiscriminate use of bone marrow transplants at this time would undoubtedly be disastrous and only serve to slow down progress in the development of this potentially useful procedure.

Pressure on space required the deletion by the publisher of contributed material on the functional anatomy of cells in the myeloid and lymphoid systems. The reader is referred to reviews by McCulloch[58] and Osoba (p. 319) and to specific references 6, 13, 16, 17, 28, 30, 47, 57, 59, 60, 63, 69, 71, 73, 74, 76, 80–83, 95–98, and 104–107.

ACKNOWLEDGMENTS

We wish to thank the following individuals who provided us with unpublished data and recent information concerning their patients: Dr. F. Bach, Dr. R. H. Buckley, Dr. K. A. Dicke, Dr. E. Gelfand, Dr. R. A. Good, Dr. G. Mathé, Dr. G. Santos, and Dr. E. D. Thomas.

REFERENCES

1. Albertini, R. J., and Bach, F. H.: Quantitative assay of antigenic disparity at HLA—the major histocompatibility locus in man. J. Exper. Med., 128:639–651, 1968.
2. Amato, D., Bergsagel, D. E., Clarysee, A. M., Cowan, D. H., Iscove, N. N., McCulloch, E. A., Miller, R. G., Phillips, R. A., Ragab, A. H., and Senn, J. S.: Review of bone marrow transplants at the Ontario Cancer Institute. Transplant. Proc., 3:397–399, 1971.
3. Amato, D., Cowan, D. H., and McCulloch, E. A.: Separation of immunocompetent cells from human and mouse hemopoietic cell suspensions by velocity sedimentation. Blood, in press.
4. Amos, D. B., Seigler, H. F., Southworth, J. G., and Ward, F. E.: Skin graft rejection between subjects genotyped for HLA. Transplant. Proc., 1:342–346, 1969.
5. August, C. S., Rosen, F. S., Filler, R. M., Janeway, C. A., Markowski, B., and Kay, H. E. M.: Implantation of a fetal thymus, restoring immunological competence in a patient with thymic aplasia (diGeorge's syndrome). Lancet, 2:1210–1211, 1968.
6. Austin, P. E., McCulloch, E. A., and Till, J. E.: Characterization of the factor in L-cell conditioned medium capable of stimulating colony formation by mouse marrow cells in culture. J. Cellular Physiol., 77:121–134, 1971.
7. Bach, F. H.: Transplantation: Problems of histocompatibility testing. Science, 159:1196–1198, 1968.
8. Bach, F. H., Albertini, R. J., Joo, P., Anderson, J. L., and Bortin, M. M.: Bone marrow transplantation in a patient with Wiskott-Aldrich syndrome. Lancet, 2:1364–1366, 1968.
9. Bain, B., Vas, M. R., and Lowenstein, L.: The development of large immature mononuclear cells in mixed leucocyte cultures. Blood, 23:108–116, 1964.
10. Barnes, B. A., Murray, J. E., and Atkinson, J. C.: Transplant survival and patient activity data from the human kidney transplant registry. Transplant. Proc., 3:303–307, 1971.
11. Batchelor, J. R., Ellis, F., French, M. E., Bewick, M., Cameron, J., and Ogg, C. S.: Immunological enhancement of human kidney graft. Lancet, 2:1007–1010, 1970.
12. Beilby, J. O. W., Cade, I. S., Jelliffe, A. M., Parkin, D. M., and Stewart, J. W.: Prolonged

survival of a bone marrow graft resulting in a blood group chimera. Brit. Med. J., *1*:96–99, 1960.

13. Bernstein, S. E.: Tissue transplantation as an analytic and therapeutic tool in the treatment of hereditary anemias. Amer. J. Surg., *119*:448–451, 1970.

14. Boranić, M.: The time pattern of the anti-leukemic effect of the graft-versus-host reaction. Transplant. Proc., *3*:394–396, 1971.

15. Bortin, M. M.: A compendium of reported human bone marrow transplants. Transplantation, *9*:571–587, 1970.

16. Bradley, T. R., and Metcalf, D.: The growth of mouse bone marrow cells *in vitro*. Austr. J. Exper. Biol. Med. Sci., *44*:287–300, 1966.

17. Bradley, T. R., and Sumner, M. A.: Stimulation of mouse bone marrow colony growth *in vitro* by conditioned medium. Austr. J. Exper. Biol. Med. Sci., *46*:607–618, 1968.

18. Bruce, W. R.: The action of chemotherapeutic agents at the cellular level and the effects of these agents on hematopoietic and lymphomatous tissue. Can. Cancer Conf., *7*:53–64, 1967.

19. Bruce, W. R., Meeker, B. E., and Valeriote, F. A.: Comparison of the sensitivity of normal hematopoietic and transplanted lymphoma colony-forming cells to chemotherapeutic agents administered *in vivo*. J. Nat. Cancer Inst., *37*:233–245, 1966.

20. Buckley, R. H.: Reconstitution: Grafting of bone marrow and thymus. *In* Progress in Immunology. New York, Academic Press, in press.

21. Buckley, R. H., Amos, D. B., Kremer, W. P., and Stickel, D. L.: Incompatible bone marrow transplantation in lymphopenic immunologic deficiency. New Eng. J. Med., *285*:1035–1042, 1971.

22. Cleveland, W. W., Fogel, B. J., Brown, W. T., and Kay, H. E. M.: Fetal thymic transplant in a case of diGeorge's syndrome. Lancet, *2*:1211–1214, 1968.

23. Congdon, C. C.: Cooperative group on bone marrow transplantation in man. Transplant. Proc., *2*:342–360, 1970.

24. Cowan, D. H.: Unpublished data.

25. Cudkowicz, G., and Bennett, M.: Peculiar immunobiology of bone marrow allografts. I. Graft rejection by irradiated responder mice. J. Exper. Med., *134*:83–102, 1971.

26. de Koning, J., Dooren, L. J., van Bekkum, D. W., van Rood, J. J., Dicke, K. A., and Radl, J.: Transplantation of bone marrow cells and fetal thymus in an infant with lymphopenic immunological deficiency. Lancet, *1*:1223–1227, 1969.

27. Dicke, K. A.: Personal communication.

28. Dicke, K. A., Platenburg, M. G. C., and van Bekkum, D. W.: Colony formation in agar: *In vitro* assays for hemopoietic stem cells. Cell and Tissue Kinetics, in press.

29. Dicke, K. A., van Hooft, J. I. M., and van Bekkum, D. W.: The selective elimination of immunologically competent cells from bone marrow and lymphatic cell mixtures. II. Mouse spleen fractionation on a discontinuous albumin gradient. Transplantation, *6*:571–586, 1968.

30. Edwards, G. E., Miller, R. G., and Phillips, R. A.: Differentiation of rosette-forming cells from myeloid stem cells. J. Immunol., *105*:719–729, 1970.

31. Fialkow, J., Thomas, E. D., Bryant, J. I., and Neiman, P. E.: Leukemic transformation of engrafted human marrow cells *in vivo*. Lancet, *1*:251–255, 1971.

32. Ford, C. E., Hamerton, J. H., Barnes, W. H., and Loutit, J. F.: Cytological identification of radiation chimeras. Nature, *177*:452–454, 1956.

33. Gatti, R. A., and Good, R. A.: The immunological deficiency diseases. Med. Clin. N. Amer., *54*:281–307, 1970.

34. Gelfand, E. W., and Rosen, F. S.: Personal communication.

35. Gowans, J. L.: The fate of parental strain small lymphocytes in F1 hybrid hosts. Ann. N. Y. Acad. Sci., *99*:432–455, 1962.

36. Graff, R. J., Hildeman, W. H., and Snell, G. D.: Histocompatibility genes in mice. VI. Allografts in mice congenic at various non-H-2 histocompatibility loci. Transplantation, *4*:425–437, 1966.

37. Graul, E. H., Schaumloffel, E., Hundeshagen, H., Wilmanns, H., and Simon, G.: Metabolism of radioactive cyclophosphamide: Animal tests and clinical studies. Cancer, *20*:896–899, 1967.

38. Graw, R. G., Levinthal, B. C., Yankee, R. A., Rogentine, G. N., Whang-Peng, J., Ginnif, M. H., Herzig, G. P., Halterman, R. H., and Henderson, E. S.: HLA and mixed leucocyte culture matched allogeneic bone marrow transplantation in patients with acute leukemia. Transplant. Proc., *3*:405–408, 1971.

39. Graw, R. G., Whang-Peng, J., Kruger, G., Buckner, C. D., Levinthal, B. G., Berard, C., and Henderson, E. S.: Complications of bone marrow transplantation. Graft-versus-host disease resulting from chronic-myelogenous-leukemia leukocyte transfusions. Lancet, *2*:338–341, 1970.

40. Greenberg, M. L., Chanana, A. D., Cronkite, E. P., Schiffer, L. M., and Stryckmans, P. A.: Extracorporeal irradiation of blood in man: Radiation resistance of circulating platelets. Radiation Res., *35*:147–154, 1968.

41. Hamilton-Fairley, G.: The treatment of acute myeloblastic leukemia. Brit. J. Haematol., 20:567–570, 1970.

42. Hellström, K. E., and Hellström, I.: Immunological enhancement as studied by cell culture techniques. Ann. Rev. Microbiol., 24:373–398, 1970.

43. Hellström, I., Hellström, K. E., Storb, R., and Thomas, E. D.: Colony inhibition of fibroblasts from chimeric dogs mediated by the dogs' own lymphocytes and specifically abrogated by their serum. Proc. Nat. Acad. Sci., 66:65–71, 1970.

44. Hewitt, H. B., and Wilson, C. W.: Survival curve for mammalian leukemic cells irradiated *in vivo* (implications for treatment of mouse leukemia by whole-body irradiation). Brit. J. Cancer, 13:69–75, 1959.

45. Hong, R., and Bach, F. H.: Bone marrow transplantation. Aggravating factors in graft-versus-host disease. Transplantation, 10:192–194, 1970.

46. Hume, D. M., Leo, J., Rolley, R. T., and Williams, G. M.: Some immunological and surgical aspects of kidney transplantation in man. Transplant. Proc., 1:171–177, 1969.

47. Iscove, N. N., Senn, J. S., Till, J. E., and McCulloch, E. A.: Colony formation by normal and leukemic human marrow cells in culture: Effect of conditioned medium from human leukocytes. Blood, 37:1–5, 1971.

48. Jose, D. G., Choi, Y. S., Gatti, R. A., Kersey, J. H., Biggar, W. P., and Good, R. A.: Humoral antagonism of cellular immunity in children with immune deficiency disease reconstituted by bone marrow transplantation. Lancet, 2:841–844, 1971.

49. Levey, R. H., Klemperer, M. R., Gelfand, E. W., Sanderson, A. R., Batchelor, J. R., Berkel, A. I., and Rosen, F. S.: Bone marrow transplantation in severe combined immunodeficiency syndrome. Lancet, 2:571–575, 1971.

50. Lorenz, E., Congdon, C., and Uphoff, D.: Modification of acute radiation injury in mice and guinea pigs by bone marrow injection. Radiology, 58:863–877, 1952.

51. Mathé, G., Amiel, J. L., and Schwarzenberg, L.: Bone marrow transplantation. *In* Rapaport, F., and Dausset, J., eds.: Human Transplantation. New York, Grune and Stratton, 1968, pp. 284–303.

52. Mathé, G., Amiel, J. L., and Schwarzenberg, L.: Bone Marrow Transplantation and Leucocyte Transfusions. Springfield, Illinois, Charles C Thomas, 1971.

53. Mathé, G., Amiel, J. L., Schwarzenberg, L., Cotton, A., Schneider, M., de Vries, M. J., Tubiana, M., Lalanne, C., Binet, J. L., Papiernik, M., Seman, G., Matsukura, M., Mery, A. M., Schwarzmann, V., and Flaisler, A.: Successful allogeneic bone marrow transplantation in man: Chimerism, induced specific tolerance and possible antileukemic effects. Blood, 25:179–195, 1965.

54. Mathé, G., Amiel, J. L., Schwarzenberg, L., Choay, J., Trolard, P., Schneider, M., Hayat, M., Schlumberger, J. R., and Jasmin, C.: Bone marrow graft in man after conditioning by antilymphocyte serum. Transplant. Proc., 3:325–332, 1971.

55. Mathé, G., Amiel, J. L., Schwarzenberg, L., Schneider, M., Cotton, A., Schlumberger, J. R., Nouza, K., and Hrask, Y.: Bone marrow transplantation in man. Transplant. Proc., 1:16–24, 1969.

56. Mathé, G., Jammet, H., Pendic, B., Schwarzenberg, L., Duplan, J. F., Marjsin, B., Laterjet, L., Larrieu, M. J., Kalic, D., and Djukic, Z.: Transfusions et greffes de moelle osseuse homologue chez des humains irradiés à haute dose accidentuellement. Rev. Franc. Etudes Clin. Biol., 4:226–238, 1959.

57. McCool, D., Miller, R. J., Painter, R. H., and Bruce, W. R.: Erythropoietic sensitivity of rat bone marrow cells separated by velocity sedimentation. Cell and Tissue Kinetics, 3:55–65, 1970.

58. McCulloch, E. A.: Control of hematopoiesis at the cellular level. *In* Gordon, A. S., ed.: Regulation of Hematopoiesis. New York, Appelton-Century-Crofts, 1970, vol. 1, pp. 133–159.

59. McCulloch, E. A., Siminovitch, L., and Till, J. E.: Spleen-colony formation in anemic mice of genotype W/W^v. Science, 144:844–846, 1964.

60. McCulloch, E. A., Siminovitch, L., Till, J. E., Russell, E. S., and Bernstein, S. E.: The cellular basis of the genetically determined hemopoietic defect in anemic mice of genotype S1/S1^d. Blood, 26:399–410, 1965.

61. McCulloch, E. A., and Till, J. E.: Repression of colony-forming ability of C57BL hematopoietic cells transplanted into nonisologous hosts. J. Cell. Comp. Physiol., 61:301–308, 1963.

62. Metcalf, D., Bradley, T. R., and Robinson, W.: Analysis of colonies developing *in vitro* from mouse bone marrow cells stimulated by kidney feeder layers or leukemic serum. J. Cell. Physiol., 69:93–108, 1967.

63. Meuwissen, H. J., Rodney, G., McArthur, J., Pabst, H., Gatti, R., Chilgren, R., Hong, R., Frommel, D., Coifman, R., and Good, R. A.: Bone marrow transplantation - Therapeutic usefulness and complications. Amer. J. Med., 51:513–532, 1971.

64. Micklem, H. S., Ford, C. E., Evans, E. P., and Gray, J.: Interrelationships of myeloid and lymphoid cells: Studies with chromosome-marked cells transfused into lethally irradiated mice. Proc. Roy. Soc. (London). Ser. B., 167:78–102, 1966.

65. Micklem, H. S., and Loutit, J. F.: Tissue Grafting and Radiation. New York, Academic Press, 1966.
66. Miller, D. G., and Diamond, H. D.: The biological basis and clinical application of bone marrow transplantation. Med. Clin. N. Amer., 45:711–731, 1961.
67. Möller, G.: Studies on the mechanism of immunological enhancement of tumour homografts. I. Specificity of immunological enhancement. J. Nat. Cancer Inst., 30:1153–1175, 1963.
68. Muller-Bérat, C. N., van Putten, L. M., and van Bekkum, D. W.: Cytostatic drugs in the treatment of secondary disease following homologous bone marrow transplantation: Extrapolation from the mouse to the primate. Ann. N. Y. Acad. Sci., 129:340–354, 1966.
69. Nowell, P. C., Hirsch, B. E., Fox, D. H., and Wilson, D. B.: Evidence for the existence of multipotential lympho-hematopoietic stem cells in the adult rat. J. Cell. Physiol., 75:151–158, 1970.
70. Perkins, E. H., Nettesheim, P., and Morita, T.: Radioresistance of the engulfing and degradative capacities of peritoneal phagocytes to kiloroentgen x-ray doses. J. Reticuloendothelial Soc., 3:71–82, 1966.
71. Phillips, R. A.: The immune response as a model system for studies on cellular differentiation. In Warren, K. B., ed.: Differentiation and Immunology. Symposia of the International Society for Cell Biology. New York, Academic Press, 1968, vol. 7, pp. 111–122.
72. Phillips, R. A., and Miller, R. G.: Physical separation of hemopoietic stem cells from cells causing graft-versus-host disease. I. Sedimentation properties of cells causing graft-versus-host disease. J. Immunol., 105:1168–1174, 1970.
73. Pillow, R. P., Epstein, R. B., Buckner, C. D., Giblett, E. R., and Thomas, E. D.: Treatment of bone marrow failure by isogeneic marrow infusion. New Eng. J. Med., 275:94–97, 1966.
74. Pluznik, D. H., and Sachs, L.: The cloning of normal "mast" cells in tissue culture. J. Cell. Comp. Physiol., 66:319–324, 1965.
75. Rogentine, G. N., Rosenberg, S., Merritt, C. B., Yankee, R. A., Levinthal, B. G., Graw, R. G., Greipp, P., Whang-Peng, J., and Fahey, J. L.: Successful allogeneic bone marrow transplantation in aplastic anemia (abstract). Blood, 36:829, 1970.
76. Russell, E. S.: Problems and potentialities in the study of genic action in the mouse. In Burdette, W. J., ed.: Methodology in Mammalian Genetics. San Francisco, Holden-Day, Inc., 1963, pp. 217–232.
77. Santos, G. W.: Application of marrow grafts in human disease: its problems and potential. In Hanna, M. G., ed.: Current Problems in Immunobiology. New York, Plenum Publishing Corp., in press.
78. Santos, G. W., Burke, P. J., Sensenbrenner, L. L., and Owens, A. A., Jr.: Rationale for the use of cyclophosphamide as immunosuppression for marrow transplants in man. In Bertolli, A., and Monaco, A. P., eds.: International Symposium on Pharmacologic Treatment in Organ and Tissue Transplantation, Milan, Italy, 1969. Amsterdam, Excerpta Medica Foundation, 1970, pp. 24–31.
79. Santos, G. W., Sensenbrenner, L. L., Burke, P. J., Colvin, M., Owens, A. H., Jr., Bias, W. B., and Slavin, R. E.: Marrow transplantation in man following cyclophosphamide. Transplant. Proc., 3:400–404, 1971.
80. Senn, J. S.: Personal communication.
81. Senn, J. S., and McCulloch, E. A.: Kinetics of regeneration after cyclophosphamide in human marrow assessed by a culture method (abstract). Exper. Hematol., 20:8–9, 1970.
82. Senn, J. S., McCulloch, E. A., and Till, J. E.: Comparison of colony-forming ability of normal and leukemic human marrow in cell culture. Lancet, 2:597–598, 1967.
83. Siminovitch, L., McCulloch, E. A., and Till, J. E.: The distribution of colony-forming cells among spleen colonies. J. Cell. Comp. Physiol., 62:327–336, 1963.
84. Singal, D. P., Mickey, M. R., and Terasaki, P. I.: Serotyping for homotransplantation. XXII. Analysis of kidney transplants from parental versus sibling donors. Transplantation, 7:246–258, 1969.
85. Solberg, C. O., Meuwissen, H. J., Needham, R. N., Good, R. A., and Matsen, J. M.: Infectious complications in bone marrow transplant patients. Brit. Med. J., 1:18–23, 1971.
86. Speck, B., Dooren, L. J., de Koning, J., van Bekkum, D. W., Eernisse, J. G., Elkerbout, F., Vossen, J. M., and van Rood, J. J.: Clinical experience with bone marrow transplantation: failure and success. Transplant. Proc., 3:409–413, 1971.
87. Storb, R., Epstein, R. B., Rudolf, R. H., and Thomas, E. D.: The effect of prior transfusion on marrow grafts between histocompatible siblings. J. Immunol., 105:627–633, 1970.
88. Stuart, F. P., Saitoh, T., and Fitch, F. W.: Rejection of renal allografts: specific immunologic suppression. Science, 160:1463–1465, 1968.
89. Thomas, E. D., Buckner, C. D., Rudolf, R. H., Fefer, A., Storb, R., Neiman, P. E., Bryant, J. I., Chard, R. L., Clift, R. A., Epstein, R. B., Fialkow, P. J., Funk, D. D., Giblett, E. R., Lerner, K. G., Reynolds, F. A., and Slichter, S.: Allogeneic marrow grafting for hematologic malignancy using HLA matched donor-receipient sibling pairs. Blood, 38:267–287, 1971.

90. Thomas, E. D., Herman, E. C., Jr., Greenough, W. B., III, Hager, E. B., Cannon, J. H., Sahler, O. D., and Ferrebee, J. W.: Irradiation and marrow infusion in leukemia. Arch. Intern. Med., 107:829–845, 1961.

91. Thomas, E. D., Kasakura, S., Cavino, J. A., Swisher, S. N., and Ferrebee, J. W.: Significance of blood groups in homotransplantation of marrow in the dog. Ann. N. Y. Acad. Sci., 120:362–366, 1964.

92. Thomas, E. D., Rudolf, R. H., Fefer, A., Storb, R., Slichter, S., and Buckner, C. D.: Isogeneic marrow grafting in man. Exper. Hematol., in press.

93. Thomas, E. D., and Storb, R.: Technique for human marrow grafting. Blood, 36:507–515, 1970.

94. Till, J. E.: Personal communication.

95. Till, J. E.: Cellular differentiation in the hemopoietic system. In Cole, A., ed.: Theoretical and Experimental Biophysics, New York, Marcel Dekker, vol. 3, in press.

96. Till, J. E., and McCulloch, E. A.: A direct measurement of the radiation sensitivity of normal mouse bone marrow. Radiation Res., 14:213–222, 1961.

97. Trentin, J. J.: Influence of hematopoietic organ stroma (hematopoietic inductive microenvironment) on stem cell differentiation. In Gordon, A. S., ed.: Regulation of Hematopoiesis. New York, Appleton-Century-Crofts, 1970, vol. 1, pp. 161–186.

98. Trentin, J. J., Wolf, N., Cheng, V., Fahlberg, W., Weiss, D., and Bonhag, R.: Antibody production by mice repopulated with limited numbers of clones of lymphoid cell precursors. J. Immunol., 98:1326–1337, 1967.

99. Uphoff, D. W., and Law, L. W.: An evaluation of some genetic factors influencing irradiation protection by bone marrow. J. Nat. Cancer Inst., 22:229–241, 1959.

100. van Bekkum, D. W.: Bone marrow transplantation. Transplant. Proc., 3:53–57, 1971.

101. van Bekkum, D. W., and deVries, M. J.: Radiation Chimeras. London, Logos Press, Ltd., 1967.

102. van Putten, L. M., Balner, H., Muller-Bérat, C. N., deVries, M. J., and van Bekkum, D. W.: Progress in the treatment and prevention of secondary disease after homologous bone marrow transplantation in monkeys. Effects of chemotherapy and of donor selection by histocompatibility testing. Bibliotheca Haematol., 29:574–586, 1968.

103. Voisin, G. A., Kinsky, R., and Maillard, J.: Protection against homologous disease in hybrid mice by passive and active immunological enhancement facilitation. Transplantation, 6:187–202, 1968.

104. Worton, R. G., McCulloch, E. A., and Till, J. E.: Physical separation of hemopoietic stem cells from cells forming colonies in culture. J. Cell. Physiol., 74:171–182, 1969.

105. Wu, A. M., Till, J. E., Siminovitch, L., and McCulloch, E. A.: Cytological evidence for a relationship between normal hemopoietic colony-forming cells and cells of the lymphoid system. J. Exper. Med., 127:455–463, 1968.

106. Wu, A. M., Till, J. E., Siminovitch, L., and McCulloch, E. A.: A cytological study of the capacity for differentiation of normal hemopoietic colony-forming cells. J. Cell. Physiol., 69:177–184, 1967.

107. Wu, A. M., Siminovitch, L., Till, J. E., and McCulloch, E. A.: Evidence for a relationship between mouse hemopoietic stem cells and cells forming colonies in culture. Proc. Nat. Acad. Sci., 59:1209–1215, 1968.

Department of Medicine
Ontario Cancer Institute
500 Sherbourne Street
Toronto, Ontario
Canada
(Dr. Cowan)

The Future of Transplantation Immunology

Erwin Diener, Ph.D.,* and Dennis Jirsch, M.D.**

During recent years much attention has been focused on clinical organ transplantation. While the communications media have extensively publicized the achievements of transplantation surgery, the scientific community remains aware of the persistent obstacle of the transplantation barrier. The modest success in organ transplantation so far achieved is the result of sophisticated surgical techniques and the judicious use of cytotoxic drugs in conjunction with tissue-typing genetics, rather than the clinical application of what one might call, "immunological engineering." Each of the immunosuppressive agents currently used—azathioprine, corticosteroid drugs, and antilymphocyte globulin—causes its own toxicity problems, and all these agents seriously diminish the patient's resistance to the microbial environment.

Ideally, the practicing physician must be provided with a technique which will specifically block the recipient's immune response to the grafted tissue but will maintain the vanguard of defense mechanisms necessary to combat infection. Research is aiming toward this goal by investigating mechanisms which govern the immune reaction at the cellular and molecular levels so that subsequent manipulation of these reactions may become possible.

In this review we will briefly discuss highlights of immune function, evaluate the present success of organ transplantation and then speculate about current and future developments.

BASIC MECHANISMS OF IMMUNE REACTIONS

Antigen Recognition

The body's lymphoreticular system is concerned with defense mechanisms which are selectively directed against substances foreign to it-

From the M.R.C. Transplantation Unit, and the Departments of Pathology and Surgery, University of Alberta, Edmonton, Alberta, Canada

*Professor of Pathology, Co-Director, MRC—Transplantation Unit, Faculty of Medicine, University of Alberta
**Resident in Thoracic and Cardiovascular Surgery, and Fellow, Medical Research Council of Canada, Faculty of Medicine, University of Alberta

self. Thus the initiation of an immune reaction requires the discrimination between "self" and "foreign" and may lead to either antibody production or, in the case of graft rejection, to the appearance of "killer cells" which destroy transplanted tissue by direct contact. From the incisive experiments of Gowans and colleagues[8, 11, 12] we have come to regard the lymphocyte as the "spearhead" in the immunologic mechanism. In graft rejection a proportion of small lymphocytes differentiate into large cells which begin to proliferate. These progeny represent the cell population which is concerned with the actual destruction of the transplant. To initiate these events there must have existed lymphocytes which were specifically triggered by the presence of foreign molecular components of the graft.

What are these cellular entities which discriminate between "self" and "foreign," and what are the means by which this recognition is controlled? Evidence now suggests that the surface membrane of the lymphocyte can be regarded as a switchboard from which specific signals are transmitted to the cell's interior. These signals originate from molecular entities, the "switches," for which there are specific "keys." At the surface of a lymphocyte these "switches," called "recognition sites," are stereo specifically complementary to "keys" which are represented by antigen molecules. Recognition sites have been identified as protein molecules identical in basic structure with antibody. Since antigen recognition is highly specific, there must exist a control mechanism which allows the lymphocyte to interact with only one type of antigen at a time. It is evident that such a control mechanism must be exerted at the genetic level, i.e., the molecular structure of the recognition site must be coded in the genome of the lymphocyte concerned. To understand the most important consequences of this conclusion, we should recall some of the fundamental steps of protein synthesis.

It is generally accepted that the basic mechanisms of protein synthesis in bacteria are also applicable to the mammalian cell. Thus a unique sequence of amino acids which constitutes the chemical specificity of a polypeptide chain is determined by a transfer of information from the nuclear DNA through messenger RNA, ribosomal RNA, and transfer RNA. This dogma of modern biochemistry, when applied to the phenomenon of antigen recognition by a lymphocyte, postulates a code for a recognition site which is specific for a particular antigenic structure.

These conclusions have led to a serious problem: since there are several thousand different antigenic structures, each lymphocyte must bear the genetic information for the synthesis of several thousand different recognition sites. Such a consequence is inconsistent with current genetic concepts.

A theory which has provided an elegant solution to the problem suggests the existence of a few genes which undergo random somatic mutation during lymphopoiesis to give rise to very large numbers of mutant lymphocytes, each genetically programmed to recognize a different specific antigenic structure.[4] Thereafter, the capacity to synthesize recognition sites complementary to a specific antigen is the property of a single clone of cells. The antigen is thought to act as a selective force for the relevant cell clone to initiate a specific immune response. This theory, known as "the clonal selection theory of immunity,"[4] has been regarded as a basic working hypothesis in immunology for over a decade.

Origin of Immunocompetent Cells

A lymphocyte which has acquired the capacity to recognize a particular antigen is called an "immunocompetent cell." What is the origin of these cells? This question was regarded as of academic interest until it became relevant to the problem of bone marrow transplantation. The grafting of bone marrow into an animal which has suffered lethal x-irradiation (and in consequence has had its own blood-forming tissue destroyed) is a life-saving procedure. After a period of approximately 3 weeks animals display a full complement of blood-forming cells.

Indeed repopulation studies by Ford,[7] by Micklem and colleagues,[18] and by Globerson[10] have conclusively shown that bone marrow has the capacity to recolonize not only bone marrow but also thymus and peripheral lymphoid tissues such as lymph nodes and spleen. There is now strong evidence pointing to the existence of self-perpetuating bone marrow stem cells as the origin of the lymphoid tissue and similarly, the capacity for self-renewal of erythropoietic and granulopoietic tissue is thought to be controlled by stem cells.

Whether erythropoietic and granulopoietic stem cells are identical with lymphoid stem cells is not yet clear. Somewhere along the developmental pathway from a few precursor cells to the immensely large pool of specific immunocompetent cells in lymphoid tissue there occurs a critical phase during which the capacity for antigen recognition becomes

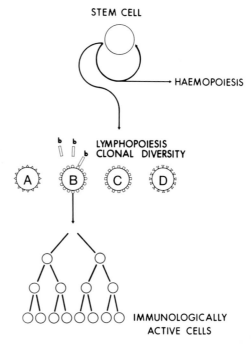

Figure 1. Origin of immunocompetent cells. A, B, C, and D are immunocompetent cells belonging to different cell clones. Each clone possesses recognition sites specific for only one antigen. b, specific antigen interacting with an immunocompetent cell.

diversified. The end product of this selective differentiation is the mature immunocompetent cell with exposed recognition sites specific for a given antigen (Fig. 1).

CLINICAL ORGAN TRANSPLANTATION

Current Methods to Minimize Rejection

Unqualified success in organ transplantation has eluded us because of inadequate knowledge in organ preservation techniques and the limitation of current means of restraining the allograft reaction (immune reaction against a transplant from an unrelated individual of the same species). The surgical techniques necessary for organ transplantation are generally well developed, and the most pressing problem remains that of organ rejection. The severity of graft rejection depends upon the antigenic differences between host and recipient and this has led to efforts to match major histocompatibility antigens.

Methods are now available for determining so-called transplantation or histocompatibility antigens, the genetically determined tissue proteins important in provoking an immune response, so that the matching of donor with recipient can be achieved. The procedure is analogous to blood typing but is more demanding since parenchymal grafts are intended to last indefinitely and minor incompatibilities become more significant. In man, the major histocompatibility antigens are represented on nucleated cells, and leukocyte typing therefore permits a direct approach to histocompatibility testing.

Studies indicate that there exists a single genetic locus, the HL-A locus, displaying multiple alleles and several subloci. The large number of alleles at the HL-A locus and their random distribution make the chance of finding an HL-A identical cadaver donor poor. Consequently the great majority of cadaver organ donors and recipients are HL-A incompatible and it is therefore necessary to suppress the natural immune defenses of the graft recipient.

Four main techniques of immune suppression are currently in use: (1) x-irradiation, (2) mechanical lymphoid cell depletion, (3) chemotherapy, and (4) treatment with antilymphocyte serum.

These are all nonspecific in that they constitute a frontal attack on the entire immune system and not on that limited number of specific immunocompetent cells engaged in recognizing and destroying the foreign tissue. Because of this nonspecificity, these techniques share common disadvantages of variable direct toxicity and severe reduction in host resistance to infection. In addition to these problems, they are usually unable to permanently eliminate graft rejection. There is thus an urgent need for an alternative, more specific means of inhibiting the host's immune response to the donor transplantation antigens.

Whole body irradiation of the host has been discarded as a means of immunosuppression because of its dangers but local irradiation of the graft can modestly prolong survival,[15] apparently by destroying "killer" lymphocytes attacking the graft and perhaps interfering with sensitization of circulating lymphocytes. Extracorporeal irradiation of the recipient's blood may also be useful in this regard.[29] Surgical removal of lymphoid organs has proven ineffective. Adult thymectomy, splenectomy, and lymphadenectomy produce no measurable effect in graft prolongation.

Chemical immunosuppression has been largely responsible for the present level of success of graft survival. Since the cells engaged in antibody snythesis and graft destruction divide and differentiate after contact with antigen, cancer chemotherapeutic agents which inhibit cell differentiation or division can effectively inhibit the immune response.[3] The basic drug in current use is azathioprine, an analogue of 6-mercaptopurine which is a purine antagonist disrupting nucleic acid synthesis. The polyfunctional alkylating agents are also effective and inhibit both differentiation and proliferation of cells through action on nucleic acids. These drugs comprise the nitrogen mustards, of which cyclophosphamide appears to be most effective. The corticosteroids are usually employed along with azathioprine in immunosuppressive regimens, and prednisone, the drug used most often, is especially effective in acute rejection crises. Although the mode of action of corticosteriod drugs is unclear, high doses can inhibit antibody synthesis both in vivo and in vitro. In addition corticosteroids are potent anti-inflammatory agents and this effect may be most important.

Antilymphocyte serum, used clinically, is an antiserum raised in a foreign species, usually the horse, against human lymphocytes. The biologic activity of such serum resides in the globulin fraction. Antilymphocyte globulin (ALG) is a general immunosuppressant. It has high specifity for lymphoid cells without the general cellular toxicity of drugs. It appears that ALG depresses both cellular hypersensitivity and antibody production and can markedly prolong the survival of skin allografts in experimental animals.[20] The mechanism of action of ALG is not known with certainty but inhibition or destruction of those lymphocytes responsible in initiating graft rejection is suggested.[16]

Since ALG is invariably used in conjunction with immunosuppressive drugs its clinical efficacy has been difficult to assess. It appears however, that ALG in conjunction with azathioprine has simplified the control of rejection in kidney transplantation, especially from related living donors.[25] Like the immunosuppressive drugs, ALG has significant adverse effects:[14] thrombocytopenia and febrile reactions are common. Most ALG preparations induce antibody formation against the foreign (e.g., horse) serum proteins they contain, and this raises the problems of anaphylaxis and serum sickness. Prolonged experimental use in animals has caused forms of glomerulonephritis. Perhaps most important, the natural immunologic defenses, particularly antiviral responses, are depressed, and a degree of susceptibility to infection analogous to that encountered with immunosuppressant drugs may be produced. There is mounting evidence, moreover, that the incidence of malignancies, particularly lymphomas, is higher among patients who have received ALG in conjunction with chemical immunosuppression.[24]

Experiences in the Transplantation of Different Organs

Allografting parenchymal organs in which rejection is a major obstacle is a relatively recent event in contrast to the long successful clinical use of bone and cornea. Extensive experience has accumulated in renal transplantation, and well over 3000 cases are recorded with the Kidney Transplant Registry.[2] Of these, approximately half involved kidneys removed from living related donors. A kidney transplant from an unrelated cadaver donor has a 40 per cent, 2 year success rate, but kidneys removed from matched related donors have a 2 year survival rate of up to 80 per cent, and kidneys exchanged between identical twins enjoy near permanent survival.[21] Failure of transplantation is due to rejection of the kidney consequent upon the antigenic disparity between host and recipient, or to opportunistic infection or the systemic toxicity of immunosuppressive chemotherapy. Current means of immunosuppression have been able to diminish the rejection reaction and even reverse ongoing acute rejection episodes, but chronic rejection damage of the grafted kidney has not been prevented.

Experience with liver grafts has been much less extensive. The liver is technically more difficult to transplant than the kidney and there is no routine method for assisting hepatic function from external sources, as there is for the kidney. Experience with heart and lung grafts has illustrated perhaps most forcefully the inadequacies of current immunosuppression, as survival is poor for both organs. The transplanted heart functions surprisingly well in the early postoperative period, responding to exercise and catecholamines, but rejection failure within several months is common, with a 6 per cent one year survival rate.[1] The reason for this accelerated rejection in comparison with the kidney experience is poorly understood. Organ-specific immune reactions against heart muscle or autosensitization of the recipient during the pre-existing heart disease have been raised as possibilities.

Wildevuur,[28] in a review of 23 lung transplants, underscores the difficulties with pulmonary allografting. Infection is a major obstacle in an exposed organ, and early functional adequacy of the transplanted lung has been difficult to achieve. The lung is very susceptible to hypoxic damage and during exchange the presence of a contralateral diseased lung with a fixed high vascular resistance may contribute to subnormal pulmonary function. For both the lung and heart there is again no means for long term extracorporeal support, and donor-recipient histocompatibility matching may be poor.

Bone marrow transplantation has posed specific difficulties owing to the fact that this organ is of the donor's immune system, thus capable of an immune attack against the recipient (graft-versus-host reaction). The fact that bone marrow is the prime source for stem cells able to replenish the haemopoietic as well as the lymphopoietic system, has led to efforts to isolate stem cells from their lymphoid contaminant before grafting. This possibility holds great potential in a variety of hematologic disorders and some immune deficiency diseases.

PROGNOSIS

Present restrictions on organ transplantation result from our inability to manipulate the immune response because of two main problems.

We are hampered not only by a limited knowledge of basic mechanisms of immunity but also by the inaccessability of the immune system, comprising a vast number of cells, each in a precise functional environment. However, research on various aspects of these problems is advancing at a rate which justifies optimism. Clearly the aim of our efforts is to abolish immune activity against the graft while maintaining full immunocompetence towards microorganisms and neoplasms. Let us now briefly explore the present state of basic research in immunology relevant to the hopes of the near future.

Immunologic Tolerance

SELF TOLERANCE. There is now good evidence that lymphoid cells have a limited life span and the immune system must be permanently replenished by bone marrow stem cells. This requires the continuous development of new immunocompetent cells and thus random mutation, implying that self-reactive cell clones are generated as part of the process, ensuring recognition of a large number of different antigens. The general lack of self reactivity is probably acquired by those lymphocytes which happen to carry recognition sites complementary to a self antigen. Although the actual mechanism of self tolerance induction is unknown, evidence suggests that it must occur before the relevant cells have reached complete immunocompetence.

This may best be illustrated by the following experiment (Fig. 2):[13] two groups of mice of strain A/A are lethally irradiated in order to destroy their entire lymphopoietic and hemopoietic tissue. The mice will die within a few days if we do not reconstitute them with bone marrow from the same strain A/A. Group I receives whole bone marrow consisting of stem cells as well as granulopoietic and lymphopoietic cells (including immunocompetent cells). Group II receives stem cells only (all other cells are removed by physical methods to be discussed later). At the same time transplantation is carried out of embryonic hearts from mouse strain B/B into the two groups of A/A mice. Such a graft is easily performed by the implantation of an embryonic heart into the subcutaneous tissue of the outer ear where it will become vascularized. Electrocardiograms are then recorded from all the grafted hearts in both groups at frequent intervals (Fig. 2).

As expected A/A recipients reconstituted with whole A/A bone marrow reject the B/B hearts owing to the presence of immunologically active lymphocytes in the reconstituting bone marrow. In contrast, the B/B hearts in A/A recipients, reconstituted with A/A bone marrow stem cells only, are permanently accepted as self. This clearly implies that tolerance was induced by the tiny heart graft at some time point during maturation of lymphoid cells from their stem cell ancestors. The question as to how this state of naturally acquired tolerance is induced remains a great challenge to immunologists. Its answer may well provide the future means for artificial tolerance induction in clinical organ transplantation.

EXPERIMENTALLY INDUCED TOLERANCE. Although still lacking fundamental knowledge about naturally occurring tolerance inducing mechanisms to self antigens, research on induction of tolerance for clinical application is concentrated on a phenomenon which we may call ex-

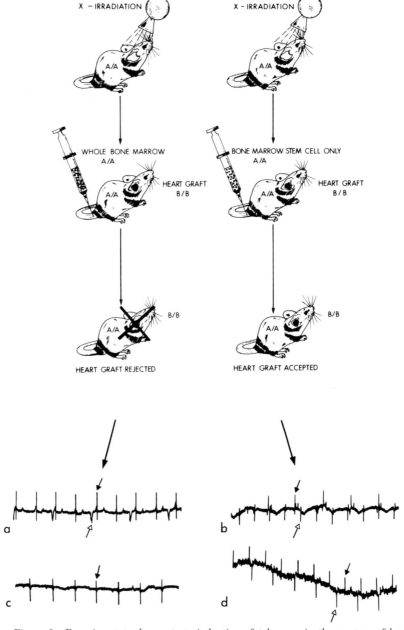

Figure 2. Experiment to demonstrate induction of tolerance in the progeny of bone marrow stem cells (for explanation see text). Electrocardiograms: open arrow = graft electrical activity; closed arrow = host's own heart. *a, b,* initial acceptance of graft showing rhythmic electrical activity; *c,* rejection of graft with cessation of rhythmical electrical activity; *d,* continued graft survival with no electrocardiographic evidence of rejection, 60 days following transplantation.

perimentally induced tolerance. Certain antigens, when injected in a specified amount into an experimental animal, may cause specific unresponsiveness upon subsequent attempts to immunize.

Ever since the early experiments by Smith and Bridges[23] it has been realized that two factors are of paramount importance in tolerance-induction: concentration and molecular structure of the antigen used. A direct analysis of these factors and of their relationship with tolerance-inducing mechanisms at the single cell level has become possible through models of tolerance-induction in the test tube.[5, 6] This has enabled us to analyze critically in a direct way the interaction between antigen molecules and the surface receptors of immunocompetent cells which eventually leads to tolerance. The data gained by work carried out over the last 3 years may be summarized as follows: (i) Tolerance results from direct interaction of immunocompetent cells with antigen molecules. (ii) This interaction involves the attachment of antigen molecules to recognition sites of immunocompetent cells. (iii) The conditions under which an immunocompetent cell is rendered immune or tolerant may be defined in terms of degree of interlinking of recognition sites by antigen.

Such interlinking, up to a critical threshold level, causes immunization, whereas beyond this threshold level it results in tolerance induction. Interlinking is best achieved by polymeric antigens which contain repetitive units to combine with the cell's antigen recognition sites.

These findings have now made it possible to transform monomeric nontolerance inducing antigens into polymeric tolerogens by either chemically induced polymerization or by creating linear *antigen-antibody complexes*. Clearly the aim of future research on tolerance induction is to chemically isolate tissue antigens (transplantation antigens) and modify them to become tolerogens. Should this prove possible we would be a great step closer to our goal, although still faced with the task of applying the *in vitro* model to the *in vivo* situation. Ideally one hopes for a situation in which the recipient of a graft would be made tolerant to the donor's antigens prior to transplantation.

Selective Depletion of Immunocompetence by Physical Means

Depletion of immunocompetence by various laboratory techniques has become one of the most promising developments in the field of bone marrow transplantation. This involves the removal of lymphoid cells from donor bone marrow prior to transplantation into a bone marrow-deficient recipient. This procedure is required because normal bone marrow is contaminated with immunocompetent cells which are capable of becoming immunologically active against the host, thus causing graft-versus-host disease.

As mentioned earlier, the cells remaining after bone marrow separation contain multipotential stem cells which can replenish the entire hemopoietic as well as the lymphopoietic system of the recipient. The lymphoid progeny of stem cells are expected to become tolerant of the host tissue in essentially the same way as happens in the developing fetus. To date the methods used to separate bone marrow stem cells are based on differences between different cell classes with respect to size and density.[19, 27] Other prospective methods make use of differences in the surface charge between cells. So far these methods, although successful in laboratory experiments, have yielded little success when applied to clinical purposes. There is however good reason to believe that further research in technology of cell separation will eventually yield positive results.

Deletion of Immunocompetence by Pharmacologic Means

Research in the use of pharmacologic agents to eliminate graft-versus-host responsive cells in bone marrow promises to become a major area of interest in bone marrow transplantation. The argument for drug use is as follows: immunocompetent cells in bone marrow can be stimulated by specific antigens or nonspecific mitogens such as PHA and concanavalin A. The consequent proliferation of responding cells renders them susceptible to pharmacologic attack by drugs which are incorporated into nucleic acids. The cellular toxicity of these drugs results in selective removal of cells responsive to a given stimulus.

In recent ingenious[22, 30] experiments both radioactive tritiated thymidine and 5 bromodeoxyuridine (BUdR) have been used to effectively remove stimulated lymphocytes from cell cultures. The incorporation of BUdR, a uridine analog, into DNA of dividing cells renders them light-sensitive so that cell death occurs upon exposure to light in the visible or near visible region.

It is likely that the more well known antineoplastic drugs such as 5 fluorouracil and cyclophosphamide can be added to stimulated lymphoid cell cultures to selectively remove cells which are responsive to antigens such as transplantation antigens. Such cultures, deprived of selected immunocompetent cells, should retain stem cell activity, because most of them are not in cycle and are thus unaffected by the drug. Transplantation of marrow cell cultures depleted of donor-responsive cells could thus circumvent the forbidding problem of graft-versus-host disease.

Immunologic Enhancement

Immunologic enhancement refers to the enhanced survival of histoincompatible grafts owing to the presence of humoral antibody directed against graft antigens. The mechanism whereby this antibody protects the graft is unclear, but experimentation in rats[9, 26] has convincingly demonstrated prolonged and even indefinite survival of incompatible kidney grafts in recipients treated with antigraft antiserum. Such antiserum may coat the graft and prevent recognition and attack or, alternately, may centrally depress the immune response. Enhancement requires further evaluation in other experimental animals and for other graft tissues but promises to be one specific means of immunosuppression. Knowing that multiparous women often contain antibodies directed against their husband's histocompatibility antigens, it may be possible to establish panels of enhancing antisera for specific HL-A specificities. If rat experimentation is valid the use of appropriate antisera directed toward known HL-A specificities could prove invaluable in selectively protecting grafts in clinical situations.

There are thus a number of ways in which we can experimentally modify antigenic responses and the possibilities will no doubt extend in the coming years as researchers unravel further the secrets of lymphoid function. That the intriguing mechanisms controlling participation of antigen, antibody, and lymphocyte in the immune response will be sufficiently understood as to permit manipulation in the clinical situation is one of the brightest horizons in modern biology.

REFERENCES

1. ACS/NIH Organ Transplant Registry, Chicago, Illinois. Quoted by J. Bergan in J. Thorac. Cardiovasc. Surg., 60:319, 1970.
2. Advisory Committee of the Human Kidney Transplant Registry: Seventh report of the Human Kidney Transplant Registry. Transplantation, 8:721–728, 1969.
3. Berenbaum, M. C.: Immunosuppressive agents and allogeneic transplantation. (Symposium on Tissue and Organ Transplantation.) J. Clin. Path., 20 (Suppl.): 471–498, 1967.
4. Burnet, F. M.: The Clonal Selection Theory of Acquired Immunity. Cambridge, Massachusetts, Vanderbilt University Press, 1959.
5. Diener, E., and Feldmann, M.: Relationship between antigen and antibody induced suppression of the immune response. Tranplant. Rev., in press.
6. Diener, E., Feldmann, M., and Armstrong, W. D.: Induction in vitro of immunological tolerance to the H-antigens of Salmonella adelaide. Ann. N.Y. Acad. Sci., 181:119, 1971.
7. Ford, C. E.: Traffic of lymphoid cells in the body In Wolstenholme, G. E. W., and Porter, R., eds.: The Thymus: Experimental and Clinical Studies. Ciba Foundation Symposium. London, Churchill, 1966, p. 131.
8. Ford, W. L., Gowans, J. L., and McCullagh, P. J.: The origin and function of lymphocytes. In Wolstenholme, G. E. W., and Porter, R. eds.: The Thymus. Experimental and clinical studies. Ciba Foundation Symposium. London, Churchill, 1966, p. 58.
9. French, M. E., and Batchelor, J. R.: Immunological enhancement of rat kidney grafts. Lancet, 2:1103, 1969.
10. Globerson, A.: In vitro studies on radiation lymphoid recovery of mouse spleen. J. Exper. Med., 123:25, 1966.
11. Gowans, J. L., and McGregor, D. D.: The immunological activities of lymphocytes. Prog. Allerg., 9:1, 1965.
12. Gowans, J. L., McGregor, D. D., Cowen, D. M., and Ford, C. E.: Initiation of immune responses by small lymphocytes. Nature, 196:651–655, 1962.
13. Jirsch, D., and Diener, E.: Unpublished data.
14. Kashiwagi, N.: Clinical reactions and serologic changes after adiministration of heterologous antilymphocyte globulin to human recipients of renal homografts. Ann. Intern Med., 68:275, 1968.
15. Kauffman, H. M. Jr., Cleveland, R. J., Divger, J. J., et al.: Prolongation of renal homograft function by local graft irradiation. Surg. Gynec. Obstet., 120:49–58, 1965.
16. Levey, R. H., and Medewar, P. B.: Nature and mode of action of antilymphocytic antiserum. Proc. Nat. Acad. Sci., U.S.A., 56:1130–1137, 1966.
17. Medawar, P. B.: Theories of immunological tolerance. In Ciba Foundation Symposium: Cellular Aspects of Immunity. London, Churchill, 1960, p. 134.
18. Micklem, H. S., Ford, C. E., Evans, E. P., and Gray, J.: Interrelationships of myeloid and lymphoid cells: Studies with chromosome-marked cells transfused into lethally irradiated mice. Proc. Roy. Soc. (Biol)., 165:78, 1966.
19. Miller, R. G., and Phillips, R. A.: Separation of cells by velocity sedimentation. J. Cell Physiol. 73:191, 1969.
20. Monaco, A. P., Wood, M. L., Gray, J. G., et al.: Studies on heterologous antilymphocyte serum in mice. II. Effect on the immune response. J. Immunol., 96:229–238, 1966.
21. Murray, J. E.: Sixth report of the human Kidney Transplant Registry. Transplantation, 6:944, 1968.
22. Salmon, S. E., Krakauer, R. S., and Whitmore, W. F.: Lymphocyte stimulation: selective destruction of cells during blastogenic response to tranplantation antigens. Science, 172:490, 1971.
23. Smith, R. J., and Bridges, R. A.: Immunological unresponsiveness in rabbits produced by neonatal injection of defined antigens. J. Exper. Med., 108:227, 1958.
24. Starzl, T. E., Porter, K. A., Andres, G., Halgrimson, C. G., Hurwitz, R., Giles, G., Terasaki, P. I., Penn, I., Schroter, G. T., Lilly, J., Starkie, S. J., and Putnam, G. W.: Long-term survival after renal transplantation in humans, with special reference to histocompatibility matching, thymectomy, homograft glomerulonephritis, heterologous ALG and recipient malignancy. Ann. Surg., 172:437–472, 1970.

25. Starzl, T. E., Porter, K. A., Twasaki, Y., et al.: The use of heterologous antilymphocyte globulin in human renal homo-transplantation. In Wolstenholme, G. E. W., ed.: Antilymphocyte Serum. (Ciba Foundation Study Group No. 29.) Boston, Little Brown and Company, 1967, pp. 4–40.
26. Stuart, R. F.: Rejection of renal allografts: specific immunologic suppression. Science, *160*:1463, 1968.
27. Turner, R. W. A., Siminovitch, L., McCullough, E. A., and Till, J. E.: Density gradient separation of hemopoietic colony forming cells. J. Cell Physiol., *69*:73, 1967.
28. Wildevuur, C. R. H., and Benfield, J. R.: A review of 23 human lung transplantations by 20 surgeons. Ann. Thorac. Surg., *9*:489–515, 1970.
29. Wolf, J. S., and Hune, D. M.: Prolongation of renal homograft survival by external radiation of renal arterial blood. Fed. Proc., *24*:573, 1965.
30. Zoschke, D. C., and Bach, F. H.: Specificity of allogeneic cell recognition by human lymphocytes in vitro. Science, *172*:1380, 1971.

Department of Pathology
University of Alberta
Edmonton, Alberta
Canada

Transfer of Immune Responsiveness

W. H. Marshall, M.D., Ph.D.[*]

The deliberate transfer of immune responsiveness is becoming commoner in medicine. There are three situations where transfers are used. Of particular interest are the *immunodeficiency diseases* where the aim of a transfer is to reconstitute the immune mechanism. Trials of transfer in these diseases are presently helping to throw light on the nature of the underlying deficiencies. In *infectious disease,* transfer has been used successfully to destroy an invading microorganism. Finally, the discovery that *tumors* may be antigenic to the host in which they are growing suggests that a powerful immune response against such antigens could be produced in the patient, perhaps by transfer, in order to eliminate the tumor.

There are alternative means of producing powerful immune responses that do not involve transfer of immunity; these are outside the scope of this paper. Such methods are direct immunization, the use of adjuvants, and the elimination of inhibitors of effective immune responses. Also outside its scope is a discussion of the transfer of immunity with serum antibody. The emphasis of this paper will be upon transfer of cells or cell extracts.

HISTORICAL DEVELOPMENT

Landsteiner and Chase in 1942[42] were the first to show that an immune response could be transferred with live lymphoid cells. They transferred contact sensitivity to simple chemicals in guinea pigs with viable lymphoid cells. The finding has since been confirmed in many species, including man, and with many different antigens.[14, 21]

The first demonstration of the transfer of transplantation immunity with lymphoid cells was made by Mitchison in 1954,[63] working with a transplantable tumor in mice. He coined the term "adoptive immunity" to describe this sort of transfer. In the same year, Harris et al.[36] reported the successful transfer, with lymphoid cells, of antibody-forming capability in rabbits.

---

[*]Professor of Immunology, Faculty of Medicine, Memorial University of Newfoundland, St. John's, Newfoundland, Canada

When Lawrence began performing experimental transfers of delayed hypersensitivity in man, he discovered in 1954[43, 44] that, contrary to expectation, delayed hypersensitivity could be transferred by killed or even disrupted cells. This curious finding and the subsequent work of Lawrence and others on this "transfer factor" is summarized below, and has been reviewed in detail elsewhere by Lawrence.[45, 46, 49, 50]

PROBLEMS ARISING FROM CELL TRANSFER

There are two major problems that can be encountered if live lymphoid cells are transferred from one individual to another. The transferred cells, being immunologically competent, may mount an immune response against the host; alternatively, the grafted cells may be rejected by the host's own immune mechanism.

Graft-Versus-Host Disease

If the host's rejection mechanisms are absent, as for example in congenital T-cell deficiency, then the grafted lymphoid cells will survive and may themselves undertake a rejection reaction, rejecting the host in which they reside. This "graft-versus-host" (GVH) reaction is often fatal.

The fact that grafted lymphoid cells can actually attack the host in which they reside has been recognized in experimental animals for more than a decade. The extensive literature has been concisely summarized by Billingham.[13] The requirements for production of a graft-versus-host reaction are that graft and host differ antigenically, that the grafted lymphocytes are not destroyed in the host, and that a sufficiently large dose of cells is grafted. An important point, emerging from a study in rodents of the requirement for antigenic difference, is that there must be a major histocompatibility antigen involved, that is to say, an H-2 locus difference in mice or an Ag-B locus difference in rats. It is impossible to produce a lethal graft-versus-host reaction if one transfers cells between animals who share the same major antigens. The single exception to this statement is when the grafted cells are taken from an animal that has already been sensitized to host antigens; such "primed" cells can, and do, mount a graft-versus-host reaction against minor histocompatibility antigens.

Graft-versus-host reactions are now being recognized in human beings,[62] but, as will be evident later, man appears to be different from laboratory rodents. Bone marrow cells grafted between subjects who are apparently identical at the presumed major histocompatibility locus, HL-A, have unfortunately caused fatal graft-versus-host disease. The alternative interpretation of this conflict between findings in man and animals, although radical at this late stage, is that the main HL-A antigens in man have not yet been demonstrated; this challenging proposition has come from Snell, one of the most experienced workers in the field.[78]

Destruction of the Grafted Cells

If grafted cells contain an antigen which is foreign to the host into which they have been grafted, they will usually be destroyed by the host immune response, a transplantation response. In the case of a free cell suspension, which in fact we are considering for the most part, there is the added hazard that serum antibody and complement may immediately destory the injected cells. Antibodies of this sort can easily be induced by prior transfusion or pregnancies.

Methods of Avoiding Unwanted Transplantation Reactions

The unwanted transplantation reactions – rejection of the graft and graft-versus-host disease – can be avoided in animal experiments by a number of strategies, and it is instructive to review some of them now so that the principles for solving similar problems in clinical situations become clear.

The transplantation response can be avoided completely, both for graft rejection and for graft-against-host reactions, if the animals are from the same inbred strain, that is to say, if there are no antigenic differences between the tissues of donor and recipient. In clinical practice as it stands today, a perfect match of this sort is found only between identical twins. However, the matching even of unrelated donor and recipient can, on rare occasions, be remarkably good.[29] Such matching is best achieved by a combination of serologic methods and the mixed leukocyte reaction.

Maneuvers that abolish the transplantation response can be listed in sequence according to the degree to which they achieve the specific result that is wanted. For example, whole-body X-irradiation and radiomimetic drugs are quite nonspecific. Corticosteroids spare many tissues but kill lymphocytes and depress inflammatory reactions. X-irradiation of the blood in an extracorporeal circuit,[20] on the other hand, will kill only blood cells and in so doing will sterilize the circulating lymphocytes. Cannulation of the thoracic duct with the formation of a chronic fistula is another way of getting rid of circulating lymphocytes;[54, 55] chronic local x-irradiation of the spleen does an even better job of destroying circulating lymphocytes.[31] Antilymphocyte serum destroys lymphocytes in both blood and tissues and, if the serum is monospecific, the other blood cells will be spared.[85] Finally, the induction of specific immunologic tolerance inactivates only those particular cells in the body which have the capability to respond to the antigen in question.

A completely different approach can be made with a specific "enhancing" antiserum.[11] Evidently, an appropriate serum against a transplantation antigen can hinder the access of lymphocytes to that antigen and thus prevent a transplantation response.

In experimental animals the above solutions can be used to overcome transplantation barriers, but in clinical medicine there are ethical problems as well since it is not easy to accept that a *donor* should be pretreated (although this has been done[59]) with drugs or antigen or x-irradiation, and so alternative methods have been sought. Cell separation by biophysical methods is presently being developed, the aim being to remove, from an inoculum, cells with unwanted activities. For example, potential graft-versus-host cells need to be removed if the inoculum is being injected into a patient with deficient cellular immunity.

It will be noted in the subsequent sections how much room there still is for improvements in cell transfer techniques simply by applying principles already well established in animal experimentation.

TRANSFER WITH SUBCELLULAR MATERIALS

Lawrence's transfer factor has the great advantage over inocula of live cells in that it will not produce graft-versus-host disease. However, the biological significance of transfer factor is still obscure and, as Burnet[19] recently wrote, the material poses "one of the outstanding conundrums of immunology." Since the original discovery that a state of sensitivity for delayed reactions could be transferred from one person to another with extracts of killed leukocytes, Lawrence has relentlessly repeated the experiment in a series of different systems, and has varied the experimental design in many ways, in order to meet the requests of his critics. However, because of the conceptual difficulties involved, it is likely that critics will remain until the chemical nature of transfer factor has been elucidated and its mechanism of action demonstrated.

Lawrence has performed transfers of sensitivity for a number of bacterial products, the prototype and the most easily transferred being tuberculin sensitivity; but, in spite of many years of careful work, the nature of the active material remains unknown. The reason for the delay is that there has been no laboratory animal in which transfer with disrupted cells can be achieved; in experiments in small laboratory mammals the cells must be alive for transfer to occur. Thus all analytical experiments have had to be made in human volunteers, and it is evident that if one uses tuberculin sensitivity, there will be rather few useful subjects (i.e., true tuberculin negative reactors) even in a large batch of volunteers. Whilst a biochemist might like to have a hundred tuberculin negative volunteers every week for assays, in practice it is usually possible to get negative subjects only in ones and twos.

So far as they have gone, experiments done to elucidate the chemical nature of transfer factor have simply added to the puzzle. For example, the material will pass through a dialysis membrane, which indicates that it has a molecular weight of less than 10,000, and in fact trials with chromatography suggest that it may be nearer to 5,000 M.W.[3, 9, 10, 47] This is very small for a specific "informational" molecule. Studies with enzymes have shown that transfer factor activity was not lost after incubation with either RNAse, DNAse, or trypsin. These treatments do not exclude the idea that transfer factor is low molecular weight double-stranded RNA; this appears to be the favorite hypothesis at present.

Lawrence has pursued the idea that transfer factor may be replicated within the body. In the first place, this could be suggested because the number of lysed leukocytes used for transfer is relatively small, the cells derived from 500 ml. of blood or less. This amount obviously represents only a tenth of the circulating blood and a very much smaller proportion of the total lymphoid tissue of the body, and yet this small amount of material converts the whole body of the recipient to a fair state of sensitivity. Lawrence has deliberately set out to find how long such a state of transferred sensitivity lasts, and in some cases of transfer of tuberculin sensitivity it lasted for the duration of the experiment, i.e., more than a year. This finding again points to the idea of self-replication. Finally, he has performed a few serial transfers to a third party and has been able to transfer tuberculin and streptococcal M substance sensitivities in this way.[45] Thus the concept of a small, highly specific, self-replicating molecule has gained ground. The only known molecules with the informational and replicating properties required are nucleic acids. In the case of transfer factor, the molecular weight is so small that only a few bases could be contained in each molecule, and that number would not be sufficient to dictate the required range of specificities, or any specificity for that matter if the conventional genetic code were employed for defining a conventional and complete antigen receptor site.

It is a curious finding that not all specificities are transferred with the same ease. There is in fact a rank order of antigens for the ease with which they are transferable. Tuberculin sensitivity is by far the easiest to transfer; in an intermediate category are diphtheria toxoid and streptococcal M substance sensitivity. Coccidioidin sensitivity is more difficult to transfer in spite of the fact that donors from endemic areas show very vigorous cutaneous reactions. In his study of transfer of coccidioidin sensitivity,[72] Lawrence only obtained regular success in transfer when he mixed equal quantities of positive transfer factor with coccidioidin itself. Such a maneuver looks suspiciously like immunization; however, Lawrence obtained evidence that the transfer factor did play a specific role, since, when he used truly negative transfer factor, there was no sensitization with a coccidioidin-transfer factor mixture. Homograft sensitivity similarly presented problems when Lawrence tried transfers after sensitizing a leukocyte donor with a skin graft.[48] He eventually found it was possible to transfer homograft sensitivity only by taking leukocytes from the donor during the process of rejection of the fourth of a series of skin grafts. Finally, when we come to consider contact chemical sensitivity in which prior skin testing of the recipient is excluded and which is a classic sensitivity transferable by cells in the guinea pig, it must be admitted that a serious attempt by Brandriss[16] to transfer this sensitivity in man, with dialysed transfer factor, showed absolutely no transfer. This result was despite successful concurrent transfer of tuberculin sensitivity to the test subjects with the same transfer factor preparation. Whether this represents a more "difficult" sensitivity to transfer or whether there is a qualitative difference is unknown; it is possible that, since the sensitivity is to a chemical sensitizer bound to tissue, there may be important antigenic differences between the tissue of the donor in whom the sensitivity was clearly demonstrable and the recipient who failed to show sensitivity. It is known that the "carrier" of a hapten has to be identical to that used for immunization for there to be demonstrable delayed hypersensitivity to a hapten-protein conjugate on cutaneous testing.

The present attack on the transfer factor problem is being carried on *in vitro*. For example, Baram and Condoulis[8] have been able to induce nonsensitized cells to behave as if they had been sensitized, by culturing them together with a lysate of sensitive cells; so far, though, they have had no positive results using the small molecular weight material prepared by dialysis. In Lawrence's laboratory, Valentine[82] had negative or minimally positive results in attempts to alter the reactivity of cultured lymphocytes by adding dialysable transfer factor, but he has now discovered that sensitive cells can release a material into the culture medium which in its action is tantalizingly like transfer factor. The experiment involves culturing sensitive leukocytes with antigen and then taking the culture medium and placing it in a fresh culture tube together with some lymphocytes which are known to be not sensitive to the antigen in question. These nonsensitive leukocytes are now found to respond to the antigen by growing into lymphoblasts which divide. Valentine has done the experiment in various ways to show that the response is both antigen dependent and antigen specific. Further analyses of this experiment are awaited with interest.

There is a whole branch of scientific literature devoted to the laboratory artifact of adding nucleic acids to cells of a certain genetic constitution and watching them perform differently under the influence of the added genetic information. Experiments of this sort involving immune systems have been reviewed in a symposium,[71] and it suffices to describe one recent experiment to indicate what can happen. Bell and Dray[12] took normal spleen cells from a rabbit and incubated them in the presence of RNA extracted from another rabbit spleen at the height of an immune response against sheep red blood cells. Presumably some of the RNA entered these normal spleen cells because a large number of antibody-forming cells appeared which were making antibody against sheep red cells. That the antibody synthesis had been directed by the donor RNA was neatly demonstrated by showing that the antibody was of the allotype appropriate to the donor spleen rather than to the normal spleen cells. Whether the donated RNA becomes transmitted to subsequent generations of cells is an open question, but the existence in transformed lymphocytes of an enzyme capable of making new DNA from an RNA template[70] would allow such a genetic transformation to occur.

It is sometimes argued that both the transfer factor experiments and the *in vitro* experiments with RNA are artifacts of the experimentalist and bear no relationship to biological reality. That may be, but from a therapeutic point of view a successfully transferred response is what is aimed at, no matter if it is an artificial or unnatural maneuver.

TREATMENT OF CONGENITAL IMMUNODEFICIENCY BY TRANSFER

If one excludes from this discussion defects of nonspecific immunity (e.g., complement or phagocytosis defects), one is left with congenital defects in specific immunity, of which there are three main groups: (1) agammaglobulinemia, (2) absence of specific cell-mediated immunity typified by the DiGeorge syndrome, and (3) combined deficiency where there is a lack both of immunoglobulins and of specific cell-mediated immunity. Agammaglobulinemia has been reasonably effectively treated with replacement injections of immunoglobulin,[51, 60] and there has been little justification for trials of cell transfer; this group of diseases will therefore receive no further mention, except to note that in one revealing case, a patient was treated with bone marrow transfusions from an identical twin, with no lasting restoration.[23] The treatment of the latter two syndromes has been primarily by transfer of immune responsiveness, and it is pertinent to review what has been achieved. At the end of this section the Wiskott-Aldrich syndrome will also be considered.

DiGeorge Syndrome

Attempts to treat the DiGeorge syndrome are recent and make an exciting story. In 1968, two cases were treated, both in the United States.

The Miami case[22] involved an infant who had had recurrent infections and diarrhea as well as a troublesome hypocalcemia. No thymic shadow was demonstrable even by pneumomediastinography. A fetal thymus was transplanted into the rectus abdominis muscle. By the next day the lymphocyte count had risen from 1300 to 5600. Subsequently it was found that dinitro-chlorobenzene (DNCB) sensitivity appeared spontaneously (earlier attempts at sensitization had failed) and "within a few weeks after the transplant, diarrhoea and rhinorrhoea ceased." The boy was observed for 18 months and remained restored and well.

The Boston case[5] was a typical case of DiGeorge syndrome with absence of thymus on x-ray, right-sided aortic arch. and other anomalies. In this patient, as in the Miami case, DNCB sensitivity and other delayed sensitivities appeared spontaneously after transplantation of a thymus from a 16-week fetus. The lymphocyte responses to phytohemagglutinin (PHA) were studied extensively; there was a minimal response before transplantation, which was restored to normal 4 days after transplantation. Of great interest was the finding, by use of the sex chromosome marker, that the cells responding to PHA were the patient's own; in some fashion, possibly hormonal, the thymus transplant had endowed his own lymphocytes with the ability to respond to PHA. This patient, too, has been followed for over a year and remains well and fully restored.[4]

Combined Immunodeficiency

Treatment of this malignant condition has proved to be difficult, and it is interesting to review chronologically the published attempts, since they show the way in which ideas have developed.

A patient was treated in Boston by thymic transplant as early as 1962,[74] only a year after the first description of the effect of neonatal thymectomy in mice. A piece of thymus from a 5 month old child, obtained during a heart operation, was transplanted but without any effect. In 1965 Swiss workers[37] treated two patients by transplantation of fetal thymus. The results in one patient showed that such a transplant could survive, since healthy thymus was later found at necropsy after two thymuses and some fetal bone marrow cells had been administered without effect. The second patient had a total of 11 fetal thymuses transplanted and on one occasion some fetal liver cells. The fetal liver injection was followed by restoration of the blood lymphocyte count, but DNCB sensitization was not possible, the cells failed to respond in culture to PHA, and the patient died at 6 months of age.

In 1966 a group in Oslo[35] transplanted a thymus from a 16 week old fetus. A monoclonal gammopathy developed in the patient subsequently, and this protein was thought, from Gm typing, to have originated from cells of the donor and not of the patient. However, the patient became ill with an erythematous rash and died. The French experience with thymus transplantation in one case was equally disappointing.[56]

In 1966 and 1967, 2 patients in the United States were given injections of maternal bone marrow cells. One child[62] developed a fulminant graft-against-host syndrome (which was beginning to be recognized by this time) and died. The other child's[75] lymphocyte count rose 1 week after transplantation, with more than half of the cells being of infant origin as shown by sex chromosome analysis. Furthermore, the child developed a cutaneous sensitivity to Monilia antigen. However, the patient died some 13 days after transplantation, from multiple causes, including infection.

In 1968 a similar case was reported from Minnesota.[39] The infant was given fetal thymus and liver cells plus a transfusion of fresh maternal blood. Within days there was evidence of immunologic restoration, but this was shortly followed by a recognizable graft-versus-host syndrome, and the patient died.

It was evident from these cases of graft-versus-host disease that better histocompatibility matching would be needed, and it was hoped that a complete match at the main locus (HL-A) would be sufficient[38] (see above). HL-A-compatible siblings were considered to be the most promising sources of compatible bone marrow.

In 1969, after 7 years of failures, there were at last sporadic successes. A patient was treated in Minnesota[61] by sibling bone marrow and was apparently restored by a second marrow transplant after the first had induced a state of aplastic anemia. A patient was treated in Holland[26] with HL-A-compatible sibling bone marrow; however, the Dutch workers introduced a further modification in the procedure, namely, the "purification" of the bone marrow cell suspension on a density gradient to remove the majority of graft-versus-host cells. The patient had a mild graft-versus-host reaction with a morbilliform rash but ultimately did well. Two further patients have been treated; in one[41] a bone marrow transplant from a sibling caused a fatal graft-versus-host reaction; the other was treated by The Ontario Cancer Institute group,[1] who attempted to remove graft-versus-host cells by a cell separation method involving differential sedimentation. While there was no restoration of the defect in the Canadian patient, there was no graft-versus-host disease either.

An atypical case of combined deficiency was recently managed[2] successfully with two marrow transplants from an HL-A identical sibling. A delayed graft-versus-host reaction resolved spontaneously, and the child has done well for a year.

The occurrence of graft-versus-host reaction, even with bone marrow grafts from HL-A compatible siblings, encouraged further trials of fetal liver cells but these have met with no success.[33, 34]

Another interesting approach is mentioned in a recent World Health Organization report;[83] in 2 patients an enhancing antiserum was injected into the bone marrow recipient in order to prevent the grafted cells from mounting a graft-versus-host response, the idea being that the antibody conceals the host's transplantation antigens.

Thus, at the time of writing, despite many years of unfruitful experiment, the outlook is now good. Several patients have evidently been cured with bone marrow transplants, and we can expect that further technical refinements will soon allow many more persons to be cured.

The Wiskott-Aldrich Syndrome

This syndrome is characterized by eczema, thrombocytopenia, and recurrent infections. Both bone marrow transplantation and injections of Lawrence's transfer factor have been tried in order to correct this condition. Bach et al.[7] gave HL-A compatible marrow from a sibling and apparently effected both a cure and the establishment of a chimeric state as regards the blood cells. The patient's eczema cleared, infections regressed, and the platelet count rose from about 7500 per cu. mm. to around 17,500, and he has apparently remained well for nearly 2 years.[6]

An interesting approach was that of Levin and Spitler and their colleagues,[52, 53, 79] who prepared transfer factor from healthy individuals and injected it into patients with this syndrome. In 3 out of 5 cases there was marked improvement in the clinical state although the platelet counts were not dramatically altered. In the remaining 2 patients there was no response. Further trials of this safe and simple form of treatment are awaited with interest.

TREATMENT OF INFECTIOUS DISEASE BY TRANSFER

When an infection overwhelms an individual there is, almost by definition, an immunologic deficit in the sense that the immune response is inadequate to the task of destroying the infectious agent. Thus the consideration of infections as separate from immune deficiency states is somewhat artificial; however, there are several well documented instances where transfer of immunity has been used in the treatment of specific infections, so that is is convenient to consider these separately. It is probable that the use of cell transfer to overcome troublesome infections is commoner than the literature would suggest, since many instances of leukocyte transfusions may go unreported. For example, an overwhelming infection with varicella virus in a patient with leukemia or lymphoma can sometimes be cured by giving the patient a transfusion of blood leukocytes or bone marrow from a healthly individual – preferably, of course, one who has recently emerged from the convalescent period after an attack of chicken pox.

Generalized Vaccinia

Kempe[40] has reported a dramatic case in which generalized vaccinia occurred in a child following smallpox vaccination and progressed to the lethal stage termed vaccinia necrosum. There was no improvement after huge doses of hyperimmune globulin, and the child's arm eventually needed amputation. The generalized infection continued unabated until buffy coat leukocytes from three recently vaccinated adult donors were injected locally round the amputation site and the cells from three lymph nodes from similar donors were given intravenously and a further three lymph nodes were implanted in the rectus abdominis muscle. Kempe amply documents the regression of the infection and reports that there was no recurrence during the succeeding year.

O'Connell et al.[67] treated an elderly lady with progressive vaccinia which involved skin and mucous membranes. After other measures, including immune globulin, had failed, they gave her an injection of washed leukocytes from 250 ml. of blood obtained from a recently vaccinated donor. This transfer was apparently responsible for regression of the lesions and return of the patient to good health. A recurrence of one lesion on the foot occurred a month later, and was treated with a second injection of washed leukocytes with the same gratifying result—a huge ulcer healed almost completely in a matter of 2 weeks.

Chronic Mucocutaneous Candidiasis

This condition may be found in clearly defined immunodeficiency states such as the DiGeorge syndrome, but in many cases the nature of the underlying defect is obscure and there may be a group of different defects. The treatment for the most part remains empirical and experimental. Some success with cell transfer has been described, and attempts have been made to treat this condition with leukocyte extracts.

Buckley et al.[17] treated a 10 year old patient who had had the condition all her life. All other treatments having failed, they gave her a transfusion of bone marrow cells from her father. The result was impressive, with clearance of the candida infection and a growth spurt raising her from the third percentile to between the tenth and twenty-fifth percentiles, and she remained well for over a year.

Attempts have been made to use transfer factor, but the clinical results have been mixed. Rocklin et al.[73] gave dialysable transfer factor and showed that there was a temporary conversion of the delayed skin reaction to candida, and the patient's lymphocytes responded to the antigen in vitro by producing migration inhibition factor (MIF) but the infection did not improve. Another patient[57] was given dialysable transfer factor from very sensitive donors on 5 separate occasions, but there was no clinical improvement and no conversion of his negative skin test even after a final injection of whole leukocyte lysate. Spitler et al.,[80] on the other hand, have treated 3 patients and found clinical improvement in all of them, although extensive testing of lymphocytes before and after transfer failed to show any consistent defects or changes resulting from treatment. Similarly Schulkind et al.[77] found transfer factor to be beneficial in their patient.

Leprosy

The prognosis of leprosy is considerably better when the patient shows delayed hypersensitivity to lepromin than when such hypersensitivity is absent. It was therefore suggested[28] that transfer of immunity might be good treatment. De Bonaparte et al.[25] were able to convert 5 of 13 lepromatous patients to a sensitive state by transfer of leukocytes from positive reactors. Similarly transfer has been achieved with transfer factor.[18] In neither case is it yet possible to state whether the clinical course of the patients was significantly improved.

TREATMENT OF TUMORS BY TRANSFER

Immunotherapy of cancer, which includes the transfer of immune responsiveness as one of its techniques, acquired a sound theoretical basis once it was recognized that tumors may contain antigens not present in the host and that there may be evidence of an immune response in the host directed against the tumor. It was realized that this response could, potentially at any rate, destroy the tumor.

Methods of immunotherapy other than by transfer have been reviewed elsewhere.[30, 59, 64, 68]

The use of transfer in the treatment of human cancer is in an early stage, but there is every reason to believe that the initial approach can be refined. In general, there have been two approaches: (1) transfer normal lymphoid cells (or cell products) in the hope that these might mount an attack on the tumor; (2) remove tumor cells and use them to immunize either an animal or another human in order to obtain "immune" lymphoid cells which can then be transferred to the patient.

Transfer of Normal Cells

The pioneers of this method were Woodruff and Nolan,[86] who injected large numbers of normal spleen cells into patients with advanced or terminal cancer. The spleens were obtained from the operating room, having been removed for a variety of reasons, and were reduced to cell suspensions for intravenous or intraperitoneal injection. Despite the advanced stage of disease and despite the fact that there was no prior exposure of the spleen cells to tumor antigens, there was in every case some evidence suggestive of a temporary attack on the tumor. For example, cutaneous metastases became inflamed and partly necrotic, and in the case of peritoneal metastases there was a temporary regression in the rate of ascites formation. The authors suggested that the grafted cells had become sensitized to the tumor and had produced a destructive "graft-against-tumor" response.

Other workers have continued these experiments,[81] with the modification that they used spleen cells which had been stored frozen. Their results were essentially similar to the earlier work, but the authors were more impressed with results obtained using immunized pig lymphocytes (see below).

Mathé and his group[59] have tried inducing graft-against-tumor effects in the treatment of acute leukemia. They took 21 patients and gave them transfusions of large numbers of leukocytes from patients with chronic myeloid leukemia. They report obtaining remissions in 9 of the patients and, in 5, these were described as "complete." Subsequent attempts to produce the same remissions using vast numbers of lymphocytes from healthy volunteers were disappointing. The authors suggested that there was something particularly beneficial in the use of chronic myeloid leukemia cells for such transfusions.

Immunization of the Leukocyte Donor

Using Human Beings. Nadler and Moore[66] took pairs of patients with malignant tumors and immunized each member with a piece of the other's tumor. After about 5 days, leukocyte transfers were begun. The cells from 500 ml. blood of each member of the pair were removed and were injected into the other member of the pair, and this process was repeated daily for 3 weeks. In their series of 85 patients, 53 were considered suitable for inclusion in the final analysis of results. Of these 13 had clear objective evidence of improvement and two remarkable patients were apparently cleared completely of their disease.

Other groups are preparing to perform similar trials; for example, a group in Texas[24] has completed preliminary baseline experiments to establish satisfactory transfer routines.

USING ANIMALS. Symes et al.[81] immunized pigs with tumor biopsy material and then, at the height of a presumed immune response, removed all the draining lymph nodes and made from them a lymphocyte suspension. The cells were then injected into the patient. In the 2 patients who received this therapy, there was apparently a striking improvement which lasted 4 to 6 weeks, but ultimately both patients died of their disease.

Use of Subcellular Materials

Two trials have recently been made in the use of transfer factor for tumor immunotherapy. Brandes et al.[15] used the cross-immunization design of Nadler and Moore in 2 patients with advanced malignant melanoma, and transfer factor was exchanged between members of the pair. Significant but temporary improvement was reported. A group in New York[69] have used transfer factor from healthy middle-aged women to treat breast cancer, arguing that breast cancers are likely to arise in many women and be eliminated by an immune response in most of them. Thus anti-tumor activity could be predicted to occur in such transfer factor preparations. In 1 of their 5 patients, the progress of the disease was halted for 6 months.

POSSIBLE FUTURE TRENDS

Removal of Cells of Certain Specificities

Cell separation by biophysical methods exploits differences in cell size and cell density, but neither of these is in any sense immunologically specific. There are, however, ways of separating cells on the basis of immunologic specificity; for example, Wigzell[84] has devised *antigen-loaded columns*. He attaches an antigen to a filter material in a column and then runs a cell suspension slowly through the column and finds that cells with specific receptors for the antigen adhere to the column and can be removed from the rest of the suspension. Hopefully transplantation antigens will one day be used in this way to remove cells with a certain transplantation response capability.

Another way to remove specific cells is to use the *"hot pulse" method* devised by Dutton.[27] Here the object is to stimulate a cell suspension with an antigen and then, when specifically reactive cells have responded by starting to divide, a large dose of tritiated thymidine is added to the culture. The dividing cells will then take up a disabling or even lethal dose of radioactivity. In fact, a first attempt to use this method in a clinical situation has been briefly reported.[76] One can visualize other modifications of this general approach, for example, the large dividing cells might be separated from the rest of the suspension by a biophysical method; this, indeed, has already been done in mice by Dutton.[27]

Enriching for a Certain Specificity

In the treatment of infectious disease or tumors, one needs a large number of cells possessing one particular specificity. Since it is known that antigen-stimulated cells can form quite large clones *in vitro* by repeated division,[58] it may be possible by careful tissue culture to grow vast numbers of cells with the single required specificity and then return them to the patient. Certainly the technology has now been developed for growing phenomenal numbers of cells in culture,[65] and indeed cultured leukocytes have been found to produce an occasional cell line which divides continuously. The specific reactivity, if any, of these lines is unknown, but attempts have been made to stimulate such a line with tumor antigen before returning the cells to the patient.[65] The ineffectiveness of this treatment was presumably because the tumor antigens failed, at that late stage, to direct the immunologic activity of the cell line.

SUMMARY

It is possible to transfer immune responsiveness with cells of the lymphatic system and, in certain cases, with RNA or other material extracted from the lymphoid cells (Lawrence's transfer factor). The hazard of graft-versus-host disease is avoided if cell extracts are used, but the potency of extracts may be less than that of live cells in some cases.

In *immunodeficiency disease*, (1) thymus transplantation has been used successfully to reconstitute two patients with the DiGeorge syndrome, (2) recent developments in bone marrow transplantation are improving the outlook for treatment of the combined immunodeficiency syndrome, and (3) the Wiskott-Aldrich syndrome has been ameliorated with bone marrow cells and with transfer factor. In *infectious disease*, transfer of immunity has been valuable in progressive vaccinia, in some cases of mucocutaneous candidiasis, and it has been possible to convert lepromin negative lepers to a lepromin positive state. *Cancer immunotherapy* by cell transfer is in its early stages, but even so the results are encouraging, and there have been two cases where complete disappearance of malignant melanoma was associated with cell transfer.

Future trends will involve treatment of inocula of cells to remove cells with unwanted specificities and to enrich for cells of the required specificity.

REFERENCES

1. Amato, D., Bergsagel, D. E., Clarysse, A. M., Cowan, D. H., Iscove, N. N., McCulloch, E. A., Miller, R. G., Phillips, R. A., Ragab, A. H., and Senn, J. S.: Review of bone marrow transplants at the Ontario Cancer Institute. Transplant. Proc., 3:397–399, 1971.
2. Ammann, A. J., Meuwissen, H. J., Good, R. A., and Hong, R.: Successful bone marrow transplantation in a patient with humoral and cellular immunity deficiency. Clin. Exper. Immunol., 7:343–353, 1970.

3. Arala-Chaves, M. P., Lebacq, E. G., and Heremans, J. F.: Fraction of human leukocyte extracts transferring delayed hypersensitivity to tuberculin. Int. Arch. Allergy, 31:353–365, 1967.
4. August, C. S., Berkel, A. I., Levey, R. H., Rosen, F. S., and Kay, H. E. M.: Establishment of immunological competence in a child with congenital thymic aplasia by a graft of fetal thymus. Lancet, 1:1080–1083, 1970.
5. August, C. S., Rosen, F. S., Filler, R. M., Janeway, C. A., Markowski, B., and Kay, H. E. M.: Implantation of a foetal thymus, restoring immunological competence in a patient with thymic aplasia. Lancet, 2:1210–1211, 1968.
6. Bach, F. H.: Personal communication, cited by Levin et al.[52]
7. Bach, F. H., Albertini, R. J., Anderson, J. L., Joo, P., and Bortin, M. M.: Bone-marrow transplantation in a patient with the Wiskott-Aldrich syndrome. Lancet, 2:1364–1366, 1968.
8. Baram, P., and Condoulis, W.: Transfer of delayed hypersensitivity to rhesus monkey and human lymphocytes with transfer factor obtained from rhesus monkey peripheral white blood cells. J. Immunol., 104:769–779, 1970.
9. Baram, P., and Mosko, M. M.: A dialysable fraction from tuberculin-sensitive human white blood cells capable of inducing tuberculin-delayed sensitivity in negative recipients. Immunology, 8:461–474, 1965.
10. Baram, P., Yuan, L., and Mosko, M. M.: Studies on the transfer of human delayed-type hypersensitivity. I. Partial purification and characterization of two active components. J. Immunol., 97:407–420, 1966.
11. Batchelor, J. R., Ellis, F., French, M. E., Bewick, M., Cameron, J. S., and Ogg, C. S.: Immunological enhancement of human kidney graft. Lancet, 2:1007–1010, 1970.
12. Bell, C., and Dray, S.: Conversion of non-immune spleen cells by ribonucleic acid of lymphoid cells from an immunized rabbit to produce γy-M antibody of foreign light chain allotype. J. Immunol., 103:1196–1211, 1969.
13. Billingham, R. E.: The biology of graft-versus-host reactions. In Harvey Lectures, Series 62, 1966–1967. New York, Academic Press, 1968, pp. 21–78.
14. Bloom, B. R., and Chase, M. W.: Transfer of delayed-type hypersensitivity: A critical review and experimental study in the guinea pig. In Kallós, P., and Waksman, B. H., eds.: Progress in Allergy. Basel and New York, S. Karger, 1967, vol. X, pp. 151–255.
15. Brandes, L. J., Galton, D. A. G., and Wiltshaw, E.: New approach to immunotherapy of melanoma. Lancet, 2:293–295, 1971.
16. Brandriss, M. W.: Attempt to transfer contact hypersensitivity in man with dialysate of peripheral leukocytes. J. Clin. Invest., 47:2152–2157, 1968.
17. Buckley, R. H., Lucas, Z. J., Hattler, B. G., Jr., Zmijewski, C. M., and Amos, D. B.: Defective cellular immunity associated with chronic mucocutaneous moniliasis and recurrent staphylococcal botryomycosis: Immunological reconstitution by allogeneic bone marrow. Clin. Exper. Immunol., 3:153–169, 1968.
18. Bullock, W. E., Fields, J., and Brandriss, M.: Transfer factor therapy in lepromatous leprosy: An evaluation. J. Clin. Invest., 50:16a, 1971.
19. Burnet, M.: In Cellular Immunology. Carlton, Australia, and Great Britain, Melbourne University Press and Cambridge University Press, 1969, book 1, p. 254.
20. Chanana, A. D., Brecher, G., Cronkite, E. P., Joel, D., and Schnappauf, H.: The influence of extracorporeal irradiation of the blood and lymph on skin homograft rejection. Radiat. Res., 27:330–346, 1966.
21. Chase, M. W.: Delayed sensitivity. Med. Clin. N. Amer., 49:1613–1646, 1965.
22. Cleveland, W. W., Fogel, B. J., Brown, W. T., and Kay, H. E. M.: Foetal thymic transplant in a case of DiGeorge's syndrome. Lancet, 2:1211–1214, 1968.
23. Cruchaud, A., Girard, J.-P., Kapanci, Y., Laperrouza, C., Mégevand, R., and Schwarzenberg, L.: Agammaglobulinémie chez un seul de deux jumeaux univitellins: Description et tentatives thérapeutiques par transfusion de cellules immunocompétentes isologues. Rev. Franç. Clin. Biol., 13:245–257, 1968.
24. Curtis, J. E., Hersh, E. M., and Freireich, E. J.: Antigen-specific immunity in recipients of leukocyte transfusions from immune donors. Cancer Res., 30:2921–2929, 1970.
25. DeBonaparte, Y., Morgenfeld, M. C., and Paradisi, E. R.: Immunology of leprosy. New Eng. J. Med., 279:49, 1968.
26. DeKoning, J., van Bekkum, B. W., Dicke, K. A., Dooren, L. J., van Rood, J. J., and Rádl, J.: Transplantation of bone-marrow cells and fetal thymus in an infant with lymphopenic immunological deficiency. Lancet, 1:1223–1227, 1969.
27. Dutton, R. W., and Mishell, R. I.: Cellular events in the immune response. The in vitro response of normal spleen cells to erythrocyte antigens. Cold Spring Harbor Symposium Quant. Biol., 32:407–414, 1967.
28. Editorial: Transfer factor and leprosy. New Eng. J. Med., 278:333, 1968.
29. Eijsvoogel, V. P., Schellekens, P. T. A., Breur-Vriesendorp, B., Koning, L., Koch, C., van Leeuwen, A., and van Rood, J. J.: Mixed lymphocyte cultures and HL-A. Transplant. Proc., 3:85–88, 1971.
30. Fairley, G. H.: Immunity to malignant disease in man. In The Scientific Basis of Medicine Annual Reviews. London, Athlone Press, 1971, pp. 17–38.

31. Ford, W. L.: The mechanism of lymphopenia produced by chronic irradiation of the rat spleen. Brit. J. Exper. Path., 49:502–510, 1968.
32. Gatti, R. A., Meuwissen, H. J., Allen, H. D., Hong, R., and Good, R. A.: Immunological reconstitution of sex-linked lymphopenic immunological deficiency. Lancet, 2:1366–1369, 1968.
33. Gatti, R. A., Platt, N., Pomerance, H. H., Hong, R., Langer, L. O., Kay, H. E. M., and Good, R. A.: Hereditary lymphopenic agammaglobulinemia associated with a distinctive form of short-limbed dwarfism and ectodermal dysplasia. J. Pediat., 75:675–684, 1969.
34 Githens, J. H., Muschenheim, F., Fulginiti, V. A., Robinson, A., and Kay, H. E. M.: Thymic alymphoplasia with XX/XY lymphoid chimerism secondary to probable maternal-fetal transfusion. J. Pediat., 75:87–94, 1969.
35. Harboe, M., Pande, H., Brandtzaeg, P., Tveter, K. J., and Hjort, P. F.: Synthesis of donor type G-globulin following thymus transplantation in hypo-globulinaemia with severe lymphocytopenia. Scand. J. Haemat., 3:351–374, 1966.
36. Harris, S., Harris, T. N., and Farber, M. B.: Studies on the transfer of lymph node cells. I. Appearance of antibody in recipients of cells from donor rabbits injected with antigen. J. Immunol., 72:148–160, 1954.
37. Hitzig, W. H., Kay, H. E. M., and Cottier, H.: Familial lymphopenia with agammaglobulinaemia: An attempt at treatment by implantation of foetal thymus. Lancet, 2:151–154, 1965.
38. Hong, R., Gatti, R. A., and Good, R. A.: Hazards and potential benefits of blood-transfusion in immunological deficiency. Lancet, 2:388–389, 1968.
39. Hong, R., Kay, H. E. M., Cooper, M. D., Meuwissen, H., Allan, M. J. G., and Good, R. A.: Immunological restitution in lymphopenic immunological deficiency syndrome. Lancet, 1:503–506, 1968.
40. Kempe, C. H.: Studies on smallpox and complications of smallpox vaccination. Pediatrics, 26:176–189, 1960.
41. Kretschmer, R., Jeannet, M., Mereu, T. R., Kretschmer, K., Winn, H., and Rosen, F. S.: Hereditary thymic dysplasia: A graft-versus-host reaction induced by bone marrow cells with a partial 4a series histoincompatibility. Pediat. Res., 3:34–40, 1969.
42. Landsteiner, K., and Chase, M. W.: Experiments on transfer of cutaneous sensitivity to simple chemical compounds. Proc. Soc. Exper. Biol., New York, 49:688–690, 1942.
43. Lawrence, H. S.: The transfer of generalized cutaneous hypersensitivity of the delayed tuberculin type in man by means of the constituents of disrupted leucocytes. J. Clin. Invest., 33:951–952, 1954.
44. Lawrence, H. S.: The transfer in humans of delayed skin sensitivity to streptococcal M substance and to tuberculin with disrupted leucocytes. J. Clin. Invest., 34:219–230, 1955.
45. Lawrence, H. S.: Transfer factor. Adv. Immunol., 11:195–266, 1969.
46. Lawrence, H. S.: Transfer factor and cellular immune deficiency disease. New Eng. J. Med., 283:411–419, 1970.
47. Lawrence, H. S., Al-Askari, S., David, J., Franklin, E. C., and Zweiman, B.: Transfer of immunological information in humans with dialysates of leucocyte extracts. Trans. Assoc. Amer. Phys., 76:84–91, 1963.
48. Lawrence, H. S., Rapaport, F. T., Converse, J. M., and Tillett, W. S.: Transfer of delayed hypersensitivity to skin homografts with leukocyte extracts in man. J. Clin. Invest., 39:185–198, 1960.
49. Lawrence, H. S., and Valentine, F. T.: Transfer factor and other mediators of cellular immunity. Amer. J. Path., 60:437–451, 1970.
50. Lawrence, H. S., and Valentine, F. T.: Transfer factor in delayed hypersensitivity. Ann. N.Y. Acad. Sci., 169:269–280, 1970.
51. Leading Article: Variable immunodeficiency. Lancet, 1:959–960, 1971.
52. Levin, A. S., Spitler, L. E., Stites, D. P., and Fudenberg, H. H.: Wiskott-Aldrich syndrome, a genetically determined cellular immunologic deficiency: Clinical and laboratory responses to therapy with transfer factor. Proc. Nat. Acad. Sci., 67:821–828, 1970.
53. Levin, A. S., Spitler, L. E., Stites, D. P., and Fudenberg, H. H.: Molecular intervention in genetically determined cellular immune deficiency disorders. J. Clin. Invest., 50:59a, Abstr. 196, 1971.
54. McGregor, D. D., and Gowans, J. L.: The antibody response of rats depleted of lymphocytes by chronic drainage from the thoracic duct. J. Exper. Med., 117:303–320, 1963.
55. McGregor, D. D., and Gowans, J. L.: Survival of homografts of skin in rats depleted of lymphocytes by chronic drainage from the thoracic duct. Lancet, 1:629–632, 1964.
56. Marie, J., Hennequet, A., Jarlier, H., Cloup, M., Watchi, J.-M., and Allaneau, C.: Alymphocytose congénitale. Greffe thymique le 28ᵉ. Jour. Ann. Pediat., Paris, 13:804–811, 1968.
57. Marshall, W. H., and Darte, J. M. M.: Unpublished observations, 1971.
58. Marshall, W. H., Valentine, F. T., and Lawrence, H. S.: Cellular immunity in vitro. J. Exper. Med., 130:327–343, 1969.
59. Mathé, G.: Approaches to the immunological treatment of cancer in man. Brit. Med. J., 4:7–10, 1969.

60. Medical Research Council Special Report Series No. 310: Hypogammaglobulinaemia in the United Kingdom. London, Her Majesty's Stationery Office, 1971.
61. Meuwissen, H. J., Gatti, R. A., Terasaki, P. I., Hong, R., and Good, R. A.: Treatment of lymphopenic hypogammaglobulinemia and bone-marrow aplasia by transplantation of allogeneic marrow: Crucial role of histocompatibility matching. New Eng. J. Med., 281:691–697, 1969.
62. Miller, M. E.: Thymic dysplasia ("Swiss Agammaglobulinemia"). I. Graft versus host reaction following bone-marrow transfusion. J. Pediat., 70:730–736, 1967.
63. Mitchison, N. A.: Passive transfer of transplantation immunity. Proc. Roy. Soc., B, 142:72–87, 1954.
64. Mitchison, N. A.: Immunologic approaches to cancer. Transplant. Proc., 2:92–103, 1970.
65. Moore, G. E., and Moore, M. B.: Auto-inoculation of cultured human lymphocytes in malignant melanoma. N.Y. State J. Med., 69:460–462, 1969.
66. Nadler, S. H., and Moore, G. E.: Immunotherapy of malignant disease. Arch. Surg., 99:376–381, 1969.
67. O'Connell, C. J., Karzon, D. T., Barron, A. L., Plaut, M. E., and Ali, V. M.: Progressive vaccinia with normal antibodies: A case possibly due to deficient cellular immunity. Ann. Intern. Med., 60:282–289, 1963.
68. Oettgen, H. F., Old, L. J., and Boyse, E. A.: Human tumor immunology. Symposium on Medical Aspects of Cancer. Med. Clin. N. Amer., 55:761–785, 1971.
69. Oettgen, H., Old, L., Farrow, J., Valentine, F., Lawrence, S., and Thomas, L.: Effects of transfer factor in cancer patients. J. Clin. Invest., 50:71a, Abstr. 239, 1971.
70. Penner, P. E., Cohen, L. H., and Loeb, L. A.: RNA-dependent DNA polymerase in human lymphocytes during gene activation by phytohemagglutinin. Nat. New Biol., 232:58–60, 1971.
71. Plescia, O. J., and Braun, W., eds. Nucleic Acids in Immunology. Proceedings of a Symposium held at the Institute of Microbiology of Rutgers, The State University. New York, Springer Verlag, 1968.
72. Rapaport, F. T., Lawrence, H. S., Millar, J. W., Pappagianis, D., and Smith, C. E.: Transfer of delayed hypersensitivity to coccidioidin in man. J. Immunol., 84:358–367, 1960.
73. Rocklin, R. E., Chilgren, R. A., Hong, R., and David, J. R.: Transfer of cellular hypersensitivity in chronic mucocutaneous candidiasis monitored in vivo and in vitro. Cellular Immunol., 1:290–299, 1970.
74. Rosen, F. S., Gitlin, D., and Janeway, C. A.: Alymphocytosis, agammaglobulinaemia, homografts, and delayed hypersensitivity: Study of a case. Lancet, 2:380–381, 1962.
75. Rosen, F. S., Gotoff, S. P., Craig, J. M., Ritchie, J., and Janeway, C. A.: Further observations on the Swiss type of agammaglobulinemia (Alymphocytosis): The effect of syngeneic bone-marrow cells. New Eng. J. Med., 274:18–21, 1966.
76. Salmon, S. E., Smith, B. A., Lehrer, R. I., Mogerman, S. N., Shinefield, H. R., and Perkins, H. A.: Modification of donor lymphocytes for transplantation in lymphopenic immunological deficiency. Lancet, 2:149–150, 1970.
77. Schulkind, M. L., Adler, W. H., Altemeier, W. A., and Ayoub, E. M.: Transfer factor in the treatment of chronic mucocutaneous candidiasis. Abstracts, American Pediatric Society, Inc., and Society for Pediatric Research, 1971, p. 30.
78. Snell, G. D., Cherry, M., and Démant, P.: Evidence that H-2 private specificities can be arranged in two mutually exclusive systems possibly homologous with two subsystems of HL-A. Transplant. Proc., 3:183–186, 1971.
79. Spitler, L. E., Levin, A. S., Huber, H., and Fudenberg, H. H.: Prediction of results of transfer factor therapy in the Wiskott-Aldrich syndrome by monocyte IgG receptors. Sixth Leucocyte Culture Conference, 1971. New York, Academic Press, to be published.
80. Spitler, L. E., Levin, A. S., Stites, D., Pirofsky, B., and Fudenberg, H. H.: Transfer factor therapy in mucocutaneous candidiasis. Sixth Leucocyte Culture Conference, 1971. New York, Academic Press, to be published.
81. Symes, M. O., Riddell, A. G., Immelman, E. J., and Terblanche, J.: Immunologically competent cells in the treatment of malignant disease. Lancet, 1:1054–1056, 1968.
82. Valentine, F. T., and Lawrence, H. S.: Lymphocyte stimulation: Transfer of cellular hypersensitivity to antigen in vitro. Science, 165:1014–1016, 1969.
83. W.H.O. Committee Report: Primary immunodeficiencies. Pediatrics, 47:927–946, 1971.
84. Wigzell, H., and Andersson, B.: Cell separation on antigen-coated columns. Elimination of high rate antibody-forming cells and immunological memory cells. J. Exper. Med., 129:23–36, 1969.
85. Wolstenholme, G. E. W., and O'Connor, M., eds.: Antilymphocytic Serum. Ciba Foundation Study Group 29. Boston, Little, Brown and Co., 1967.
86. Woodruff, M. F. A., and Nolan, B.: Preliminary observations on treatment of advanced cancer by injection of allogeneic spleen cells. Lancet, 2:426–429, 1963.

Faculty of Medicine
Memorial University of Newfoundland
St. John's, Newfoundland
Canada

Circulating Humoral Antibodies in Cancer

*Martin G. Lewis, M.D., M.R.C. Path.**

The concept of the role of host mechanisms in the natural history of cancer has been suggested by several observers as far back as the turn of this century.[22, 36] Not until the 1950's, however, did Foley[27] and Prehn and Maine[73] demonstrate clearly in the laboratory that an immune mechanism was present in carcinogen-induced tumors in mice. Since this time a great deal of experimental data and clinical observation has established that immunity, both cellular and humoral, plays an important part in various aspects of malignancy, and the subject has been extensively reviewed recently.[72, 80] In this paper we will consider some of the evidence related to circulating humoral immunity; the cellular aspects are dealt with elsewhere.

CLINICAL OBSERVATIONS

The first clues which led to much of our present understanding of immunity in malignant disease came from careful clinical observation. Although the variable nature of cancer in individuals and in groups of individuals in itself led to the concept that one should consider the host's part in the interaction,[36] three main types of clinical phenomena also deserve careful consideration: (1) inappropriate response to inadequate therapy, (2) delayed metastases beyond the normal expected for a particular tumor, and (3) spontaneous regression.

Inappropriate Response to Inadequate Therapy

There have been numerous examples of this type of clinical data.[24] One is the patient who, despite surgery which clearly leaves residual tumor in a totally inoperable situation, survives longer than expected or even experiences a cure. Although reports would seem rare, when they are collected from the literature, it becomes apparent that the experiences cannot easily be disregarded or refuted.[77] The most dramatic ex-

---

*Professor and Chairman, Department of Pathology, Memorial University of Newfoundland, St. John's, Newfoundland

ample of this, however, is Burkitt's report[12, 14, 56] cases of African lymphoma in which minute doses of cyclophosphamide resulted in exceedingly rapid regression of sometimes enormous tumors. This, in itself led to a considerable advance in the concepts of host-tumor relationship, and will bè discussed later with the details of immunologic mechanisms. In addition, the response to cytotoxic drug therapy in the treatment of choriocarcinoma can also be cited.[17]

Delayed Metastases

The phenomenon of metastatic disease appearing after removal of the primary tumor, at a much later date than the normal or mean expectancy, has been established clinically in several types of cancer,[24, 34, 87] possibly the most striking being malignant melanoma.[11, 23] It is well known that in a patient with an intraocular malignant melanoma which is removed by enucleation of the eye, liver metastases can appear anywhere from 15 to 30 years later.[3, 70] In my own experience this was clearly impressive in malignant melanoma in Ugandan Africans, in whom the majority of tumors began on the sole of the foot (Fig. 1), the first metastases usually appearing in the regional groin lymph nodes[48] (Fig. 2).

Studying a large number of these patients, it soon became apparent that they could be divided into three groups:[49] Group I – patients in whom the primary tumor remained, slowly growing but localized to the sole of the foot, for many months or even years before the first metastases appeared; Group II – patients with a similar tumor arising from the sole of the foot but with extremely rapid dissemination both to the regional lymph nodes of the groin and to all the usual widespread sites to which this tumor is known to metastasize; Group III – patients in whom no primary tumor can be detected at the time that secondary tumors were apparent in the regional draining lymph nodes of the groin.[20, 49, 60] Further studies revealed that in many of these patients a primary tumor on the foot had been present months or years earlier and had spontaneously disappeared.[85]

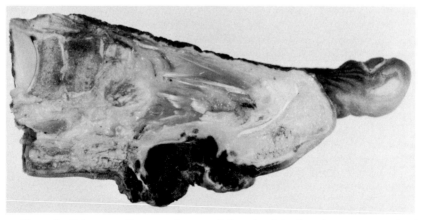

Figure 1.   Primary malignant melanoma of the sole of the foot shows extensive local invasion.

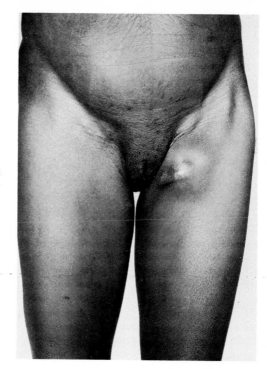

Figure 2. Secondary malignant melanoma in the groin lymph nodes in an African.

This latter phenomenon will be discussed in more detail in the next paragraph. The differences in age, sex, tribe, and histopathology were not consistent or related to these three clinically distinct biological behavior types, and it was concluded that the difference lay in the host's resistance to the tumor, resulting in delayed metastatic spread. This was followed by subsequently and will be discussed in later sections.

Spontaneous Regression

This is almost certainly the most dramatic of all phenomena seen in cancer, particularly the spontaneous disappearance of well established, widespread metastatic disease. In the experience of any individual, this is of course very rare, but when the well documented cases are examined critically there still remains a considerable body of evidence that this phenomenon is a real and established one. A classical description and analysis of this situation has been compiled by Everson and Cole[24] and by Smithers.[77]

Most of the attention has been drawn to the spontaneous regression of established metastatic disease and relatively little to the disappearance of eary primary tumors. This latter is not by any means as rare as previously considered, the main problem being that spontaneous regression or disappearance of early primary tumors is rarely seen to occur. The most convincing examples have to be in sites where such early primary tumors are visible, the skin of course being the most likely, and in this situation it is interesting to note that the disappearance of moles and nevi on the skin is by no means rare[55, 57] and can be shown in almost any individual during his lifetime.

In some recent studies we have been impressed by the more exaggerated form of disappearing mole, the so-called halo nevus.[75, 81] Immunologic tests so far would indicate its clear relationship with malignant melanoma and suggest that this might, in fact, be an example of such an early melanoma exhibiting spontaneous regression.[53] Of the numerous examples of spontaneous regression collected from the literature, whether they represent early tumors or late metastatic lesions, the following are amongst the most common: neuroblastoma, Burkitt lymphoma, malignant melanoma, choriocarcinoma, and hypernephroma. It is, I believe, by no means coincidental that these are the most clearly defined human tumors in which immune mechanisms, both cellular and humoral, have been demonstrated both in vitro and in vivo. These aspects will now be described in more detail.

LABORATORY TESTS FOR IMMUNITY TO MALIGNANT DISEASE

Some of the earliest work in this field was carried out using techniques which had recently been developed in transplantation work, namely the use of transplantable tumors in animals,[21, 32, 33] the measure of immunity being the ability of the particular animal to reject the tumor, measured in the same way that graft rejection is measured. Most refinements of this technique utilized suspensions of tumor cells, whereby definite numbers of malignant cells were injected into animals which had previously been immunized against the particular tumor, indicating an increased resistance.[44, 45, 66]

In man, these approaches are, of course, not feasible and more standard techniques such as those already developed in the field of serology have been used. The techniques used to measure circulating antibody against tumor cells and tumor antigens will now be briefly reviewed. The equivalent techniques regarding cellular immune mechanisms will be discussed in another section.

LABORATORY TESTS FOR TUMOR-SPECIFIC ANTIBODIES AND ANTIGENS

The basic principle underlying all these attempts to measure circulating antibody against tumor cells is the same, namely the interaction between a specific component of the immunoglobulins present in the serum of an individual and its reaction against either the patient's tumor or a component of such. The more direct approach will be discussed first, and the easier but less direct methods will subsequently be described.

Cytotoxicity

The subject of serum cytotoxicity against tumor cells has recently been reviewed by Arpels and Southam.[8] Antibodies reacting with the surface of cells in the presence of complement cause lysis, and this has been well established as a routine procedure in hematology where well-known red cell lysis can be produced by such antibody-antigen reactions.[15] In tumor work, however, the problems are more difficult. The tumor cells need to be obtained in a viable state, and the measure of cytotoxicity is not as easy as the well defined and easily recognizable lysis in red cells. Several attempts have been made to overcome these problems. The most commonly used means involves the ability of viable cells to prevent certain vital dyes such as Trypan blue or Eosin Y entering their cytoplasm.[76] The method therefore consists of producing a suspension of living tumor cells kept in a nutrient tissue culture medium; the particular serum containing the antibody is added, with some source of complement, and the cultures are then treated with Trypan blue. The degree of cytotoxicity is the difference between the control group and the test group in terms of the production of cells which are Trypan blue-positive. As alternatives to the use of Trypan blue, radioactive isotope-labelled metabolites of the cell can be measured. These can be released from dead cells, or measured as uptake by living cells.

Variations of this technique have been used widely throughout the field of tumor immunology and in transplantation experiments, and in a number of human tumors, cytotoxic sera have been shown to be present.[8, 37] There are, however, numerous problems associated with the test, the main one being the fact that in human tumor cells the controls as well as the tests are in fact dying and the degree of cytotoxicity can be measured only if the test cells are damaged more rapidly than the control cells. It has also been shown that Trypan blue indicates not cell death, but cell damage, and therefore this particular test, although useful in the laboratory may in fact not represent the mechanism occurring *in vivo*.

Another approach which has been demonstrated, particularly in human malignant melanoma, is the ability of circulating antibody in the presence of complement to cause tumor cells surface damage and subsequent lysis.[48] In this test again, cell suspensions are made from freshly removed tumor, and these are placed in special culture chambers with a coverslip on the top.[74] The culture chambers are then inverted so that the tumor cells (Fig. 3) drop onto the coverslip. After incubation at 37°C. for 24 to 48 hours the cultures are placed with the coverslip upmost again. The dead cells and debris float down away from the coverslip and the living cells spread out and adhere to the undersurface of the coverslip. They can then be readily observed by means of phase contrast microscopy (Fig. 4). All the coverslips can be removed and stained and examined by conventional light microscopy. The addition of serum containing antibodies and complement results in the cells becoming rounded up and falling away from the coverslip into the medium with the dead cells and debris, the difference between the test and the controls indicating the approximate degree of cytotoxicity.[50]

Although this technique may be in more senses physiologic and represent the situation in vivo, the drawbacks are the larger numbers of cells needed, the time taken and the difficulty in quantitation. To overcome this problem of cell numbers and quantitation a method using a microplate technique has been used.[83] This consists of a plastic dish containing 60

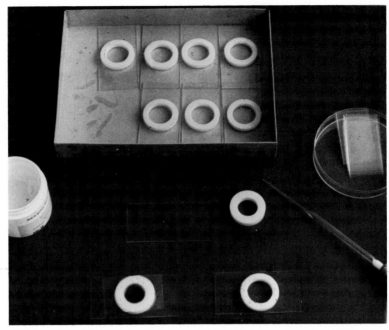

Figure 3. Tissue culture chambers, made from Teflon rings and glass slides, sterilized in metal containers. (Technique after Pulvertaft, 1959.)

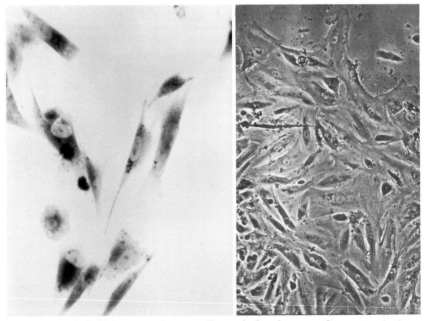

Figure 4. *Left*, Malignant melanoma cells attached to glass coverslips – grown in tissue culture. *Right*, Malignant teratoma cells in tissue culture, viewed by phase contrast microscopy.

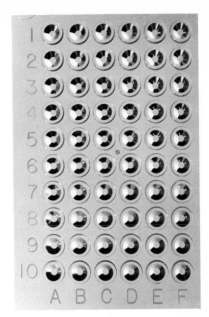

Figure 5.   Tissue culture microplate shows 60 small wells for cell culture.

wells where very small numbers of tumor cells can be seeded (Fig. 5); the serum and complement are added and after the appropriate incubation period the dishes are washed, the viable cells remaining attached, the dead cells washing away.[18] These can then be stained either in conventional methods or using Trypan blue or by means of direct phase contrast microscopy. This technique has been used with great success in lymphocyte cytotoxic tests used extensively now in the field of transplantation immunology.

Inhibition of Growth or Colony Formation

A test system whereby the ability of tumor cells to multiply and grow out from tissue fragments[13] and form colonies (Fig. 6) rather akin to that seen in bacterial cell cultures can also be used,[56, 69] and the effect of adding appropriate antibody-containing sera can be measured. This so-called colony inhibition technique has been used now with a variety of human tumors[37] and is particularly useful where the tumor has the ability to produce colonies readily and where the measurement between the control and the test is easily determined. Again, fresh tumor must be used and the procedure relies on first the establishment of reproduceable cell division or cloning.

Immunofluorescence

This technique first described by Coons and Kaplan[16] has now been used very extensively indeed throughout the field of immunology. It is based on the simple principle that antibody-antigen complexes can be detected in tissues or cells by means of adding an anti gammaglobulin which is coupled to a fluorescent reagent and, with appropriate light stimulation and filter systems, produces a specific fluorescence. The

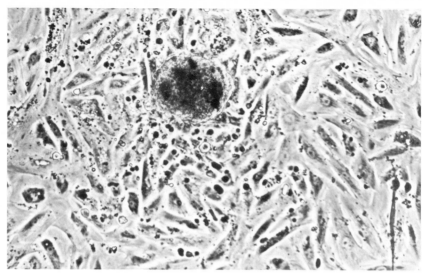

Figure 6. Phase contrast microscopy, showing an island or "clone" of cells, with extension into the surrounding media.

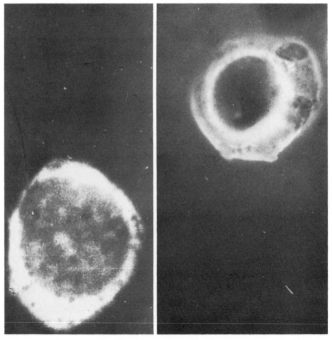

Figure 7. Examples of immunofluorescence on "fixed" tumour cells, showing fluorescence in the cytoplasmic contents.

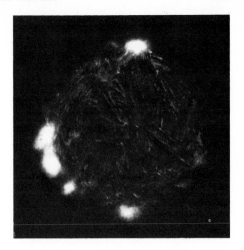

Figure 8. Immunofluorescence on the surface membrane of a living tumour cell (membrane immunofluorescence).

main problem of this technique has been the standardization of reagents, conjugates, and microscopes.[41, 64, 71] With careful control of all these factors, reliable and reproduceable results can be obtained.

This method has been applied in tumor work in a variety of ways, but the most reliable and fruitful has been its application to cells obtained from tumors and dispersed in suspension. Cells can be snap-frozen on glass with liquid nitrogen and isopentane,[65, 71] or with standard cytologic fixatives; the appropriate sera can be added or viable tumor cells in suspension can be used. In snap-frozen tumor cells, it is the cytoplasmic contents which are being tested, forming the antigen[71] (Fig. 7). On the viable tumor cell suspensions, the surface membrane of the cells reacts with the antibody[61, 71] (Fig. 8). The different patterns of fluorescence can be determined with experience.

The degree of cross-reactivity, indicating common antigenicity, in human tumors determined by means of immunofluorescent techniques varies with the type of tumor. For instance, Burkitt lymphoma,[30, 40] osteogenic sarcoma, and colonic carcinoma[29] well represent the type where multiple cross-reactivity occurs, with what appears to be common antigens, even on the surface membrane of the tumor cells. This phenomenon also occurs in virus-induced tumors in animals and has led several observers to comment on the possibility that these human tumors might have a viral aetiology.

In human malignant melanoma, although there does appear to be a common cytoplasmic antigen[50] against which most positive sera from our melanoma patient react, the surface membrane antibody-antigen reaction is patient specific and unique in type.[71] This is similar to the chemical carcinogen-induced animal tumors.[9]

Electron Microscopy

The electron microscope has been used with considerable success in locating with more accuracy the sites of antibody-antigen reactions both on the surface of tumor cells and in the cytoplasm.[6] Instead of a fluores-

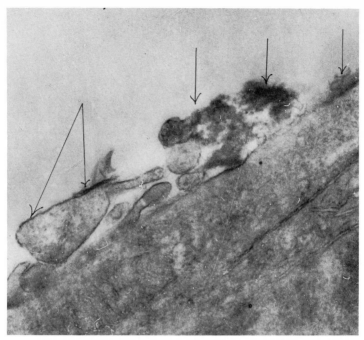

Figure 9.   Part of an electron micrograph (× 60,000) showing antibody antigen complex by means of peroxidase-labelled immunoglobulin on the cell membrane.

cent dye, ferritin-labelled antiglobulin can be used; More recently an enzyme peroxidase linked to the antiglobulin has been used. The reaction of peroxidase can then be located histochemically in or on the tumor cells by means of electron microscopy (Fig. 9). This has in fact been of considerable importance in the location of the particular sites in which these reactions occur, and will undoubtedly be used more frequently as the techniques become easier to standardize and to reproduce.

TESTS OF ANTIBODY ACTIVITY NOT REQUIRING
VIABLE TUMOR CELLS

So far, we have discussed the detection of antibody using the tumor cell itself as the indicator. More conventional immunologic tests for antibody-antigen reactions can, of course, be used and are being carried out more frequently. The problem is to obtain a suitable tumor-specific antigen. This can be produced by preparing fractions of cell membranes obtained free of cytoplasmic contents or by various extracts of whole cell homogenates. The various fractions will, of course, contain different types of antigen,[21, 86] not all of which will be tumor-specific but will in addition represent the normal tissue antigens present in all cells. Recent work has shown that in some situations common antigens are present in certain fetal tissues[51, 82] as well as tumors and that the antigen can be shown to be circulating in the blood of patients at various stages of their disease. Conventional tests for such antibody-antigen reactions, such as precipitation, immunodiffusion,[19, 51, 59] complement fixation,[7, 31] immunoelectrophoresis, hemabsorption, hemagglutination,[26, 28] and various forms of chromatography, can all be used and have shown clearly, in many human tumors, measurable antibody and antigen.

THE SPECIFICITY OF TUMOR ANTIBODY

Having obtained information suggestive of tumor antibody by any of the previously mentioned approaches, it is obviously important to establish the specificity of such reactions and to determine the significance. The specificity depends on demonstrating that the reaction in the serum is contained in the immunoglobulin fractions of the serum – in other words that it is an antibody by the usual chemical standards – then to show that its reaction is against a specific component of a tumor cell and not against normal tissues in the same patient, and finally that the antibody being measured can in some way be shown to cause damage to the cell or the death of the cell. It is arguable whether the latter is absolutely essential, since a tumor-specific antibody may in fact be present in various forms which are clearly not cytotoxic. This will be dealt with under the section "Significance of Reactions."

To illustrate some of the methods for determining specificity, some of the results obtained from the study of malignant melanoma will be used. In these studies it was shown that this substance was present not only in the gammaglobulin fraction of the serum, but within either the IgG or IgM component. This same substance did not react either by immunofluorescence or cytotoxicity with normal components of the skin.[71] In addition, it was shown that an homogenate of the patient's tumor could absorb out completely the antibody effect from the serum but similar absorption with homogenates of skin, melanin, or a variety of other normal tissues still resulted in clear antibody activity.[50, 71] Thus, in the system of human melanoma, many of the criteria for tumor specificity have been met.

The Significance of Tumor-Specific Antibody

This can best be shown in the human situation by demonstrating that the presence of antibody is related in some way to the natural history of the tumor, the ultimate significance, of course, being the demonstration that this relationship between antibody and tumor is one beneficial in some degree to the patient. In several human tumors, particularly malignant melanomas[50, 63] and colonic carcinoma,[84] the presence of detectable antibody in the serum is clearly associated with early or localized tumors. In both these examples, dissemination of the tumor with metastases is associated with a lack of detection of antibody. In human malignant melanoma, this was clearly shown in some of the early experiments carried out in East Africa where patients with a long history of localization were the ones with positive antibody and the ones with rapidly disseminating tumors showed no antibody.[49] In colonic carcinoma it has also been shown that antibodies detected against the so-called carcinoembryonic antigen found in this group of tumors was not seen in those with metastatic disease. The next question arose as to which came first, the dissemination of the tumor or the disappearance of the antibody, or indeed whether one was dealing with entirely different types of patients. This has raised the question, first, how important is circulating antibody, and secondly, why in so many systems has it been shown that antibody disappears in association with metastases.

REASONS FOR DISAPPEARANCE OF ANTIBODY WITH METASTATIC MALIGNANCY

In malignant melanoma, it has been shown that not only is the positive antibody associated with localized tumor, but that in individual patients studied over a period of time the serum activity changes from positive to negative as the tumor becomes clinically disseminated (Fig. 10). It has also been recently shown that the drop in antibody detection often precedes the appearance of such metastatic disease by weeks or even months.[52] Of equal importance, the volume or mass of tumor is not related to the antibody levels, since patients with large quantities of tumor which are still localized are antibody-positive, whereas patients with minute deposits disseminated, that is, beyond the regional draining lymph nodes, antibody-negative.[54] These factors, and the clinical relationship and antibody studies described in Ugandan Africans, clearly demonstrate that the presence of antibody in the circulation has a strong

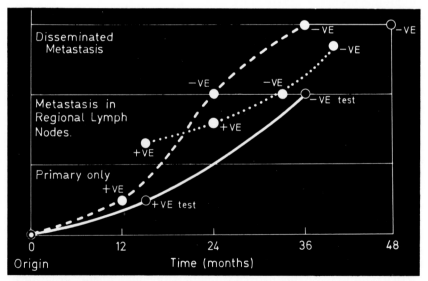

Figure 10. Diagrammatic representation of loss of antibody detection in 3 patients, during the phase from localization to dissemination of their tumors.

influence on the duration of localization, and the absence of antibody, the rapidity of spread of this tumor. It is, therefore, obvious from these comments, that it is time that the rather imprecise terms such as the "cancer patient," used so often in medical literature, be replaced with more clearly defined clinical parameters. The exact stage of the natural history and the type of tumor need to be considered in the light of such immune studies.

REASONS FOR FAILURE OF IMMUNITY IN MALIGNANCY

There are many possible mechanisms and viewpoints from which this subject can be approached. The whole problem of suppression of general immune mechanisms in patients with advanced malignancy has been examined by numerous investigators, with somewhat conflicting results, which are largely explained on the basis of the lack of detailed coordination in many of the series. The problems of lack of response of the patient against not only tumor antigens but a variety of other antigens also needs to be considered. Of particular importance in this are the abnormalities of cellular immunity. Again this subject will be considered largely in this chapter from the point of view of circulating antibody.

At this stage in the discussion it is as well to remove from the picture the situation described in very advanced malignancy where clearly generalized nonspecific suppression of immunity can be demonstrated.[46, 47, 78] Usually these are patients who are almost moribund or cachectic. The situation becomes much clearer when one examines the change from localization to dissemination, which after all is the key time in the natural history of any metastatic tumor, for it is at this moment in time that the difference exists between benignity and malignancy. It has been clearly shown that although tumor-specific immunity alters during this period of change from localization to dissemination, this is not necessarily accompanied by a general lack of immune response.[25, 88] It is therefore of paramount importance that we begin to understand the detailed mechanisms which result in a drop in antibody levels during this crucial time period.

Firstly, it has now been clearly demonstrated in a series of human tumors that the tumor cells taken from metastatic lesions are not appreciably different in their antigenic components.[42, 63] Certainly modulation of the antigenicity can occur[62] but the use of metastatic tumor cells to raise tumor-specific antibodies identical with those seen in the earlier stages of the disease clearly indicate that the main antigens are still present.

The patient's response to this process of autoimmunization with his own metastatic tumor cells with a clear rise in antibodies also shows (Fig. 11) that the individual is still capable of recognizing the antigen and responding appropriately and by a secondary type of response. This led to the investigation into the possibility that some form of specific inhibition of antibody response occurred in certain individuals.

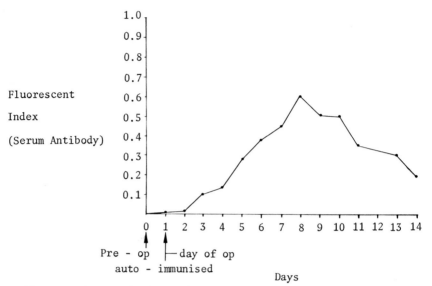

Figure 11.   An example of antibody production, by means of autoimmunisation of a patient with his own irradiated tumour cells.

INHIBITORS OF TUMOR IMMUNITY

Over the past few years, several investigators both in the field of transplantation and in tumor immunology have been impressed by the presence of certain serum factors which appear to inhibit the patient's lymphocyte and cellular response against both grafts and tumours.[4, 10, 43, 61] The fact that some of these inhibitors have been identified as immunoglobulins[38, 39] has led to a concept that circulating antibody in malignancy may in fact be far from beneficial but may represent a disadvantageous situation with blocking of cellular immunity. This has been reinforced by the idea expressed by several people that it is cellular immunity which is the most important mechanism.[72] This needs challenging, particularly since there are many well known parallels in bacterial, viral, and protozoal infections of man. Whatever immune mechanisms are in operation to protect the peripheral areas of the body, the ultimate protection must surely lie in the blood, and the well known role of circulating antibody in this respect, preventing septicemia, needs no question. If one regards circulating tumor cells in the same light, it would not be surprising that some circulating antibody might be also important in preventing such dissemination; therefore, not all antibody in tumor studies can be regarded as detrimental to the immune response, and in recent work, inhibitors of circulating antibody have also been detected.

In human malignant melanoma, for example, the serum taken during dissemination which is shown to be antibody negative against the autologous tumor cells has a specific inhibitory blocking effect on positive serum taken from the same patient following autoimmunization with the patient's tumor cells.[51] The investigation of this inhibitor is still in a preliminary stage, but it is shown to be contained in the IgG immunoglobulin component of the preimmunized or negative serum. It appears to react specifically only with the autologous positive serum taken from the same patient.

Whether this inhibitor is a complex between tumor antibody and antigen with antigen excess, thus reacting with free antibody and neutralizing it, or is in fact a specific antibody, has yet to be determined with certainty. Either way the results have certain important implications for they demonstrate that it is not the patient's inability to respond to the tumor or the lack of antigenicity in the tumor but some form of abnormal reaction in the patient himself causing inhibition of the specific immune response. This has considerable additional support from the effect on cellular immunity demonstrated by other investigators.[38, 39]

THE POSSIBILITIES OF IMMUNOTHERAPY OF MALIGNANCY

A great deal has been written about the problem of producing a form of immunotherapy which would be effective against malignant tumors. The consensus of opinion from most of the literature is that so far this has been disappointing, and many regard it as unlikely ever to succeed. On the other hand, there have been encouraging reports that some effect of the beneficial nature has been produced in some patients with certain human malignant tumors.[58, 63] but in many cases the follow-up is, as yet, not extensive enough.

The ultimate goal, of course, is to produce in the patient some form of increased responsiveness against his tumor. This could be achieved in several ways. The most ambitious of all would be to mimic the well known, though rare phenomenon of spontaneous regression mentioned earlier in this chapter. If this phenomenon has an immunologic basis, and it is highly suggestive that this is so, then a mechanism must exist and research into this must remain an important priority.

On the other hand, helping the immune response in a more limited fashion has still a value. There are many patients in whom the primary tumor can be removed at a stage when there is no detectable evidence of metastases,[11] and yet a high proportion of these patients ultimately returned with metastatic disease. If some form of immunologic exploitation can be produced during this stage between localization and dissemination, then this might ultimately be more realistic. In addition, some form of immunotherapy in conjunction with surgery, radiotherapy, and chemotherapy has already been shown to have some beneficial effect. One of the main stumbling blocks would appear to be the production of some forms of inhibition, and these may yet turn out to be more frequent and complicated than so far is indicated. There is a need, therefore, to understand and to be able to alter the production of such inhibitors, whether it be against cellular immunity, possibly in the early stage of the disease, or against the circulatory inhibitors preventing antibody from being effective in blood-borne dissemination. It is, therefore, imperative that research into the subject of the host's reaction against his tumor progress with the ultimate aim of producing a satisfactory and successful therapeutic approach.

It is most important that we do not produce artificial distinctions and competition between cellular and humoral immunity[35] but regard them as they should be, facets of a much more complete and complicated system of protection against not only the external but also the internal environment.

SUMMARY AND CONCLUSIONS

This is an attempt to summarize some aspects of tumor immunity, with particular reference to circulating tumor-specific antibodies. Such antibodies have been shown in a variety of human tumors, and their relationship to the clinical stage of the disease has been emphasized, particularly the disappearance of such antibody during the change from localization to dissemination of the tumor.

It is suggested that circulating humoral antibody is important at some stage in the natural history of malignancy in preventing rapid dissemination. The final breakdown of this mechanism is linked in some way with the production of some form of inhibition by the patient himself. The relationship between cellular and humoral immunity is complex but definitely interrelated. The final goal, to produce a successful form of immunotherapy, depends on further detailed understanding of the interplay between circulating antibody and cellular immunity, and the ways in which both are inhibited and prevented from being effective.

REFERENCES

1. Alexander, P.: Immunotherapy of cancer: experiments with primary tumors and syngeneic tumor grafts. Progr. Exper. Tumor Res., *10*:293, 1960.
2. Alexander, P., and Hamilton-Fairley, G.: Cellular Resistance to Tumors. Brit. Med. Bull., 23:86, 1967.
3. Allen, A. C., and Spitz, S.: Malignant melanoma: a clinico-pathological analysis of the criteria for prognosis and diagnosis. Cancer, 6:1, 1953.
4. Allison, A. C.: Relationship of cellular and humoral immunity in virus carcinogenesis. Life Sci., 3:1415–1422, 1964.
5. Alpert, M. E.: Alpha-fetoglobulin in the diagnosis of human hepatoma. New Eng. J. Med., 278:984, 1968.
6. Andres, G. A., Hsu, K. C., and Seegal, B. C.: Immunoferritin technique for the identification of antigens by electron microscopy. *In* Weir, D. M., ed.: Handbook of Experimental Immunology. Oxford, Blackwell Scientific Publications, 1967.
7. Armstrong, D., Henle, G., and Henle, W.: Complement-fixation tests with cell lines derived from Burkitt's lymphoma and acute leukemias. J. Bacteriol., 91:1257, 1966.
8. Arpels, C., and Southam, C. M.: Cytotoxicity of sera from healthy persons and cancer patients. Int. J. Cancer, 4:548, 1969.
9. Baldwin, R. W., and Moore, M.: Isolation of membrane-associated tumour-specific antigen from an amino-dye induced rat hepatoma. Int. J. Cancer, 4:753, 1969.
10. Batchelor, J. R.: The use of enhancement in studying tumour antigens. Cancer Res., 28:1410, 1968.

11. Bodenham, D. C.: A study of 650 observed malignant melanomas in the southwest. Ann. Roy. Coll. Surg. Eng., 43:218, 1968.
12. Burkitt, D. P., and Kyalwayi, S. K.: Spontaneous remission of African lymphoma. Brit. J. Cancer, 21:14, 1967.
13. Chatterjee, J.: Action of homologous and autologous serum and plasma on the growth of cancer cells in tissue culture. Ann. Biochem., 16:113, 1956.
14. Clifford, P., Stjernsward, J., Singh, S., and Klein, G.: Long-term survival of patients with Burkitt's Lymphoma—an assessment of treatment and other factors which relate to survival. Cancer Res., 27:2578, 1967.
15. Coombs, R. R. A., Bedford, D., and Rouilland, L. M.: A and B blood group antigens on human epidermal cells demonstrated by mixed agglutination. Lancet, 1:461, 1956.
16. Coons, A. H., and Kaplan, M. H.: Localization of antigen in tissue cells. II. Improvements in the method for the detection of antigen by means of fluorescent antibody. J. Exper. Med., 91:1, 1950.
17. Currie, G. A., and Bagshawe, K. D.: The masking of antigens on trophoblasts and cancer cells. Lancet, 1:708, 1967.
18. Currie, G. A., Lejeune, F., and Hamilton-Fairley, G.: Immunization with irradiated tumour cells and specific lymphocyte cytotoxicity in malignant melanoma. Brit. Med. J., 2:305, 1971.
19. Czajowski, N. P., Rosenblatt, M., Wolf, P. L., and Vasquez, J.: A new method for active immunization to autologous human tumour tissue. Lancet, 2:905, 1967.
20. Das Gupta, T., Bowden, L., and Berg, T. W.: Malignant melanoma of unkown primary origin. Surg. Gynec. Obstet., 117:341, 1963.
21. Davies, D. A. L.: Mouse histocompatibility isoantigens derived from normal and from tumour cells. Immunology, 11:115, 1966.
22. Ehrlich, P.: In Himmelweit, F., ed.: The collected papers of Paul Ehrlich, 1909. Vol. II. Immunology and Cancer Research. London, Pergamon Press, 1957.
23. Eve, F.: A lecture on melanoma. Practitioner, 70:165, 1903.
24. Everson, T. C., and Cole, W. H.: Spontaneous Regression of Cancer. Philadelphia, W. B. Saunders, 1966.
25. Fass, L., Herberman, R. B., Zeigler, J. L., and Kiryabwire, J. W. M.: Cutaneous hypersensitivity reactions to autologous extracts of malignant melanoma cells. Lancet, 1:116, 1970.
26. Finney, J. W., Byers, E. H., and Wilson, R. H.: Studies in tumour autoimmunity. Cancer Res., 20:351, 1969.
27. Foley, E. J.: Antigenic properties of methylcholantrene-induced tumours in mice of the strain of origin. Cancer Res., 13:835, 1953.
28. Gold, P.: Circulating antibodies against carcinoembryonic antigens of the human digestive system. Cancer, 20:1663, 1967.
29. Gold, P., and Freedman, S.: Demonstration of tumour-specific antigens in human colonic carcinomata by immunological tolerance and absorption techniques. J. Exper. Med., 121:439, 1965.
30. Goldstein, G., Klein, G., Pearson, G., and Clifford, P.: Direct membrane immunofluorescence reaction of Burkitt's lymphoma cells in culture. Cancer Res., 29:749, 1969.
31. Graham, J. B., and Graham, R. M.: The effect of vaccine on cancer patients. Surg. Gynec. Obstet., 109:131, 1959.
32. Gross, L.: The influence of sex of mice on acquired resistance to a transplantable sarcoma. Cancer Res., 1:880, 1941.
33. Haddow, A.: Immunology of the tumor cell: Tumor-specific antigens. Brit. Med. Bull., 21:133, 1965.
34. Hadfield, G.: The dominant cancer cell. Brit. Med. J., 2:607, 1954.
35. Hall, J. G.: Effector mechanisms in immunity. Lancet, 1:25, 1969.
36. Handley, W. S.: The pathology of melanocytic growths. Lancet, 1:927, 1907.
37. Hellstrom, I., Hellstrom, K. E., and Pierce, G. E.: In vitro studies of immune reactions against autochthonous and syngeneic mouse tumors induced by methylcholanthrene and plastic discs. Int. J. Cancer, 3:467, 1968.
38. Hellstrom, I.: A colony inhibition (C 1) technique for demonstration of tumor cell destruction by lymphoid cells in vitro. Int. J. Cancer, 2:65, 1967.
39. Hellstrom, I., Sjögren, H. O., Warner, G., and Hellstrom, K. E.: Blocking of cell-mediated tumor immunity by sera from patients with growing neoplasms. Int. J. Cancer; 7:226, 1971.
40. Henle, G., and Henle, W.: Immunofluorescence in cells derived from Burkitt's lymphoma. J. Bact., 91:1248, 1966.
41. Holborow, E. J.: Standardization in Immunofluorescence. Oxford, Blackwell Scientific Publications, 1970.
42. Ikonopisov, R. L., Lewis, M. G., Hunter-Craig, I. D., Bodenham, D. C., Phillips, T. M., Cooling, C. I., Proctor, J., Hamilton-Fairley, G., and Alexander, P. Autoimmunization with irradiated tumor cells in human malignant melanoma. Brit. Med. J., 2:752, 1970.
43. Kaliss, N.: The elements of immunologic enhancement: a consideration of mechanisms. Ann. N.Y. Acad. Sci., 101:64, 1962.

44. Klein, G.: Tumor-specific transplantation antigens. Cancer Res., 28:625, 1968.
45. Klein, G., Clifford, P., Klein, E., and Stjernward, J.: Search for tumor-specific immune reactions in Burkitt's lymphoma patients by the membrane immunofluorescence reaction. Proc. Nat. Acad. Sci. U.S.A., 55:1628, 1966.
46. Krant, M. J., Manskopf, G., Brandrup, C. S., and Madoff, M. A.: Immunologic alterations in bronchogenic cancer – sequential study. Cancer, 21:623, 1968.
47. Lamb, D., Pilney, F., Kelly, W. D., and Good, R. A.: A comparative study of the incidence of anergy in patients with carcinoma, leukemia, Hodgkins disease and other lymphomas. J. Immunol., 89:555, 1962.
48. Lewis, M. G.: Possible immunological host factors in human malignant melanoma. Lancet, 2:921, 1967.
49. Lewis, M. G., and Kiryabwire, J. W. M.: Malignant melanoma in Uganda, aspects of behaviour and natural history. Cancer, 21:876, 1968.
50. Lewis, M. G., Ikonopisov, R. L., Nairn, R. C., Phillips, T. M., Hamilton-Fairley, G., Bodenham, D. C., and Alexander, P.: Tumor-specific antibodies in human malignant melanoma and their relationship to the extent of the disease. Brit. Med. J., 3:547, 1969.
51. Lewis, M. G., Phillips, T. M., Cook, K. B., and Blake, J.: Possible explanation for loss of detectable antibody in disseminated malignant melanoma. Nature (London), 232:52, 1971.
52. Lewis, M. G.: The relationships between serum antibody and dissemination of malignant melanoma. Rev. de L'Institute Pasteur de Lyon, in press.
53. Lewis, M. G., Copeman, P. W. M., Phillips, T. M., and Elliott, P. G.: Immunological associations of the halo naevus with malignant melanoma. Manuscript in preparation.
54. Lewis, M. G., McCloy, E., and Blake, J.: The significance of humoral antibody in the localization of malignant melanoma. Manuscript in preparation.
55. Lunde, H. Z., and Stobbe, G. D.: The natural history of the pigment naevi: factors of age and anatomic location. Amer. J. Path., 25:1117, 1949.
56. Maledon, A., Stoh, P. B., and Talley, R. W.: Alterations in tissue culture morphology by cancerous serum. Clin. Res., 16:360, 1968.
57. Masson, P.: Les naevi pigmentaires; tumeurs nerveuses. Ann. Anat. Path. (Paris)., 3:417, 657, 1926.
58. Mathe, G., Amiel, J. L., Schwarzenberg, L., Schneider, M., Cathan, A., Schlumberger, J. R., Hayat, M., and De Vassal, P.: Active immunotherapy for acute lymphoblastic leukemia. Lancet, 1:697, 1969.
59. McKenna, J. M., Sanderson, R. P., and Blakemore, W. S.: Studies of antigens of human tumours I. Demonstration of a soluble specific antigen in HeLa cells and some human tumours. Cancer Res., 24:754, 1964.
60. Milton, G. W., Lane-Brown, M. M., and Gilder, M.: Malignant melanoma, with an occult primary lesion. Brit. J. Surg., 54:651, 1967.
61. Moller, G., and Moller, E.: In Cinnader, B., ed.: Immune Cytotoxicity and Immunological Enhancement, Antibodies to Biologically Active Molecules. Oxford, Pergamon Press, 1966.
62. Morton, D. L., and Malmgren, R. A.: Human osteosarcomas: Immunologic evidence suggesting an associated infectious agent. Science, 162:1279, 1968.
63. Morton, D. L., Eilber, R. F., Malmgren, R. A., and Wood, E. C.: Immunological factors which influence response to immunotherapy in malignant melanoma. Surgery, 68:158, 1970.
64. Nairn, R. C.: Standardization in immunofluorescence. Clin. Exper. Immunol., 3:465, 1969.
65. Nairn, R. C.: Fluorescent Protein Tracing. Edinburgh, Livingstone, 1969.
66. Old, L. J., Boyse, E. A., Clarke, D. A., and Carswell, E. A.: Antigenic properties of chemically induced tumors. Ann. N.Y. Acad. Sci., 101:80, 1962.
67. Old, L. J., and Boyse, E. A.: Prospects for immunotherapy of human cancer. Ann. Intern. Med., 69:393, 1968.
68. Osunkoya, B. O.: Various aspects of the Burkitt tumor cell in tissue culture with reference to host defences. In Burchenal, J. H., and Burkitt, D. P.: Treatment of Burkitt's Tumor. UICC Monograph, Series 8. Heidelberg, Springer-Verlag, 1967.
69. Parthenis, A., and Stone, D.: Some morphological differences in Hela Cell cultures when growth in the presence of normal or cancer sera. Brit. J. Cancer, 21:218, 1967.
70. Pack, G. T., and Miller, T. R.: Metastatic melanoma indeterminate primary site (report of two instances of long term survival). J.A.M.A., 176:55, 1961.
71. Phillips, T. M., and Lewis, M. G.: A system of immunofluorescence in the study of tumour cells. Rev. Europ. Etudes Clin. Biol., 15:1016, 1970.
72. Piessons, W. F.: Evidence for human cancer immunity: a review. Cancer, 26:1212, 1970.
73. Prehn, R. T., and Main, J. M.: Immunity to MCA induced sarcomas. J. Nat. Cancer Inst., 18:769, 1957.
74. Pulvertaft, R. J. V.: The examination of pathological tissue in a fresh state. In Collins, D. H., ed.: Modern Trends in Pathology. London, Butterworth, 1959.
75. Rolleston, H. D.: Jaundice with areas of unpigmented skin. Proc. Roy. Soc. Med., 3:195, 1910.

76. Schreck, R.: Use of eosin dye to distinguish live and dead cells. Amer. J. Cancer, 28:389, 1936.
77. Smithers, D. W.: On the Nature of Neoplasia in Man. London, Livingstone, 1964.
78. Soloway, A. C., and Rapaport, F. T.: Immunologic responses in cancer patients. Surg. Gynec. Obstet., 121:756, 1965.
79. Southam, C. M.: Immunotherapy of leukemia, theoretical and experimental. In Dameshek, W., and Dutcher, P. D., eds.: Perspectives in Leukemia. New York, Grune & Stratton, 1968.
80. Southam, C. M.: Cancer-specific antigens in man. In Samter, M., ed.: Immunological Disease. Boston, Little, Brown and Co., 2nd ed., vol. 1.
81. Sutton, R. L.: An unusual variety of vitiligo (Leukoderma acquisitum centrifugum). Report of two cases. J. Cutan. Dis., 34:797, 1916.
82. Takasugi, M., and Klein, E.: A microassay for cell-mediated immunity. Transplantation, 9:219, 1970.
83. Tatarinov, J.: Content of embryospecific gamma-globulin in fetal and neonatal sera and sera from adult humans with primary carcinoma of the liver. Vopr. Med. Khim., 11:20, 1965.
84. Thompson, D. M. P.: Diagnosis of human digestive system cancer by radioimmunoassay of carcinoembryonic antigen. Ann. Roy. Coll. Phys. Surg. Canada, July 1971.
85. Todd, D. W., Spencer-Payne, W., Farrow, G. M., and Winklmann, R. K.: Spontaneous regression of primary malignant melanoma with regional metastasis: Report of a case with photographic documentation. Proc. Mayo Clin., 41:10, 1966.
86. Viza, D. C., Degani, O., Bernard, C., and Harris, R.: Leukemia antigens. Lancet, 2:493, 1969.
87. Willis, R. A.: The Spread of Tumours in the Human Body. London, Butterworth, 1952.
88. Zeigler, J. L., Lewis, M. G., Luyombya, J. M. S., and Kiryabwire, J. W. M.: Immunological studies in patients with malignant melanoma in Uganda. Brit. J. Cancer, 23:729, 1969.

Department of Pathology
Memorial University of Newfoundland
St. John's, Newfoundland
Canada

Immune Deficiency States Associated with Malignant Disease in Man

*Jules Harris, M.D., F.R.C.P.(C), F.A.C.P.,** *
*and Ramesh C. Bagai, Ph.D.****

Patients with malignant disease may have impaired immune function.[56] This immunologic impairment is most striking and best defined with neoplasia involving the reticuloendothelial system. Malignant transformation of those cells constituting the immune apparatus provides a ready explanation for depressed immune function in these cases. Patients with nonlymphoid malignancies may also be found to have abnormal immune responses. This may occur in the absence of lymphoid replacement by malignant tissue and frequently lacks a satisfactory explanation. The picture is often further complicated by the effect of treatment. Radiation,[52, 90, 92, 150] chemotherapy,[56, 57, 65, 121] and surgery[103] have all been shown to depress immune function in man. This paper will review those malignant diseases in man known to be associated with depressed immune function. The complications which are a consequence of this depressed immune function and the management of these complications have been discussed elsewhere.[56]

HODGKIN'S DISEASE

The "Hodgkin maze"[42] has long fascinated students of tumor immunobiology. Immunodeficiency in patients with Hodgkin's disease was first described early in this century.[111] Unsuccessful attempts to establish a relationship between tuberculosis and Hodgkin's disease did demonstrate that patients with Hodgkin's disease frequently manifested cutaneous anergy to tuberculin. This observation, soon widely confirmed by other investigators, was found to be but one example in Hodgkin's

*Assistant Professor of Medicine, Division of Oncology, Faculty of Medicine, University of Ottawa, Canada

**Research Fellow, Laboratory of Immunology, Division of Oncology, Faculty of Medicine, University of Ottawa, Canada

Supported in part by Ontario Cancer Research and Treatment Foundation Grant No. 242 and Medical Research Council of Canada Operating Grant MA-3903.

disease of a more generalized unresponsiveness to antigens eliciting delayed hypersensitivity.[78] Patients with Hodgkin's disease not only may have impaired established delayed hypersensitivity, i.e., cutaneous anergy to antigens presumed to have been encountered earlier in life, but also may fail to become sensitized to newly presented contact allergens such as dinitrochlorobenzene.[1, 24]

Lymphocytopenia is a prominent feature of advanced Hodgkin's disease.[2] Patients with widespread disease and lymphocyte-depleted histopathology may present initially with lymphocytopenia.[24] In such patients cell-mediated immune responses, are markedly impaired. An adequate lymphocyte presence appears necessary for effective host response to Hodgkin's disease itself.[41, 115]

Lymphocyte responsiveness to phytohemagglutinin (PHA) has been studied in patients with Hodgkin's disease as an in vitro correlate of delayed hypersensitivity. Depressed or delayed responsiveness has been reported by a number of workers,[3, 24, 53, 64, 155] but the reliability of this test as an assay of immunocompetence in Hodgkin's disease has been questioned.[52] A factor present in the plasma of Hodgkin's patients may have an inhibitory effect on lymphocyte function.[155] Antilymphocyte antibodies have been reported in Hodgkin's disease.[50] Abnormal lymphocyte function may, however, be due at least in part to an intrinsic lymphocyte defect.[39, 54]

The PHA-stimulated lymphocytes of normal subjects have been shown to produce cytotoxic effects on L-strain fibroblasts when the two cell types are cultured together. Lymphocytes from patients with Hodgkin's disease function poorly in this test.[149] In patients with advanced Hodgkin's disease the ability of lymphocytes to produce interferon may be impaired.[10] Hodgkin's disease lymphocytes appear to have low in vitro lymphotoxin release following PHA stimulation but show spontaneous release of lymphotoxin in unstimulated culture.[123] Lymphocytes from patients with Hodgkin's disease have been observed to produce cytotoxic effects on Reed-Sternberg-like cells in vitro.[137]

Skin allograft rejection time is prolonged in active, advanced Hodgkin's disease.[49, 75] Bone marrow grafts may also survive without rejection for prolonged periods of time.[15]

Efforts to transfer delayed hypersensitivity to patients with Hodgkin's disease by means of white blood cells taken from donors with established sensitivity have been for the most part unsuccessful.[75, 96] There is, though, no abnormality in the skin of patients with Hodgkin's disease. Anergic Hodgkin's patients possess normal reactivity to histamine, and sensitivity to allergens can be produced in the skin of such patients with serum passively transferred from sensitive donors.[117, 127]

Humoral immunity is impaired in Hodgkin's disease, but the deficit is not as pronounced as that observed in studies of cell-mediated immunity.[4, 24, 46, 79, 122] Humoral immunity tends to become abnormal in more advanced stages of disease. Peak antibody titers are lower than in control subjects and the titer is poorly maintained with time.[61, 66, 127] Antibody production may be delayed and the switchover from 19S to 7S antibody formation may not occur.[61] Secondary humoral immune responses remain relatively intact.[13] The anamnestic response may be found to be normal at the same time that the antigen used fails to elicit a delayed hypersensitivity response.[66]

Patients with Hodgkin's disease may have hypogammaglobuline-mia.[156] Approximately 45 per cent of patients have low IgM levels.[85] The majority of these are in late stages of disease. In contrast, IgA and IgG levels are comparatively normal.

Macrophage function[16] is probably normal in patients with Hodgkin's disease. If anything, the phagocytic capacity of the reticuloendothelial system of patients with active disease is increased.[134] The ability of neutrophils of patients with advanced Hodgkin's disease to kill ingested Candida albicans organisms is reported to be impaired.[80] Patients with active Hodgkin's disease have significantly lower plasma bradykininogen levels than do either normal subjects or patients with inactive Hodgkin's disease.[35]

In general, the extent of immunologic impairment in Hodgkin's disease is a function of the stage of the disease and of the histopathology. Thus, the greatest immunologic derangement will be found in disseminated stage IV disease with lymphocyte-depleted histopathology. Patients with intact cellular immunity have a more favorable prognosis than do their immunologically impoverished counterparts.[25, 139] With response of the disease to therapy, immune function may recover, approximating normal. Delayed hypersensitivity responses may return,[14, 140] hypogammaglobulinemia may be corrected,[114] and normal reticuloendothelial function may be restored.[134] This is not always the case, particularly where remissions have been induced with irradiation.[52]

LYMPHOMA (OTHER THAN HODGKIN'S DISEASE)

Detailed studies of immune function similar to those carried out in patients with Hodgkin's disease are lacking for lymphosarcoma. Investigations which have been conducted, however, suggest a generalized immunologic derangement, involving both humoral and cell-mediated immunity. Patients with lymphosarcoma have impaired delayed hypersensitivity responses to microbial antigens.[78] This becomes more marked as disease progresses.

Skin allograft rejection time is prolonged in lymphosarcoma.[93] The in vitro lymphocyte response to PHA is depressed, with the most pronounced depression found in older patients with small cell lymphosarcoma.[102] Both primary and secondary humoral immune responses are abnormally low.[13, 59, 122] Hypogammaglobulinemia may be a feature in advanced stages of the disease.[9, 93] Reticuloendothelial phagocytic function is for the most part within the normal range.[51]

Patients with reticulum cell sarcoma manifest cutaneous anergy and have a decreased in vitro lymphocyte response to PHA.[63, 102] Reticulum cell sarcoma lymphocytes survive poorly in culture. A lymphotoxic plasma factor may be implicated in this phenomenon. Occasional patients, however, are found with normal in vitro lymphocyte reactivity to PHA.[12] Skin graft rejection is delayed.[93] Hypogammaglobulinemia may be a feature of the disease.[93]

Low IgM and IgG levels have been found in patients with Burkitt's lymphoma.[28, 98, 161] Adaptive immunity is, though, surprisingly unimpaired. Humoral and cell-mediated immunity are reportedly normal in American patients with this disease.[28, 162] In Uganda, patients with Burkitt's lymphoma have normal in vitro and in vivo cellular immunity but impaired primary antibody formation.[161] Patients with disseminated disease of great mass may have a decreased delayed hypersensitivity response to dinitrochlorobenzene, and an impaired in vitro response to PHA.[144]

In Kaposi's sarcoma, humoral immunity and immunoglobulin levels are normal but there is gross impairment of the delayed hypersensitivity response to dinitrochlorobenzene.[86]

CHRONIC LYMPHOCYTIC LEUKEMIA

Patients with chronic lymphocytic leukemia possess two populations of small lymphocytes. The first of these consists of normal T and B lymphocytes. The second population is comprised of leukemic cells, most likely of the B-cell type.[159] They carry immunoglobulin on their surface, albeit in lower density than do normal B-cells. Patients with chronic lymphocytic leukemia may then be said to have "B-cell leukemia."[159] The leukemic B-cells are incapable of normal immune function. It is the accumulation of these cells which will in time lead to the impaired adaptive immunity found in chronic lymphocytic leukemia.

The two classes of lymphocytes found in chronic lymphocytic leukemia may be distinguished by a number of functional characteristics. The normal cells can be eluted from the neoplastic fraction by use of a polystyrene bead column.[152] The leukemic cells have when compared to normal lymphocytes an increased sensitivity to colchicine[151] and L-asparaginase.[128] They are more resistant to radiation than are normal lymphocytes. They seem in vitro to possess the ability to adsorb bacteria on their cell membranes.[63] The leukemic lymphocytes may lack the ability to circulate between vascular and extravascular sites.[62, 146] Isoproterenol inhibits the in vitro response of leukemic lymphocytes to phytohemagglutinin; the drug fails to produce this effect with normal lymphocytes.[73] The leukemic lymphocyte in chronic lymphocytic leukemia appears unable to synthesize globulin in response to PHA[40] and is defective in its ability to cause in vitro adherence of Salmonella organisms.[22] The leukocytes in chronic lymphocytic leukemia are either more osmotically fragile or more resistant than are normal cells.[99] Leukemic lymphocytes are incapable of rosette formation with red cells coated with complement, most likely because they lack a receptor site on their surface for complement.[91] This structural feature is found on 12 to 29 per cent of blood lymphocytes obtained from normal donors. When compared to normal lymphocytes leukemic lymphocytes consume less total sugar and metabolize less carbohydrate by way of the hexose monophosphate shunt pathway.[23]

The leukemic lymphocyte in chronic lymphocyte leukemia responds poorly in vitro to both specific and nonspecific mitogens.[100] Impaired responses are especially pronounced in patients with high lymphocyte counts and low serum immunoglobulin levels.[100, 119] Immunosuppressive serum factors are not involved. Improved reactivity follows a chemotherapeutically induced reduction in the total white count.[21, 132] The peak in vitro response of leukemic lymphocytes to PHA may be delayed, although still below normal.[21, 54] This delay in response is reported to result from slow new ribosome formation; the slow new ribosome formation is linked to a defective control mechanism for the conservation of 18S subunits.[118] Phytohemagglutinin-responsive leukemic lymphocytes yield a different RNA isolation pattern from that of phytohemagglutinin-responsive normal lymphocytes.[31] There is delayed induction of tRNA methylases in leukemic lymphocytes stimulated with PHA.[112] The leukemic lymphocyte maintained in culture differs morphologically from its normal counterpart. Additional differences become evident following PHA stimulation.[27] The electron microscopic and phase microscopic examination of peripheral lymphocytes from patients with untreated chronic lymphocytic leukemia shows clear morphologic differences between them and normal lymphocytes.[129, 130]

Established delayed hypersensitivity and the ability to develop new delayed hypersensitivity reactions appear relatively intact in patients with chronic lymphocytic leukemia.[17, 29, 94, 133] Delayed hypersensitivity may be transferred to negative reactors by intramuscular or intradermal injections of leukocytes obtained from positive reacting donors. The capacity to reject skin allografts is either normal or impaired.[95] There is no clear correlation between acceptance or rejection of a graft and any of the following: serum gamma globulin level, previous treatment, humoral immunity and delayed-type skin reactivity.

Both primary and secondary humoral antibody responses are impaired in chronic lymphocytic leukemia.[29, 94, 133] Patients with normal gamma globulin levels generally give better responses than do those with hypogammaglobulinemia, but the responses of both groups are abnormally low. A good correlation exists between defective antibody formation and the incidence of bacterial infectious complications. The kinetics of the immune response in chronic lymphocytic leukemia are characterized by a prolonged induction time for IgM antibody and by a delayed switchover from IgM to IgG production.[61]

Hypogammaglobulinemia and agammaglobulinemia are frequent accompaniments of chronic lymphocytic leukemia.[71, 72, 109] The majority of patients with disease of greater than 5 years' duration develop hypogammaglobulinemia.[38] The condition is usually found in the presence of advanced disseminated disease.[157] It is irreversible. A good correlation is found between hypogammaglobulinemia and the frequency of bacterial infections[94, 133] but not with subsequent length of life.[38] IgM and IgA levels appear to be affected more often than the level of IgG.[29, 126] The impaired in vitro phagocytic and bactericidal function of leukocytes taken from patients with chronic lymphocytic leukemia is quite likely related to a lack of opsonins as the result of hypogammaglobulinemia.[124] The abnormality is in large part corrected by substituting normal serum for leukemic serum in the culture system.

MULTIPLE MYELOMA – MACROGLOBULINEMIA

Patients with a malignancy involving the cells of the plasma cell series might be expected to have disordered humoral antibody formation. This is in fact the case. Although primary humoral immune responses are impaired, in contrast to the situation in chronic lymphocytic leukemia secondary humoral antibody formation is relatively intact.[29, 37, 163]

Patients with the greatest impairment of antibody formation are the most susceptible to infectious complications. Disturbances of antibody formation are most marked in patients with the most amount of abnormal globulin. Despite the fact that occasional myeloma proteins have been shown to have antibody-like activity[108] the abnormal globulin offers no protection against infection. The response to a primary antigen in multiple myeloma is characterized by a prolonged induction time for IgM antibody with more rapid switchover than normally occurs from IgM to IgG antibody formation.[55] Total serum antibody titer declines more rapidly than it does in normal subjects and peak antibody titers are lower for both IgM and IgG antibody. A factor contributing to these latter observations is the finding that not only is gamma globulin formation impaired in multiple myeloma but that there is also an increased rate of gamma globulin catabolism.[141]

Most patients with multiple myeloma have decreased immunoglobulin levels, generally to less than 20 per cent of normal.[88, 120] Recovery of normal immunoglobulin may occur in patients with multiple myeloma who respond to chemotherapy.[5]

Patients with multiple myeloma demonstrate intact established delayed hypersensitivity responses and may be sensitized to new antigens.[29, 55] The skin allograft rejection time has been found to be delayed in patients with multiple myeloma.[82]

The in vitro lymphocyte response to PHA has been reported to be normal in multiple myeloma.[61] If, however, the lymphocytes are cultured under conditions of synchronization, the responses may be shown to be significantly less than normal.[120] Normal lymphocytes incubated in myeloma serum preserve their responsiveness to PHA. (Myeloma protein may, though, interfere with the phagocytic function of granulocytes.[104]) There is no correlation between impaired lymphocyte function and low immunoglobulin levels. The lymphocytes in patients with multiple myeloma have impaired in vitro responses to streptolysin O, streptokinase-streptodornase, and vaccinia.[55]

Patients with Waldenström's macroglobulinemia have reduced in vitro lymphocyte responses to PHA.[120] Both primary and secondary humoral antibody responses are impaired in this disease.[37, 107] Normal inflammatory responses are present.[101]

ACUTE LEUKEMIA

The immunologic deficit seen in acute leukemia does not involve adaptive immune function. Both humoral and cellular immunity are intact. The susceptability to infection seen in the disease is the direct consequence of granulocytopenia and lymphocytopenia.[18] Leukopenia results from the progression of disease and the cytotoxic effect of leukemic chemotherapy.

The primary and secondary humoral antibody responses of the patient with acute leukemia are within the normal range.[59, 60, 79, 136] Serum immunoglobulins are normal in acute leukemia.[87] Any alteration in globulin levels found are due to the effect of drug treatment.[76, 110] Reduction of serum IgG levels of unusual magnitude and rate has been reported to be associated with poor prognosis in childhood acute leukemia.[76] Similarly, in vitro lymphocyte responsiveness to PHA is unaffected in the leukemic patient except during the time when chemotherapy is being administered.[65, 147] Chemotherapy during remission induction therapy in acute leukemia may depress both established delayed hypersensitivity and humoral antibody formation.[20, 34] With maintenance therapy during remission, immunologic reactivity is relatively unaffected.

Infection in acute leukemia occurs most frequently in the presence of peripheral blood granulocytopenia and lymphocytopenia.[18] Infectious complications are seen more often with granulocytopenia alone than with lymphocytopenia alone. A critical value of 1500 granulocytes per cu. mm. has been determined.[18] Above this level there is no additional decrease in the frequency of infection.

Patients with acute leukemia have a poor inflammatory response.[19, 105, 106] This is due likely to the paucity of normal granulocytes and monocytes in the disease. The neutrophils in acute leukemia may be incapable of the normal intracellular killing of bacteria.[116] Deficient myeloperoxidase and abnormal neutrophilic bactericidal function has been reported in myelomonocytic leukemia.[30] Neutrophils from patients with acute leukemia frequently have impaired killing ability for ingested Candida albicans organisms.[80] The defect has been attributed to low levels of myeloperoxidase and lysozome activity in these cells. Their carbohydrate metabolism may be impaired.[138, 145] They may be excessively fragile.[99] All these factors could contribute to the high incidence of infectious complications.

CHRONIC MYELOID LEUKEMIA

The granulocytes in chronic myeloid leukemia have apparently normal in vitro phagocytic and bactericidal activity.[125] Impaired phagocytosis has been demonstrated, however, using a skin window technique.[153] Even allowing for slightly reduced phagocytic function on the part of individual granulocytes, total phagocyte capacity is probably normal because of the greatly expanded leukocyte mass. Granulocytes from donors with chronic myeloid leukemia have been noted to be biologically active and capable of phagocytosis when transfused into leukopenic patients with acute leukemia.[135]

SOLID TUMORS

Patients with early cancer may have normal delayed skin reactions and normal in vitro lymphocyte responses to antigen.[97] With progression of disease, cell-mediated immune function becomes impaired. Patients may have peripheral blood lymphocytopenia[160] and their lymphocytes may show ultramicroscopic abnormalities.[47] The in vitro lymphocyte response to PHA is depressed.[6, 43]

The presence in malignant disease of a serum factor which inhibits in vitro lymphocyte reactivity has been reported.[44, 45, 158] This observation has been disputed.[7, 48] Cutaneous anergy to a variety of skin test antigens develops.[69, 142] Impaired skin reactivity in cancer patients may reflect impaired delayed hypersensitivity but could indicate a poor inflammatory response.[74] The allograft rejection reaction is delayed. The lymphocyte transfer reaction is weakened[58] and patients will have reduced ability to reject implants of cancer cell lines.[143] In some instances a normal humoral antibody response may be demonstrated to an antigen which fails to elicit delayed hypersensitivity.[11] There appears to be a good correlation between patient prognosis and intact cellular immunity.[36, 77] With advanced metastatic solid tumors, cell-mediated immunity is more often affected than is humoral immunity, although both may be depressed in late stages of disease.[70, 81, 84]

Other disturbances of immune function have been reported to occur with a number of disseminated solid tumors. Reticuloendothelial function is depressed with solid tumors of the breast and colon.[33] Complement activity may be high in patients with a variety of untreated tumors arising from bowel, lung, and breast.[89] The inflammatory response in advanced malignancy is abnormal, with a diminished ability to mobilize monocytes.[32] Skin allografts from patients with cancer have a prolonged rejection time when placed on other cancer patients or on individuals who do not have malignant disease.[8, 113] A variety of immunoglobulin disturbances have been described as occurring in malignant disease.[67, 68] Cancer patients may have an increased catabolic rate for gamma globulin.[148] Paraproteinemia may be found in patients with epithelial neoplasms.[83]

Intact immune function is not a prerequisite for successful response to cancer chemotherapy in patients with malignant disease.[57] "Rebound-overshoot" recovery of immune function following chemotherapy to a level of function greater than pretreatment determinations is associated with good prognosis and responsiveness to chemotherapy.[26, 57]

SUMMARY

The various immunological derangements associated with neoplastic disease in man have been reviewed. Unique patterns of immunologic impairment characterize chronic lymphocytic leukemia, multiple myeloma, and acute leukemia. Many of the immune deficits believed to have been specific for the lymphomas may also be found as features of other solid tumors. Cell-mediated immunity is affected earlier in the course of malignant illness than is humoral immunity. Later with the development of disseminated disease both these components of adaptive immunity are depressed. The precise cause for this is unknown. It may result from the direct action of the carcinogenic agent, whether chemical or virus, or it may be due to an overriding commitment on the part of the host's immune apparatus to the tumor. Programs of treatment which envisage a combined chemotherapy-immunotherapy approach must be designed, keeping well in mind the immunological status of the patient for whom they are intended.

REFERENCES

1. Aisenberg, A. C.: Studies on delayed hypersensitivity in Hodgkin's disease. J. Clin. Invest., 41:1964, 1962.
2. Aisenberg, A. C.: Lymphocytopenia in Hodgkin's disease. Blood, 25:1037, 1965.
3. Aisenberg, A. C.: Quantitative estimation of the reactivity of normal and Hodgkin's disease lymphocytes with thymidine-2-C-14. Nature, 205:1233, 1965.
4. Aisenberg, A. C., and Leskowitz, S.: Antibody formation in Hodgkin's disease. New Eng. J. Med., 268:1269, 1963.
5. Alexanian, R., and Migliore, P. J.: Normal immunoglobulins in multiple myeloma: Effect of melphalan chemotherapy. J. Lab. Clin. Med., 75:225, 1970.
6. Al-Sarref, M., Sardesai, S., and Vaitkevicius, V. K.: Effect of homologous plasma on lymphocyte cultures in cancer patients and controls. Proc. Amer. Assoc. Cancer Res., 11:3, 1970.
7. Al-Sarref, M., Sardesai, S., and Vaitkevicius, V. K.: Effect of syngeneic and allogeneic plasma on lymphocytes from cancer patients, patients with non-neoplastic diseases and normal subjects. Cancer, 27:1426, 1971.
8. Amos, D. B., Hatler, B. G., and Shingleton, W. W.: Prolonged survival of skin-grafts from cancer patients on normal recipients. Lancet, 1:414, 1965.
9. Arends, T., Coonrad, C. V., and Rundles, R. W.: Serum proteins in Hodgkin's disease and malignant lymphoma. Amer. J. Med., 16:833, 1954.
10. Armstrong, R. W., Gurwith, M. J., Waddell, D., and Merigan, T. C.: Cutaneous interferon production in patients with Hodgkin's disease and other cancers infected with varicella or vaccinia. New Eng. J. Med., 283:1182, 1970.
11. Ashikawa, K., Motoya, K., and Sekiguchi, M.: Immune response in tumour-bearing patients and animals. II. Incidence of tuberculin anergy in cancer patients. Gann, 58:565, 1967.
12. Astaldi, G., Girando, L. C., and Marsani, F.: Lymphocytes in reticulum-cell sarcoma. Lancet, 2:410, 1968.
13. Barr, M., and Fairley, G. H.: Circulating antibodies in reticuloses. Lancet, 1:1305, 1961.
14. Bastai, P.: Ueber die klinische Bedeutung der Tuberculin-Anergie bei malignem Lymphogranuloma. Klin. Wschr., 7:1606, 1928.
15. Beilby, J. O. W., Cade, I. S., Jelliffe, A. M., Parkin, D. M., and Stewart, J. W.: Prolonged survival of a bone marrow graft resulting in a blood-group chimera. Brit. Med. J., 1:96, 1960.
16. Blaese, R. M., Oppenheim, J. J., Seeger, R., and Waldmann, T. A.: In vitro lymphocyte transformation: The restoration of purified lymphocyte responses by allogeneic macrophages from normal and anergic patients. Clin. Res., 18:422, 1970.
17. Block, J. B., Haynes, H. A., Thompson, W. L., and Neimann, P. E.: Delayed hypersensitivity in chronic lymphocytic leukemia. J. Nat. Cancer Inst., 42:973, 1969.
18. Bodey, G. P., Buckley, M., Sathe, Y. S., and Freireich, E. J.: Quantitative relationships between circulating leukocytes and infections in acute leukemia. Ann. Int. Med., 64:328, 1966.
19. Boggs, D.: The cellular composition of inflammatory exudates in human leukemias. Blood, 15:466, 1960.
20. Borella, L., and Webster, R. G.: The immunosuppressive effects of long-term combination chemotherapy in children with acute leukemia in remission. Cancer Res., 31:420, 1971.
21. Bouroncle, B. A., Clausen, K. P., and Aschenbrand, J. F.: Studies of the delayed response of phytohemagglutinin (PHA) stimulated lymphocytes in 25 chronic lymphatic leukemia patients before and during therapy. Blood, 34:166, 1969.
22. Brody, J. I., and Beizer, L. H.: Immunologic incompetence of the neoplastic lymphocyte in chronic lymphocytic leukemia. Ann. Int. Med., 64:1237, 1966.
23. Brody, J. I., Oski, F. A., and Singer, D. E.: Impaired pentose phosphate shunt and decreased glycolytic activity in lymphocytes of chronic lymphocytic leukemia. Metabolic pathway? Blood, 34:421, 1969.
24. Brown, R. S., Haynes, H. A., Foley, H. T., Godwin, H. A., Berard, C. W., and Carbone, P. P.: Hodgkin's disease: immunologic, clinical and histologic features in 50 untreated patients. Ann. Intern. Med., 67:291, 1967.

25. Chawla, P. L., Stutzman, L., Dubois, R. E., Kim, U., and Sokal, J. E.: Long survival in Hodgkin's disease. Amer. J. Med., 48:85, 1970.
26. Cheema, A. R., and Hersh, E. M.: Patient survival after chemotherapy and its relationship to in vitro lymphocyte blastogenesis. Cancer, 28:851, 1971.
27. Clausen, K. P., and Bouroncle, B. A.: The ultrastructure of phytohemagglutinin (PHA) stimulated lymphocytes of chronic lymphatic leukemia. Blood, 34:179, 1969.
28. Cohen, M. H., Bennett, J. M., Berard, C. W., Ziegler, J. L., Vogel, C. L., Sheagren, J. N., and Carbone, P. P.: Burkitt's tumor in the United States. Cancer, 23:1259, 1969.
29. Cone, L., and Uhr, J. W.: Immunological deficiency disorders associated with chronic lymphocytic leukemia and multiple myeloma. J. Clin. Invest., 43:2241, 1964.
30. Davis, A. T., Brunning, R. D., and Quie, P. G.: Polymorphonuclear leukocyte myeloperoxidase deficiency in a patient with myelomonocytic leukemia. New Eng. J. Med., 285:789, 1971.
31. Deutsch, A., and Norden, A.: Isolation and characterization of RNA from lymphocytes of chronic lymphocytic leukaemia. Scand. J. Haemat., 8:112, 1971.
32. Dizon, Q. S., and Southam, C. M.: Abnormal cellular response in skin abrasion in cancer patients. Cancer, 16:1288, 1963.
33. Donovan, A. J.: Reticuloendothelial function in patients with cancer; initial observations. Amer. J. Surg., 114:230, 1967.
34. Dupuy, J. M., Kourilsky, F. M., Fradelizzi, D., Feingold, N., Jacquillat, C., Bernard, J., and Dausset, J.: Depression of immunologic reactivity of patients with acute leukemia. Cancer, 27:323, 1971.
35. Eilam, N., Johnson, P. K., Johnson, N. L., and Creger, W. P.: Bradykininogen levels in Hodgkin's disease. Cancer, 22:631, 1968.
36. Eilber, F. R., and Morton, D. L.: Impaired immunologic reactivity and recurrence following cancer surgery. Cancer, 25:362, 1970.
37, Fahey, J. L., Scoggins, R., Utz, F. P., and Szwed, C. F.: Infection, antibody response and gamma globulin components in multiple myeloma and macroglobulinemia. Amer. J. Med., 35:698, 1963.
38. Fairley, G. H., and Scott, R. B.: Hypogammaglobulinemia in chronic lymphocytic leukemia. Brit. Med. J., 2:920, 1961.
30. Fazio, M., and Bachi, C.: Combined action of phytohemagglutinin and RNA on lymphocytes from patients with Hodgkin's disease. Nature, 215:629, 1967.
40. Forbes, I. J., and Henderson, D. W.: Globulin synthesis by human peripheral lymphocytes: In vitro measurements using lymphocytes from normals and patients with disease. Ann. Int. Med., 65:69, 1966.
41. Frenster, J. H., and Archibald, R. B.: Interactions of lymphocytes with Reed-Sternberg cells within Hodgkin's disease lymph nodes. Ann. Intern. Med., 72:794, 1970.
42. Further in the Hodgkin's maze. Lancet, 1:1053, 1971.
43. Garrioch, D. B., Good, R. A., and Gatti, R. A.: Lymphocyte response to PHA in patients with non-lymphoid tumours. Lancet, 1:618, 1970.
44. Gatti, R. A.: Serum inhibitors of lymphocyte responses. Lancet, 1:1351, 1971.
45. Gatti, R. A., Garrioch, D. B., and Good, R. A.: Depressed PHA responses in patients with non-lymphoid malignancies. In Harris, J. E., ed.: Proceedings of the Fifth Leukocyte Culture Conference. New York, Academic Press, 1970, p. 339.
46. Geller, W. A.: A study of antibody formation in patients with malignant lymphomas. J. Lab. Clin. Med., 42:232, 1953.
47. Gogate, S. A., and Von Haam, E.: Ultramicroscopic studies of lymphocytes from cancer patients. Acta Cytologica, 14:224, 1970.
48. Golob, E. K., Israsena, T., Quatrale, A. C., and Becker, K. L.: Effect of serum from cancer patients on homologous lymphocyte cultures. Cancer, 23:306, 1969.
49. Green, I., and Corso, P. F.: A study of skin homografting in patients with lymphomas. Blood, 14:235, 1959.
50. Grifoni, V., DelGiacco, G. S., Tognella, S., Spano, G., Manconi, P. E., and Rugarli, C.: Antilymph node antibodies in Hodgkin's disease (brief report). Boll. Ist. Sieroter. (Milan), 48:75, 1969.
51. Groch, G. S., Perillie, P. E., and Finch, S. C.: Reticuloendothelial phagocytic function in patients with leukemia and multiple myeloma. Blood, 26:489, 1965.
52. Han, T., and Sokal, J. E.: Lymphocyte response to phytohemagglutinin in Hodgkin's disease. Amer. J. Med., 48:728, 1970.
53. Havemann, K.: Delayed response of lymphocytes to phytohemagglutinin in Hodgkin's disease. Deutsch. Med. Wschr., 94:1867, 1969.
54. Havemann, K., and Rubin, A. D.: The delayed response of chronic lymphocytic leukemia lymphocytes to phytohemagglutinin in vitro. Proc. Soc. Exper. Biol. Med., 127:688, 1968.
55. Harris, J. E., Alexanian, R., Hersh, E. M., and Migliore, P.: Immune function in multiple myeloma: Impaired responsiveness to Keyhole limpet hemocyanin. Can. Med. Assoc. J., 104:389, 1971.

56. Harris, J. E., and Sinkovics, J. G.: The Immunology of Malignant Disease. St. Louis, C. V. Mosby Co., 1970.

57. Harris, J. E., and Stewart, T. H. M.: Recovery of mixed lymphocyte reactivity (MLR) following cancer chemotherapy in man. In Schwarz, M. R., ed.: Proceedings of the Sixth Leukocyte Culture Conference. New York, Academic Press, 1971, in press.

58. Hattler, B. G., Jr., and Amos, D. B.: Reactions obtained with transferred lymphocytes in patients with advanced cancer. J. Nat. Cancer Inst., 35:927, 1965.

59. Heath, R. B., Fairley, G. H., and Malpas, J. S.: Production of antibodies against viruses in leukemia and related diseases. Brit. J. Haemat., 10:365, 1964.

60. Hersh, E. M., Carbone, P. P., and Frereich, E. J.: Recovery of immune responsiveness after drug suppression in man. J. Lab. Clin. Med., 67:566, 1966.

61. Hersh, E. M., Curtis, J. E., Harris, J. E., McBride, C., Alexanian, R., and Rossen, R.: Host defence mechanisms in lymphoma and leukemia. In Leukemia-Lymphoma. Chicago, Year Book Medical Publishers, 1970, p. 149.

62. Hersh, E. M., Guinn, G. A., Rossen, R., Wallace, S., Rose, S., and Freireich, E. J.: Two populations of lymphocytes in chronic lymphocytic leukemia. In McIntyre, O. R., ed.: Proceedings of the Fourth Leukocyte Culture Conference. New York, Appleton-Century-Crofts, 1971, p.373.

63. Hersh, E. M., and Irwin, W. S.: Blastogenic responses of lymphocytes from patients with untreated and treated lymphomas. Lymphology, 2:150, 1969.

64. Hersh, E. M., and Oppenheim, J. J.: Impaired in vitro lymphocyte transformation in Hodgkin's disease. New Eng. J. Med., 273:1006, 1965.

65. Hersh, E. M., and Oppenheim, J. J.: Inhibition of in vitro lymphocyte transformation during chemotherapy in man. Cancer Res., 27:98, 1967.

66. Hoffman, G. T., and Rottino, A.: Studies of immunologic reactions of patients with Hodgkin's disease: Antibody reaction to typhoid immunization. Arch. Intern. Med., 86:872, 1950.

67. Hughes, N. R.: Serum group-specific (Gc) protein concentrations in patients with carcinoma, melanoma, sarcoma and cancers of hematopoietic tissues as determined by radial immunodiffusion. J. Nat. Cancer Inst., 46:665, 1971.

68. Hughes, N. R.: Serum concentrations of IgG, IgA, IgM immunoglobulins in patients with carcinoma, melanoma and sarcoma. J. Nat. Cancer Inst., 46:1015, 1971.

69. Hughes, L. E., and MacKay, W. D.: Suppression of the tuberculin response in malignant disease. Brit. Med. J., 2:1346, 1965.

70. Humphrey, L. J., Lincoln, P. M., and Griffen, W. O., Jr.: Immunologic response in patients with disseminated cancer. Ann. Surg., 168:374, 1968.

71. Jim, R. T. S.: Serum gamma globulin levels in chronic lymphocytic leukemia. Amer. J. Med. Sci., 234:44, 1959.

72. Jim, R. T. S., and Reinhard, E. H.: Agammaglobulinemia and chronic lymphocytic leukemia. Ann. Int. Med., 44:790, 1956.

73. Johnson, L. D., and Abell, C. W.: The effects of isoproterenol and cyclic aldenosine 3¹, 5¹-phosphate on phytohemagglutinin-stimulated DNA synthesis in lymphocytes obtained from patients with chronic lymphocytic leukemia. Cancer Res., 30:2718, 1970.

74. Johnson, M. W., Maibach, H. I., and Salmon, S. E.: Skin reactivity in patients with cancer: Impaired delayed hypersensitivity or faulty inflammatory response. New Eng. J. Med., 284:1255, 1971.

75. Kelly, W. D., Lamb, D. L., Varco, R. L., and Good, R. A.: An investigation of Hodgkin's disease with respect to the problems of homotransplantation. Ann. N.Y. Acad. Sci., 87:187, 1960.

76. Kiran, O., and Gross, S.: The G-immunoglobulins in acute leukemia in children. Hematologic and immunologic relationships. Blood, 33:198, 1969.

77. Krant, M. J., Manskopf, G., Brandrup, C. S., and Madoff, M. A.: Immunologic alterations in bronchogenic cancer, sequential study. Cancer, 21:623, 1968.

78. Lamb, D., Pilney, F., Kelly, W. D., and Good, R. A.: A comparative study of the incidence of anergy in patients with carcinoma, leukemia, Hodgkin's disease and other lymphomas. J. Immunol., 89:555, 1962.

79. Larson, D. L., and Tomlinson, L. J.: Quantitative antibody studies in Man. III. Antibody response in leukemia and other malignant lymphomas. J. Clin. Invest., 32:317, 1953.

80. Lehrer, R. I., and Cline, M. J.: Leukocyte candidacidal activity and resistance to systemic candidiasis in patients with cancer. Cancer, 27:1211, 1971.

81. Levin, A. G., Cunningham, M. P., Steers, A. K., Miller, D. G., and Southam, C. M.: Production of 19S and 7S antibodies by cancer patients. Clin. Exper. Immunol., 7:839, 1970.

82. Linton, A. L., Dunnigan, M. G., and Thomson, J. A.: Immune responses in myeloma. Brit. Med. J., 2:86, 1963.

83. Lynch, W. J., and Joske, R. A.: The occurrence of abnormal serum proteins in patients with epithelial neoplasms. J. Clin. Path., 19:461, 1966.

84. Lytton, B., Hughes, L. E., and Fulthorpe, A. J.: Circulating antibody response in malignant disease. Lancet, 1:69, 1964.

85. Malpas, J. S., Blandford, G., and White, R. J.: Remote effects of non-endocrine cancer on the blood. Proc. Roy. Soc. Med., 61:463, 1968.
86. Master, S. P., Taylor, J. F., Kyalwazi, S. K., and Ziegler, J. L.: Immunological studies in Kaposi's sarcoma in Uganda. Brit. Med. J., 1:600, 1970.
87. McKelvey, E., and Carbone, P. P.: Serum immune globulin concentrations in acute leukemia during intensive chemotherapy. Cancer, 18:1292, 1965.
88. McKelvey, E. M., and Fahey, J. L.: Immunoglobulin changes in disease: Quantitation on the basis of heavy polypeptide chains, IgG (gamma G), IgA (gamma A), and IgM (gamma M), and of light polypeptide chains type K (I) and type L (II). J. Clin. Invest., 44:1178, 1965.
89. McKenzie, D., Colsky, J., and Hetrick, D.: Complement reactivity of cancer patients; measurements by immune hemolysis and immune adherence. Cancer Res., 27:2386, 1967.
90. Meyer, K. K.: Radiation-induced lymphocyte-immune deficiency. A factor in the increased visceral metastases and decreased hormonal responsiveness of breast cancer. Arch. Surg., 101:114, 1970.
91. Michlmayr, G., and Huber, H.: Receptor sites for complement on certain human peripheral blood lymphocytes. J. Immunol., 105:670, 1970.
92. Millard, R. E.: Effect of previous irradiation on the transformation of blood lymphocytes. J. Clin. Path., 18:783, 1965.
93. Miller, D. G.: The association of immune disease and malignant lymphoma. Ann. Int. Med., 66:507, 1967.
94. Miller, D. G., and Karnofsky, D. A.: Immunologic factors and resistance to infection in chronic lymphatic leukemia. Amer. J. Med., 31:748, 1961.
95. Miller, D. G., Lizardo, J. G., and Snydermann, R. K.: Homologous and heterologous skin transplantation in patients with lymphomatous disease. J. Nat. Cancer Inst., 26:569, 1961.
96. Muftuoglu, A. U., and Balkur, S.: Passive transfer of tuberculin sensitivity to patients with Hodgkin's disease. New Eng. J. Med., 277:126, 1967.
97. Nelson, H. S.: Delayed hypersensitivity in cancer patients: Cutaneous and in vitro lymphocyte response to specific antigens. J. Nat. Cancer Inst., 42:765, 1969.
98. Ngu, V. A., McFarland, H., Osunkoya, B. O., and Udeozo, I. O. K.: Immunoglobulins in Burkitt's lymphoma. Lancet, 2:414, 1966.
99. Nir, E., Efrati, P., and Danon, D.: The osmotic fragility of human leucocytes in normal and in some pathological conditions. Brit. J. Haemat., 18:237, 1970.
100. Oppenheim, J. J., Whang, J., and Frei, E., III.: Immunologic and cytogenetic studies of chronic lymphocytic leukemic cells. Blood, 26:121, 1965.
101. Pachter, M. R., and Havey, Q. G.: Antibody deficiency in macroglobulinemia. Amer. J. Clin. Path., 37:248, 1962.
102. Papac, R. J.: Lymphocyte transformation in malignant lymphomas. Cancer, 26:279, 1970.
103. Park, S. K., Wallace, H. A., Brody, J. I., and Blakemore, W. S.: Immunosuppressive effect of surgery. Lancet, 1:53, 1971.
104. Penny, R., and Gatton, D. A. G.: Studies on neutrophil function. II. Pathological aspects. Brit. J. Haemat., 12:633, 1966.
105. Perillie, P. E., and Finch, S. C.: The local exudative cellular response in leukemia. J. Clin. Invest., 39:1353, 1960.
106. Perillie, P. E., and Finch, S. C.: Quantitative studies of the local exudative cellular reaction in acute leukemia. J. Clin. Invest., 43:425, 1964.
107. Pitts, N. C., and McDuffie, F. C.: Defective synthesis of IgM antibodies in macroglobulinemia. Blood, 30:767, 1967.
108. Potter, M.: Myeloma proteins (M-components) with antibody-like activity. New Eng. J. Med., 284:831, 1971.
109. Prasad, A.: The association of hypogammaglobulinemia and chronic lymphatic leukemia. Amer. J. Med. Sci., 236:610, 1958.
110. Ragab, A. H., Lindquist, J., Vietti, T. J., Choi, S. C., and Osterland, C. K.: Immunoglobulin pattern in childhood leukemia. Cancer, 26:890, 1970.
111. Reed, D. M.: Pathological changes in Hodgkin's disease with special reference to its relation to tuberculosis. Johns Hopkins Hosp. Rep., 10:133, 1902.
112. Riddick, D. H., and Gallo, R. C.: The transfer RNA methylases of human lymphocytes. II. Delayed induction by PHA in lymphocytes from patients with chronic lymphocytic leukemia. Blood, 37:293, 1971.
113. Robinson, E., Ben-Hur, N., Shulman, J., Hochman, A., and Neuman, Z.: Comparative study of skin homografts of normal donors and donors with malignant neoplasia in a host with malignant disease: A preliminary report. J. Nat. Cancer Inst., 34:185, 1965.
114. Roe, R. H., Gable, S. E., and Jarrold, T.: Hypogammaglobulinemia in Hodgkin's disease treated with nitrogen mustard. Arch. Intern. Med., 118:199, 1966.
115. Rosenthal, S. R.: Significance of tissue lymphocytes in prognosis of lymphogranulomatosis. Arch. Path., 21:628, 1936.

116. Rosner, F., Valmont, I., Kozinn, P. J., and Caroline, L.: Leukocyte function in patients with leukemia. Cancer, 25:835, 1970.

117. Rostenberg, A., Jr., McCraney, H. C., and Bluefarb, S. M.: Immunologic studies in lymphoblastomas. II. Ability to develop sensitization to simple chemicals and ability to accept passive transfer antibody. J. Invest. Derm., 26:209, 1956.

118. Rubin, A. D.: In vitro evaluation of lymphocyte proliferation in lymphoproliferative disorders. In Harris, J. E.: Proceedings of the Fifth Leukocyte Culture Conference. New York, Academic Press, 1970, p. 239.

119. Rubin, A. D., Havemann, K., and Dameshek, W.: Studies in chronic lymphocytic leukemia: Further studies of the proliferative abnormality of the blood lymphocyte. Blood, 33:313, 1969.

120. Salmon, S. E., and Fudenberg, H. H.: Abnormal nucleic acid metabolism of lymphocytes in plasma cell myeloma and macroglobulinemia. Blood, 33:300, 1969.

121. Santos, G. W., Owens, A. H., and Sensenbrenner, L. L.: Effects of selected cytotoxic agents on antibody production in man: A preliminary report. Ann. N.Y. Acad. Sci., 114:404, 1964.

122. Saslaw, S., Carlisle, H. O., and Bouroncle, B.: Antibody response in hematologic patients. Proc. Soc. Exper. Biol. Med., 106:654, 1961.

123. Savel, H., and Mohring, T.: Lymphotoxin production in human neoplasia. Proc. Soc. Exper. Biol. Med., 137:374, 1971.

124. Sbarra, A. J., Shirley, W., Selvaraj, R. J., Ouchi, E., and Rosenbaum, E.: The role of the phagocyte in host-passive interactions. I. The phagocytic capabilities of leukocytes from lymphoproliferative disorders. Cancer Res., 24:1958, 1964.

125. Sbarra, A. J., Shirley, W., Selvaraj, R. J., and Rosenbaum, E.: The role of the phagocyte in host-parasite interactions. III. The phagocytic capabilities of leukocytes from myeloproliferative and other neoplastic disorders. Cancer Res., 25:1199, 1965.

126. Scamps, R. A., Streeter, A. M., and O'Neill, B. J.: Immunoglobulin levels in chronic lymphocytic leukaemia. Med. J. Austr., 1:535, 1971.

127. Schier, W. W.: Cutaneous anergy and Hodgkin's disease. New Eng. J. Med., 250:353, 1954.

128. Schrek, R., Dolowy, W. C., and Ammeraal, R. N.: L-asparaginase; toxicity to normal and leukemic human lymphocytes. Science, 155:329, 1967.

129. Schrek, R., Knospe, W. H., and Trobaugh, F. E., Jr.: Chromatin and other cytologic indices in chronic lymphocytic leukemia. J. Lab. Clin. Med., 75:217, 1970.

130. Schumacher, H. R., Maugel, T. K., and Davis, K. D.: The lymphocyte of chronic lymphatic leukemia. I. Electron microscopy-onset. Cancer, 26:895, 1970.

131. Selvaraj, R. J., McRipley, R. J., and Sbarra, A. J.: The metabolic activities of leukocytes from lymphoproliferative and myeloproliferative disorders during phagocytosis. Cancer Res., 27:2287, 1967.

132. Sharman, C., Crossen, P. E., and Fitzgerald, P. H.: Lymphocyte number and response to phytohemagglutinin in chronic lymphocytic leukemia. Scand. J. Haemat., 3:375, 1966.

133. Shaw, R. K., Szwed, C., Boggs, D. R., Fahey, J. L., Frei, E., Morrison, E., and Utz, J. P.: Infection and immunity in chronic lymphocytic leukemia. Arch. Int. Med., 106:467, 1960.

134. Sheagren, J. N., Block, J. B., and Wolff, S. M.: Reticuloendothelial system phagocytic function in patients with Hodgkin's disease. J. Clin. Invest., 46:855, 1967.

135. Shohet, S. B.: Morphologic evidence for the in vivo activity of transfused chronic myelogenous leukemia cells in a case of massive staphylococcal septicemia. Blood, 32:111, 1968.

136. Silver, R. T., Utz, J. P., Fahey, J., and Frei, E., III.: Antibody response in patients with acute leukemia. J. Lab. Clin. Med., 56:634, 1960.

137. Sinkovics, J. G., Shirato, E., Cabiness, J. R., and Shullennerger, C. C.: Cytotoxic lymphocytes in Hodgkin's disease. Brit. Med. J., 1:172, 1970.

138. Skeel, R. T., Yankee, R. A., and Henderson, E. S.: Hexose monophosphate shunt activity of circulating phagocytes in acute lymphocytic leukemia. J. Lab. Clin. Med., 77:975, 1971.

139. Sokal, J. E., and Aungst, C. W.: Response to BCG vaccination and survival in advanced Hodgkin's disease. Cancer, 24:128, 1969.

140. Sokal, J. E., and Primikirios, N.: The delayed skin test response in Hodgkin's disease and lymphosarcoma: Effect of disease activity. Cancer, 14:597, 1961.

141. Solomon, A., Waldmann, T. A., and Fahey, J. L.: Metabolism of normal 6.6S γ-globulin in normal subjects and in patients with macroglobulinemia and multiple myeloma. J. Lab. Clin. Med., 62:1, 1963.

142. Solowey, A. C., and Rapaport, F. T.: Immunologic responses in cancer patients. Surg. Gynec. Obstet., 121:756, 1965.

143. Southam, C. M., Moore, A. E., and Rhoads, C. P.: Homotransplantation of human cell lines. Science, 125:158, 1957.

144. Stjernsward, J., Clifford, P., and Svedymr, E.: General and cellular tumour-specific immunological reactivity of Burkitt's lymphoma patients. In Burkitt, D., and Wright, D., eds.: Burkitt's Lymphoma. Edinburgh, Livingstone, 1969.

145. Stjernholm, R. L., Dimitrov, N. V., and Zito, S.: Carbohydrate metabolism in leukocytes. XIII. Differentiation by metabolism of leukemic leukocytes into three groups. J. Reticuloend. Soc., 7:539, 1970.
146. Stryckmans, P. A., Chanana, A. D., Cronkite, E. P., Greenberg, M. L., and Schiff, L. M.: Studies on lymphocytes. IX. The survival of autotransfused labeled lymphocytes in chronic lymphocytic leukemia. Europ. J. Cancer, 4:241, 1968.
147. Sutherland, R. M., Inch, W. R., and McCredie, J. A.: Phytohemagglutinin (PHA)-induced transformation of lymphocytes from patients with cancer. Cancer, 27:574, 1971.
148. Tee, D. E. H., and Watkins, J.: Catabolism of serum γG-globulins in a cancer patient and a normal volunteer. Brit. Med. J., 4:210, 1967.
149. Thomas, J. W., Boldt, W., and Horrocks, G.: Lymphocyte transformation by phytohemagglutinin. III. In vitro cytotoxicity. Canad. Med. Assoc. J., 99:303, 1968.
150. Thomas, J. W., Coy, P., Lewis, H. S., and Yuen, A.: Effect of therapeutic irradiation on lymphocyte transformation in lung cancer. Cancer, 27:1046, 1971.
151. Thomson, A. E. R., and Robinson, M. A.: Cytocidal action of colchicine in vitro on lymphocytes in chronic lymphocytic leukemia. Lancet, 2:868, 1967.
152. Thomson, A. E. R., Robinson, M. A., and Wetherley-Mein, G.: Heterogeneity of lymphocytes in chronic lymphocytic leukemia. Lancet, 2:200, 1966.
153. Tornyos, K.: Phagocyte activity of cells of the inflammatory exudate in human leukemia. Cancer Res., 27:1756, 1967.
154. Trinick, R. H.: Lymphocytes and intravascular hemolysis. Lancet, 1:225, 1949.
155. Trubowitz, S., Masek, B., and Del Rosario, A.: Lymphocyte response to phytohemagglutinin in Hodgkin's disease, lymphatic leukemia and lymphosarcoma. Cancer, 19:2019, 1966.
156. Ultmann, J. E., Cunningham, J. K., and Gellhorn, A.: The clinical picture of Hodgkin's disease. Cancer Res., 26:1047, 1966.
157. Ultmann, J. E., Fish, W., Osserman, E., and Gellhorn, A.: The clinical implications of hypogammaglobulinemia in patients with chronic lymphocytic leukemia and lymphocytic lymphosarcoma. Ann. Intern. Med., 51:501, 1959.
158. Whittaker, M. G., Rees, K., and Clark, C. G.: Reduced lymphocyte transformation in breast cancer. Lancet, 1:892, 1971.
159. Wilson, J. D., and Nossal, G. J. V.: Identification of human T and B lymphocytes in normal peripheral blood and in chronic lymphocytic leukaemia. Lancet, 2:788, 1971.
160. Zacharski, L. R., and Linman, J. W.: Lymphocytopenia: its causes and significance. Mayo Clin. Proc., 46:168, 1971.
161. Ziegler, A. L., Cohen, M. H., Morrow, R. H., Kyalwazi, S. K., and Carbone, P. P.: Immunologic studies in Burkitt's lymphoma. Cancer, 25:734, 1970.
162. Ziegler, J. L., Cohen, M. H., Vogel, C. L., Sheagren, J. M., and Carbone, P. O.: Immunologic studies in American patients with Burkitt-like lymphoma. Cancer Res., 27:2527, 1967.
163. Zinneman, H. H., and Hall, W. H.: Recurrent pneumonia in multiple myeloma and some observations on immunologic response. Ann. Intern. Med., 41:1152, 1954.

Faculty of Medicine
University of Ottawa
Ottawa, Ontario
Canada

Immunologic Mechanisms in Neurologic Diseases

*R. M. Armstrong, M.D.**

There are several areas of interest common to neurology and immunology. Experimental allergic encephalomyelitis and experimental allergic neuritis are established as experimental models of autoimmune disease in which the nervous system is the target. On the basis of clinical and pathologic similarities to these experimental models, it has been suggested that acute disseminated encephalomyelitis, acute hemorrhagic leukoencephalitis, idiopathic polyneuritis, and multiple sclerosis may be the result of autoimmune reactions in the nervous system. The association of thymic abnormalities and the often beneficial effect of thymectomy in myasthenia gravis suggest that some abnormality of the immunologic system is of significance in this disease. Some immunologic aspects of these conditions will be discussed.

In addition to the above there are several subacute or chronic progressive diseases of the nervous system which are caused by or presumed to be caused by viral infection. Progressive multifocal leukoencephalopathy, subacute sclerosing panencephalitis, Kuru disease, and Jakob-Creutzfeldt disease are conditions which may be of this type. The effect on the central nervous system may be the result of an atypical or inadequate immunologic reaction of the host. As yet the immunologic factors which determine when and how these slow or latent viruses become pathogenic remain unknown.[29, 35] Ataxia telangiectasia and myotonia dystrophica are associated with specific immunologic defects, but no causal relation between the immunologic and neurologic abnormalities has been defined.[14]

Patients maintained on long-term immunosuppressive therapy after organ transplantation may develop neoplasms. Many of these are tumours of the reticuloendothelial system, and a disproportionate number of these involve the brain. The explanation for this is unknown.[76]

---

*Associate, Department of Medicine (Neurology); Lecturer, Department of Pathology (Neuropathology); Faculty of Medicine, University of Toronto; Attending Physician, Toronto General Hospital

EXPERIMENTAL ALLERGIC ENCEPHALOMYELITIS

Experimental allergic encephalomyelitis can be produced readily in a wide variety of animals by injecting myelinated central nervous system tissue with complete Freund's adjuvant subcutaneously.[27,34,54,61] One to 3 weeks after immunization the animals develop tremor, ataxia, hypotonia, seizures, and paralysis. Lesions are present throughout the central nervous system but are more frequent in the white matter. Microscopic in size, they consist of multiple foci of inflammatory cells in and around the small vessels. The cells are predominantly mononuclear leukocytes: small lymphocytes, histocytes, and plasma cells. The proportions of these cell types change somewhat with the age of the lesion. Within and adjacent to these areas there is swelling, fragmentation, and loss of myelin and an increase in the number of microglia and astrocytes. Rarely the lesions are hemorrhagic and large enough to be seen macroscopically.[1,87]

Adjuvant is not essential for the production of experimental allergic encephalomyelitis, but the disorder is more easily and regularly produced with complete Freund's adjuvant.[27,34] There is wide variability in the susceptibility of species and strains to the induction of experimental allergic encephalomyelitis, and in the severity of the disease.[65] The antigen is organ specific but not species specific. Isogeneic, syngeneic, or xenogeneic mammalian myelinated central nervous system tissue is effective as antigen in mammalian animals.[61,65,74] The disease has been produced with non-mammalian central nervous system tissue in Lewis rats, which are highly susceptible to allergic encephalomyelitis.[42] Subcutaneous injection of antigen is more effective than intraperitoneal, intravenous or intracerebral administration.[61]

In some animals a more severe or "hyperacute" form of allergic encephalomyelitis with necrosis and hemorrhage in the lesions occurs when pertussis vaccine is used as an ancillary adjuvant. Pertussis vaccine can also effect a reactivation in a previously sensitized animal.[43]

Several groups have isolated and analyzed the *encephalitogenic component* (basic protein) of myelin.[23,36,39,45,47,48,55,71,88] It can be extracted from de-fatted central nervous system tissue with aqueous solutions of low pH, and has been prepared from the tissue of a number of species. It is generally agreed that the protein is basic in nature, has a molecular weight in the range of 18,000 and has no significant secondary or tertiary conformational characteristics. It is likely the encephalitogenic activity results from the primary structure (amino acid sequence) of the protein, and this is why the activity is retained even after treatment with freeze-thawing, boiling 8M urea, etc. Polypeptides of 8 to 10 amino acids which have encephalitogenic activity have been isolated and analyzed.[23] The basic protein may contain more than one encephalitogenic region, and these regions may differ from one another in their primary structure. This possibility and variations in the systems used to assay encephalitogenic activity may account for differences reported in the structure of the encephalitogenic fragments.

Many features of experimental allergic encephalomyelitis indicate that it is a *cell-mediated* immune response. It is most readily induced by intracutaneous injection of antigen with complete Freund's adjuvant. Excision of the injection site 1 hour after injection does not prevent the occurrence of allergic encephalomyelitis, but excision of the regional lymph nodes up to 4 or 5 days after immunization prevents the disease.[20, 28]

The disease can be transferred to histocompatible nonsensitized animals with a suspension of living lymph node cells from sensitized animals but not with sera.[62, 65] Lymphocytes from diseased animals are cytotoxic and myelinoclastic for central nervous system tissue in tissue culture.[11] The lymphocytes become cytotoxic for fibroblast monolayers in tissue culture when stimulated with basic encephalitogenic protein.[24] Brain extracts inhibit the migration of peritoneal exudate cells from sensitized animals.[22] Node or spleen lymphocytes preferentially bind allergic encephalomyelitis antigen after sensitization.[36]

Rats which have been neonatally thymectomized are less vulnerable to induction of allergic encephalomyelitis in adulthood and these animals also have impaired antibody production.[5] In birds, bursectomy results in impaired antibody production but it does not protect the bird from allergic encephalomyelitis, whereas thymectomy protects the bird from the disease but does not affect the antibody formation.[33] Cutaneous hyperreactivity to nerve tissue occurs in sensitized animals.[27, 85] These observations indicate that cell-mediated immunity is a major factor in the production of this disorder.

Circulating *antibodies* may also have a significant role in producing or modifying allergic encephalomyelitis. Sera from diseased animals is cytotoxic for cerebellar tissue grown in vitro. The cytotoxic factor is a gamma globulin associated with the IgG fraction. It binds to myelin and the reaction is complement dependent.[2, 11] The sera produces a reversible block of the synaptic transmission of electrical impulses in spinal cord preparations in tissue culture.[10] The cytotoxic effect of the sera is maximal after the onset of neurologic signs, a time when lymphocytes are least effective in the transfer of the disease. Deposition of antibody in brain tissue may precede the appearance of the mononuclear lymphocyte at the sites of lesion.[57]

Antibody which binds encephalitogenic protein has been demonstrated in some animals with experimental allergic encephalomyelitis.[36] The antigenic determinants for this antibody are at sites on the basic encephalitogenic protein which are separate from those determining encephalitogenic activity. It is not known whether this antibody is the same as that producing the cytotoxic and electrophysiologic effects.

Some animals sensitized with central nervous system tissue and adjuvant develop circulating complement-fixing anti-brain antibody. The antibody is organ specific but cross reacts with central nervous system tissue of several species. The antigens for this antibody can be extracted from myelin with ethanol and thus differ from the encephalitogenic antigen. The appearance of the complement-fixing anti-brain antibody correlates inversely with the development of experimental allergic encephalomyelitis in some species.[81] Lewis rats are extremely susceptible to the disease and do not produce complement-fixing anti-brain antibody. Wistar rats are resistant to the disease and produce complement-fixing antibody. Administration of Wistar rat sera containing complement-fixing antibody protects Lewis rats from allergic encephalomyelitis.[64]

Suppression of experimental allergic encephalomyelitis has been attempted with different techniques. In addition to thymectomy, removal of regional lymph nodes after immunization and the administration of sera with complement-fixing anti-brain antibody, there are other methods which prevent or suppress the development of encephalomyelitis. Central nervous system antigen, given to neonatal rats, protects them from encephalomyelitis when sensitization is subsequently attempted at age 6 to 8 weeks.[60] Repeated administration of small amounts of antigen prior to sensitization,[20] a very large amount of antigen at the time of immunization,[12] or administration of antigen after sensitization may suppress the disease.[77] Induction of tolerance, immunologic paralysis, and desensitization are the mechanisms ascribed to these manoeuvres respectively. Antilymphocyte serum[86] and x-irradiation[63] prior to sensitization are both effective in suppressing the disorder. X-irradiation after sensitization does not. Nitrogen mustard,[41] chlorambucil,[80] methotrexate,[15] 6-mercaptopurine, and cyclophosphamide have all been used successfully in suppressing the disease, but often it occurs soon after the immunosuppressive drug is stopped. Cyclophosphamide is of interest in that its suppressive effect persists for up to 6 weeks after cessation of treatment with the drug.[67]

EXPERIMENTAL ALLERGIC NEURITIS

Experimental allergic neuritis is an immunologically induced peripheral neuritis which is similar in many respects to experimental allergic encephalomyelitis.[84] Following immunization with peripheral nerve and complete Freund's adjuvant, sensorimotor polyneuropathy develops within 1 to 2 weeks. In the small veins of the affected nerves, lymphocytes undergo blast transformation, penetrate the endothelium of the vessels, move across the cell wall, and pass through the basement membrane to lie within the nerve. Myelin breakdown begins and phagocytic cells appear in the area. The lesions are confined to the peripheral nervous system. There is segmental demyelination, and multiple foci of mononuclear inflammatory cells are found along the course of the nerve.[9]

The antigens which cause allergic neuritis have not been isolated. There is cross reaction between several species. As with allergic encephalomyelitis, the disease can be transferred with sensitized lymphocytes.[8] Lymph node or buffy coat lymphocytes are myelinoclastic for peripheral nerve in tissue culture. Sera is less effective.[6] The role of antibody in experimental allergic neuritis is not established.

RELATIONSHIP OF CLINICAL DISEASES TO EXPERIMENTAL ALLERGIC ENCEPHALOMYELITIS AND NEURITIS

In these two disorders, cell-mediated immunologic responses are critical to the production of the diseases, but circulating antibodies and chemical mediators may have a significant role in their pathogenesis. In several clinical conditions immunologic factors may be of significance, and attempts have been made to relate these to the experimental models and to investigate immunologic function in these conditions.

Acute disseminated encephalomyelitis (post-infectious, para-infectious, or post-vaccinal encephalomyelitis) is a neurologic condition which may occur in relation to a number of viral infections (mumps, measles, varicella, rubella, influenza), following immunization with rabies or small pox vaccine, with foreign serums, or without any known precipitating event or illness. Neurologic signs appear several days after immunization. When associated with viral infections, the neurologic disease may occur at the time of, after, or without the appearance of clinical signs of the viral infection. The neurologic symptoms are varied depending upon the sites and severity of the lesions in the central nervous system. Confusion, convulsions, coma, paralysis, and focal neurologic deficits occur. The process may be acutely or subacutely progressive, resulting in death, or there may be recovery. A significant proportion of surviving patients are left with neurologic deficits.

There are several similarities between experimental allergic and acute disseminated encephalomyelitis. Both usually follow an incident of immunization or infection. Neurologic signs develop after a latency of several days, and the disease is usually marked by a single episode. Pathologically the lesions are the same.[44] The encephalomyelitis induced by rabies vaccine results from sensitization to central nervous system antigens in the vaccine. With viral infections or small pox vaccination the cause is not known. Several possibilities have been suggested.[32] Viral damage to host cells may release antigens and provoke an immunologic response to the host tissue. Host antigens may be incorporated into the viral capsule and become immunogenic or the virus may produce changes in the host cell membranes rendering them antigenic or vulnerable to immunologic reaction.

Acute disseminated encephalomyelitis is not a common disease. As a result of this, as well as the difficulties in diagnosis and the relatively brief course of the disease, there is no information about the immunologic responses of these patients during the acute phase.

There is evidence that steroids given early in the course of the disease may moderate and shorten the course of the episode.[52] The use of more vigorous immunosuppressive therapy is not at present indicated.

Acute hemorrhagic leukoencephalitis is a rare condition characterised by a clinical course similar to acute disseminated encephalomyelitis but it is more severe and is usually fatal within several days. A preceding minor nonspecific infection is frequently described. The lesions are located mainly in the white matter and are hemorrhagic and necrotic. Cases have been described which appear to be transitional between acute disseminated encephalomyelitis and acute hemorrhagic leukoencephalitis. It may be an accelerated or hyperacute form of acute disseminated disease, analogous to the hyperactive form of experimental allergic encephalomyelitis which can be induced with pertussis.[43,73]

Multiple sclerosis is a common neurologic disease.[48a] Its clinical features will not be discussed here, but it is often a chronic relapsing illness. The lesions are predominantly in the white matter of the central nervous system. There are multiple foci of demyelination and glial scarring. The foci are frequently adjacent to small veins and in white matter surrounding the walls of the ventricular system. In acute lesions mononuclear inflammatory cells may be present. The chronic relapsing course and histologic differences in the lesions make multiple sclerosis a less satisfactory analog of experimental allergic encephalomyelitis than acute disseminated encephalomyelitis. The similarities are sufficient to warrant careful consideration of multiple sclerosis in its relationship to allergic encephalomyelitis and investigation of the immunologic aspects of the disease.

The rate of *lymphocyte* blast transformation in response to myelin encephalitogenic protein is the same in individuals with multiple sclerosis as it is in controls. Comparing cases of multiple sclerosis in varying stages of activity, there are no detectable differences in transformation rate.[38] Increased transformation rates of lymphocytes cultured with homologous or autologous cerebral spinal fluid have been reported in patients with multiple sclerosis.[26] Others were unable to confirm this but reported that lymphocytes from normals and patients with multiple sclerosis responded more to multiple sclerosis and autologous fluid than to pooled control fluid. Lymphocytes from patients with multiple sclerosis may be cytotoxic to glial cells in tissue culture.[38] Lymphocytes from patients with multiple sclerosis which are cultured with central nervous system antigen produce migration inhibition factor, as do lymphocytes from hosts having other neurologic diseases.[18, 72]

Attempts to demonstrate anti-brain *antibody* in multiple sclerosis have not been successful. Antibodies to the basic encephalitogenic protein can be demonstrated using a technique which detects ^{131}I antigen-antibody complexes[16] or with passive hemagglutination,[25] but the levels are the same in individuals with multiple sclerosis as in the controls.

Serum from patients with multiple sclerosis is myelinoclastic in vitro. The reaction is complement-dependent and the active factor in the sera appears to be an antibody of the IgG class. Remyelination may occur if the serum is removed from the culture system. The sera of patients with active multiple sclerosis are more myelinoclastic than the sera from patients whose disease is in remission. Sera of patients with motor neurone disease are also myelinoclastic.[2] In vitro, sera from individuals with multiple sclerosis will block synaptic electrical transmission between neuronal cells before demyelination occurs. This too is complement-dependent and reverses with removal of the serum.[10]

Cerebrospinal fluid protein may be increased in patients with multiple sclerosis, but more common is a disproportion in the amount of γ globulin in the cerebrospinal fluid. The globulin fraction is normally less than 13 to 15 per cent of the total cerebrospinal fluid protein but in a high percentage of patients with multiple sclerosis this proportion is increased. This globulin is probably synthesized within the central nervous system. Its significance in the pathogenesis of multiple sclerosis is unknown, but it is a useful diagnostic indicator if the serum proteins are normal and syphilitic infection or subacute sclerosing panencephalitis are excluded.[81]

Immunosuppressive *therapy* has been used in the management of multiple sclerosis. The role of steroids remains controversial. They may moderate single episodes but do not appear to have a significant effect on the ultimate course of the disease,[48] and maintenance therapy is not an established treatment. Trials of treatment with antilymphocyte globulin or chemotherapy have been established but there is insufficient data to evaluate the effect of these forms of treatment, and their use is considered as experimental.

Infectious polyneuritis (Guillain-Barré Syndrome) and experimental allergic neuritis are similar in many respects. Following immunization or infection, there is an incubation period of 1 to 2 weeks, and then the appearance of a sensorimotor polyneuritis. Elevation of the cerebrospinal fluid protein is common in both. The pathologic changes in the peripheral nervous system are similar. Infectious polyneuritis is usually a monophasic illness, with the majority of patients having complete or nearly complete and permanent recovery. Occasional relapses occur and in some cases a chronic relapsing course may develop.[7]

Peripheral *lymphocytes* from patients with infectious polyneuritis are myelinoclastic for peripheral nerve in tissue culture.[7] Increased numbers of transforming lymphocytes are present in the peripheral blood of patients with infectious polyneuritis.[21, 89] Lymphocytes cultured with central or peripheral nervous system antigen inhibit the migration of peritoneal macrophages in an electrophoretic field.[17] *Sera* from patients with infectious polyneuritis are also myelinoclastic. This action is complement-dependent and appears to be due to an antibody, but sera from patients with other peripheral neuropathies contain this as well. Serum is less effective than lymphocytes. In half the cases of infectious polyneuritis there is antibody which reacts with saline extract of peripheral nerve tissue.[50]

The use of immunosuppressive *therapy* in the treatment of infectious polyneuritis is not established. In the majority of cases the illness is monophasic and the prognosis is excellent. In the less common relapsing cases steroids may be of value in maintaining remission.[7]

MYASTHENIA GRAVIS

It is well established that thymectomy is beneficial in the management of myasthenia gravis.[59, 68] Recognition of this and the immunologic role of the thymus indicate that a defect of the immunologic system may be a significant factor in the pathogenesis of myasthenia gravis.

The thymus is considered to be abnormal in 80 per cent of myasthenics without thymoma who undergo thymectomy. The abnormality "thymic hyperplasia" consists of the presence of germinal centres in the medullary region of the thymus.[19] This change is not unique to myasthenia gravis. It is found in association with other "autoimmune" disorders (systemic lupus erythematosus, thyroiditis, Addison's disease) and may be found in normal individuals. In one series, germinal follicles were present in the thymuses of young adults dying sudden traumatic deaths.[51] Ten per cent of cases of myasthenia gravis are associated with thymomas and a third of thymomas are associated with myasthenia gravis.[25a]

Thymic lymphocytes prepared from the thymus or the thymoma of patients with myasthenia gravis are functionally abnormal. Their rate of blast transformation in response to phytohemagglutinin is greater than normal.[3, 40] With phytohemagglutinin stimulation they are cytotoxic for muscle cells grown in tissue culture. Their migration from capillary tubes is inhibited by muscle and thymus antigen.[3] In each of these test systems thymic lymphocytes from patients with myasthenia gravis differ from the normals.

Peripheral Lymphocytes from myasthenic patients with or without thymectomy show no abnormality of blast transformation in response to muscle or thymus homogenates.[31] Spontaneous cytotoxicity for muscle cells in tissue culture and inhibition of lymphocyte migration with muscle or thymus antigens are sometimes demonstrable during exacerbation.[4] Injection of lymphocytes from individuals affected with myasthenia gravis into mice produces a higher mortality rate than normal lymphocytes. This effect can be suppressed with azathioprine.[56]

The above observations indicate that in myasthenia gravis the thymus tissue contains lymphocytes which are abnormally responsive to phytohemagglutinin stimulation and have been sensitized to muscle and thymus antigens. This suggests that cell-mediated immunologic responses may be significant in the pathogenesis of myasthenia gravis.

Antibodies to skeletal muscle are present in 30 per cent of patients with myasthenia gravis, 95 per cent of patients with thymoma and myasthenia gravis, and 24 per cent of patients with thymoma but without myasthenia gravis.[78] They are IgG globulins which bind specifically to the skeletal muscle and to thymic epithelial cells. They cross react with other species, but rarely occur except in association with myasthenia gravis or thymoma. While highly specific for myasthenia gravis, their presence or their titre does not correlate with the clinical state. They have no apparent role in producing the neuromuscular block of myasthenia gravis. Attempts to demonstrate antibody binding at the neuromuscular junction have not been successful.[49]

Association of other "autoimmune" disorders with myasthenia gravis has been reported. Systemic lupus erythematosus, pernicious anemia, hemolytic anemia, rheumatoid arthritis, and Addison's disease have been reported in association with myasthenia gravis but it is not established that there is significantly increased incidence of these conditions with myasthenia gravis. Thyrotoxicosis, thyroiditis, and hypothyroidism may be immunologic disorders and occur with significantly increased frequency in patients with myasthenia gravis.[67]

An *experimental model* of myasthenia gravis has been developed.[30] Rats or guinea pigs are sensitized with syngeneic or xenogeneic thymic tissue or muscle and complete Freund's adjuvant. They develop an inflammatory reaction in the thymus (thymitis). Immunofluorescent studies demonstrate antibodies in the thymus and in some of the animals a defect in neuromuscular transmission develops. Thymectomy before sensitization prevents development of the transmission defect. It is proposed that as a result of the thymitis, a material "thymin" is released which causes the defect in neuromuscular transmission. The thymic lymphocytes of sensitized animals have an abnormally high blast transformation rate in response to phytohemagglutinin stimulation but other parameters of immunologic function of the thymic or peripheral lymphocytes have not been examined. Successful production of the model has been reported by two groups, but several others have not succeeded.[34a, 82]

Anticholinesterase medication is the mainstay of *therapy* in myasthenia gravis. Thymectomy reduces morbidity and mortality from myasthenia gravis. It is usually reserved for the myasthenic with fairly widespread weakness who is poorly controlled on medication, but technical advances in surgery and postoperative care have made thymectomy a practical consideration in many more patients with myasthenia gravis.[59] No significant immunologic defect has been reported as a result of thymectomy in the adult human being.

Immunosuppressive drugs have been used. Steroids are of value in the management of myasthenic crises. ACTH given in large doses (1000 units per day) for 7 to 10 days results in rapid severe deterioration in strength. Five to 10 days after the course of ACTH, a significant proportion of patients enjoy partial or almost complete remission, which may last several weeks to several months. This therapy can be given only where facilities are adequate for the maintenance of the patient during crisis.[83a] Other immunosuppressive drugs (6-mercaptopurine, cyclophosphamide, azathioprine) have been used in myasthenia gravis but their use should still be considered as experimental.

SUMMARY

The information about immunologic disorders of the nervous system is incomplete, but considerable advances have occurred in the past decade. Continued investigation of the experimental models and clinical neurologic diseases in which immunologic features are significant should lead to definition of basic mechanisms in their pathogenesis. This will allow the formulation of rational and effective treatment of several diseases in which, at present, we can only document the natural history and speculate as to cause.

REFERENCES

1. Adams, R. D.: A comparison of the morphology of the human demyelinative diseases and experimental "allergic" encephalomyelitis. *In* Kies, M., and Alvord, E., eds.: "Allergic" Encephalomyelitis. Springfield, Illinois, Charles C Thomas, 1959.
2. Appel, S. H., and Bornstein, M. B.: The application of tissue culture to the study of experimental allergic encephalomyelitis. II. Serum factors responsible for demyelination. J. Exper. Med., 119:303–312, 1964.
3. Armstrong, R. M., Nowak, R., Falk, J., and Falk, R. E.: In vitro assessment of thymus cells and thymoma cells in myasthenia gravis. *In* Schwartz, R., ed.: Proceedings of the Sixth International Leukocyte Culture Conference, New York, Academic Press, in press.
4. Armstrong, R. M.: Unpublished data
5. Arnason, B. G., Jankovic, B. D., Waksman, B. H., and Wennerstein, C.: Role of the thymus in immune reactions in rats. II. Suppressive effect of thymectomy at birth on reactions of delayed (cellular) hypersensitivity and the circulating small lymphocyte. J. Exper. Med., 116:177–186, 1962.
6. Arnason, B. G. W., Winkler, G. F., and Hadler, N. M.: Cell-mediated demyelination of peripheral nerve in tissue culture. Lab. Invest., 21:1–10, 1969.

7. Arnason, B. G. W.: Idiopathic polyneuritis (Landry-Guillain-Barré-Strohl syndrome) and experimental allergic neuritis: A comparison. *In* Neurological Disorders of the Nervous System. Res. Publ. Ass. Nerv. Ment. Dis., *49*:156-175, 1971.
8. Astrom, K. E., and Waksman, B. H.: The passive transfer of experimental allergic encephalomyelitis and neuritis with living lymphoid cells. J. Path. Bact., *83*:89-106, 1962.
9. Astrom, K. E., Webster, H. De F., and Arnason, B. G.: The initial lesion in experimental allergic neuritis. A phase and electron microscope study. J. Exper. Med., *128*:469-495, 1968.
10. Bornstein, M. B., and Crain, S. M.: Function studies of cultured brain tissues as related to "demyelinative disorders". Science, *148*:1242-1244, 1965.
11. Bornstein, M. B., and Iwanami, H.: Experimental allergic encephalomyelitis. In vitro demyelination produced by sensitized rat lymph node cells and serum. J. Neuropath. Exper. Neurol., *29*:146-147, 1970.
12. Billingham, R. E., Brent, L., and Medawar, P. B.: Quantitative studies on tissue transplantation immunity. III. Actively acquired tolerance. Phil. Trans. Roy Soc. London (B), *239*:357-414, 1956.
13. Berg, O., and Källen, B.: Gliotoxic effect of serum from patients with neurological diseases. Lancet, *1*:1051-1052, 1962.
14. Bigner, D. D., and McFarlin, D. E.: Neurological disorders with abnormalities of immunoglobulin metabolism. *In* Immunological Disorders of the Nervous System. Res. Publ. Ass. Nerv. Ment. Dis., *49*:260-274, 1971.
15. Brandriss, M. W.: Methotrexate: Suppression of experimental allergic encephalomyelitis. Science, *140*:186-187, 1963.
16. Caspary, E. A.: Precipitating antibody in multiple sclerosis and experimental allergic encephalomyelitis. Specific binding of radio-iodinated encephalitogenic factor. J. Neuro. Neurosurg. Psychiat., *29*:103-106, 1966.
17. Caspary, E. A., Currie, S., Walton, J. N., and Field, E. J.: Lymphocyte sensitization to nervous tissues and muscle in patients with the Guillain-Barré syndrome. J. Neurol. Neurosurg. Psychiat., *34*:179-181, 1971.
18. Caspary, E. A., and Field, E. J.: Sensitization of blood lymphocytes to possible antigens in neurological disease. Europ. Neurol., *4*:257, 1970.
19. Castleman, B.: The pathology of the thymus gland in myasthenia gravis. Ann. N.Y. Acad. Sci., *135*:496-504, 1966.
20. Condie, R. M., and Good, R. A.: Experimental allergic encephalomyelitis: its production, prevention and pathology as studied by light and electron microscopy. *In* Korey, S. R., Ed.: Biology of Myelin. New York, Hoeber Div., Harper and Row, 1959, pp. 321-384.
21. Cook, S. D., and Dowling, P. C.: Neurologic disorders associated with increased DNA synthesis in peripheral blood. Arch. Neurol. (Chicago), *19*:583-590, 1968.
22. David, J. R., and Paterson, P. Y.: In vitro demonstration of cellular sensitivity in allergic encephalomyelitis. J. Exper. Med., *122*:1161-1171, 1965.
23. Eylar, E. H.: Basic A1 protein of myelin: Relationship to experimental allergic encephalomyelitis. *In* Immunological Disorders of the Nervous System. Publ. Ass. Nerv. Ment. Dis., *49*:50-75, 1971.
24. Ellison, G. W., Waksman, B. H., and Ruddle, N. H.: Experimental autoallergic encephalomyelitis and hypersensitivity in vitro. Neurology (Mpls), *21*:778-782, 1971.
25. Field, E. J.: Some observations on the clinical immunology of multiple sclerosis. *In* Slow, Latent, and Temperate virus infections. Washington, D.C., National Institute of Neurological Disease and Blindness, Monograph No. 2, 1965, pp. 187-192.
25a. Fisher, E. R.: The thymus in immunology. *In* Good, R. A., and Gabrielson, A. C., eds.: The Thymus in Immunobiology. New York, Harper and Rowe, 1964.
26. Fowler, I., Morris, C. E., and Whitley, T.: Lymphocyte transformation in multiple sclerosis induced by cerebrospinal fluid. New Eng. J. Med., *275*:1041-1044, 1966.
27. Freund, J., Stern, E. R., and Pisani, T. M.: Isoallergic encephalomyelitis and radiculitis in guinea pigs after one injection of brain and mycobacteria in water-in-oil emulsion. J. Immunol., *57*:179-194, 1947.
28. Freund, J., and Lipton, M. M.: Experimental allergic encephalomyelitis after excision of the injection site of antigen-adjuvant emulsion. J. Immunol., *75*:454, 1955.
29. Gibbs, C. J., Jr., and Gajdusek, D. C.: Transmission and characterization of the agents of spongiform encephalopathies. Kuru, Creutzfeldt-Jakob disease, scrapie and mink encephalopathy. *In* Immunological Disorders of the Nervous System. Res. Publ. Ass. Nerv. Ment. Dis., *49*:383-408, 1971.
30. Goldstein, G., and Hofmann, W. W.: Experimental myasthenia gravis. *In* Immunological Disorders of the Nervous System. Res. Publ. Ass. Nerv. Ment. Dis., *49*:241-252, 1971.
31. Housley, J., and Oppenheim, J. J.: Lymphocyte transformation in thymectomized and non thymectomized patients with myasthenia gravis. Brit. Med. J., *2*:679-681, 1967.
32. Harter, D. H., and Choppin, P. W.: Possible mechanisms in the pathogenesis of "postinfectious" encephalomyelitis. *In* Immunological Disorders of the Nervous System. Res. Publ. Ass. Nerv. Ment. Dis., *49*:342-354, 1971.

33. Jankovic, B. D., and Isvaneski, M.: Experimental allergic encephalomyelitis in thymectomized, bursectomized and normal chickens. Int. Arch. Allergy, 23:188–206, 1963.
34. Kabat, E. A., Wolf, A., and Bezer, A. E.: Rapid production of acute disseminated encephalomyelitis in rhesus monkeys by injection of heterologous and homologous brain tissue with adjuvants. J. Exper. Med., 85:117–130, 1947.
34a. Kaufman, B. M., Rushworth, G., and Wright, R.: Experimental studies related to autoimmunity in myasthenia gravis. J. Neurol. Psychiat., 40:281–289, 1969.
35. Katz, M., and Koprowski, H.: Subacute sclerosing panencephalitis, measles, rabies and progressive multi-focal leukoencephalopathy. In Immunological Disorders of the Nervous System. Res. Publ. Ass. Nerv. Ment. Dis., 49:373–380, 1971.
36. Kibler, R. F., and Barnes, A. E.: Antibody studies in rabbit encephalomyelitis induced by a water soluble protein fraction of rabbit cord. J. Exper. Med., 116:807–825, 1962.
37. Kibler, R. F.: Large dose corticosteroid therapy of experimental and human demyelinating diseases. Ann N.Y. Acad. Sci., 135:469–478, 1966.
38. Kibler, R. F., Paty, D. W., and Sherr, V.: Immunology of multiple sclerosis. In Immunological Disorders of the Nervous System. Res. Publ. Ass. Nerv. Ment. Dis., 49:95–105, 1971.
39. Kies, M. W., and Alvord, E. C., Jr.: "Allergic" Encephalomyelitis. Springfield, Illinois, Charles C Thomas, 1959.
40. Knight, S., Bradley, J., Oppenheim, J. J., and Ling, N. R.: The in vitro transformation of thymocytes and lymphocytes from humans, rabbits and guinea pigs and from thymomas. Clin. Exper. Immunol., 3:323–341, 1968.
41. Kolb, L. C., Karlson, A. G., and Sayre, G. P.: Prevention of experimental allergic encephalomyelitis by various agents. Trans. Amer. Neurol. Assoc., 77:117–121, 1952.
42. Levine, S., and Wenk, E. J.: Encephalitogenic potencies of nervous system tissues. Prac. Soc. Exper. Biol. Med., 114:220–222, 1963.
43. Levine, S., and Wenk, E. J.: Exacerbation and transformation of allergic encephalomyelitis by pertussis vaccine. Proc. Soc. Exper. Biol. Med., 122:115–118, 1966.
44. Levine, S.: Relationship of experimental allergic encephalomyelitis to human disease. In Immunological Disorders of the Nervous System. Res. Publ. Ass. Nerv. Ment. Dis., 49:33–46, 1971.
45. Lipton, M. M., and Steigman, A. J.: Allergic encephalomyelitis. The extraction of highly active fractions from bovine spinal cord. J. Immunol., 82:409–414, 1959.
46. Lipton, M. M., and Steigman, A. J.: Experimental allergic encephalomyelitis in the chicken. J. Immunol., 86:445–451, 1961.
47. Lumsden, C. E., Robertson, D. M., and Blight, R.: Chemical studies on experimental allergic encephalomyelitis. Peptide as the common denominator in all encephalitogenic "antigens". J. Neurochem., 13:127–162, 1966.
48. Martenson, R. E., Deibler, G. E., and Kies, M. W.: Microheterogeneity and species related differences among myelin basic proteins. In Immunological Disorders of the Nervous System. Res. Publ. Ass. Nerv. Ment. Dis., 49:76–93, 1971.
48a. McAlpine, D., Lumsden, C. E., and Acheson, E. D.: Multiple sclerosis, A Reappraisal. London, E. and S. Livingstone, 1965.
49. McFarlin, D. E., Engel, W. K., and Strauss, A. J. L.: Does myasthenic serum bind to the neuromuscular junction? Ann. N.Y. Acad. Sci., 135:656–663, 1966.
50. Melnick, S. C.: Thirty-eight cases of Guillain-Barré syndrome: An immunological study. Brit. Med. J., 1:368–373, 1963.
51. Middleton, G.: The incidence of follicular structures in the human thymus at autopsy. Aust. J. Exper. Biol. Med. Sci., 45:189–199, 1967.
52. Miller, H. G.: Acute disseminated encephalomyelitis treated with ACTH. Brit. Med. J., 1:177, 1953.
53. Miller, H. G., and Gibbons, J. L.: Acute disseminated encephalomyelitis and acute multiple sclerosis, results of treatment with ACTH. Brit. Med. J., 2:1345, 1953.
54. Morgan, I.: Allergic encephalomyelitis in monkeys in response to injection of normal monkey nervous tissue. J. Exper. Med., 85:131–140, 1947.
55. Nakao, A., and Roboz-Einstein, E.: Chemical and immunochemical studies with a dialyzable encephalitogenic compound from bovine spinal cord. Ann N.Y. Acad. Sci., 122:171–179, 1965.
56. Namba, T., Arimori, S., and Grob, D.: Effect on mice of intravenous administration of lymphocytes from normal subjects and from patients with myasthenia gravis. Neurology (Minn.), 19:461–468, 1969.
57. Oldstone, M. B., and Dixon, F. J.: Immunohistochemical study of allergic encephalomyelitis. Amer. J. Path., 52:251, 1968.
58. Oppenheim, J. J., and Goldstein, G.: Enhanced thymic lymphocyte response to phytohemagglutinin in experimental autoimmune thymitis. Nature, 222:192–193, 1969.
59. Papatestas, A. E., Alpert, L. J., Osserman, K. E., Osserman, R. S., and Kark, A. E.: Studies in myasthenia gravis. Effects of thymectomy. Results in 185 patients with nonthymomatous and thymomatous myasthenia gravis, 1941–1969. Amer. J. Med., 50:465–474, 1971.

60. Paterson, P. Y.: Studies of immunological tolerance to nervous tissue in rats. Ann. N.Y. Acad. Sci., 73:811–817, 1958.
61. Paterson, P. Y.: Organ-specific tissue damage induced by mammalian tissue-adjuvant emulsions. *In* Lawrence, H. S., ed.: Cellular and Humoral Aspects of the Hypersensitive States. New York, Hoeber, Harper and Row, 1959, pp. 469–503.
62. Paterson, P. Y.: Transfer of allergic encephalomyelitis in rats by means of lymph node cells. J. Exper. Med., 111:119–136, 1960.
63. Paterson, P. Y., and Busaw, N. E.: Effect of whole body X-irradiation on induction of allergic encephalomyelitis in rats. J. Immunol., 90:532–539, 1963.
64. Paterson, P. Y., Hanson, M. A., and Gerner, E. W.: Complement-fixing antibrain antibodies and allergic encephalomyelitis. II. Further studies concerning their protective role. Ann. N.Y. Acad. Sci., 124:292–298, 1965.
65. Paterson, P. Y.: Experimental allergic encephalomyelitis and autoimmune disease. Advances Immunol., 5:131–208, 1966.
66. Paterson, P. Y., Hanson, M. A., and Gerner, E. W.: Cyclophosphamide inhibition of experimental allergic encephalomyelitis in Wistar rats. Proc. Soc. Exper. Bio. Med., 124:928–932, 1967.
67. Penn, A. Schotland, D. L., and Rowland, L. P.: Immunology of muscle disease. *In* Immunological Disorders of the Nervous System. Res. Publ. Ass. Nerv. Ment. Dis., 49:215–240, 1971.
68. Perlo, V. P., Poskanzer, D. C., Schwab, R. S., Viets, H. R., Osserman, K. E., and Genkins, G.: Myasthenia gravis: Evaluation of treatment in 1335 patients. Neurology (Minn.), 16:431–439, 1966.
69. Rivers, T. M., Sprunt, D. H., and Berry, G. P.: Observations on attempts to produce acute disseminated encephalomyelitis in monkeys. J. Exper. Med., 58:39–54, 1933.
70. Rivers, T. M., and Schwentker, F. F.: Encephalomyelitis accompanied by myelin destruction experimentally produced in monkeys. J. Exper. Med., 61:689–702, 1935.
71. Roboz-Einstein, E., Robertson, D. M., Di Caprio, J. M., and Moore, W.: The isolation from bovine spinal cord of a homogeneous protein with encephalitogenic activity. J. Neurochem., 9:353–361, 1962.
72. Rocklin, R. E., Sheremata, W. A., Feldman, R. G., Kies, M. W., and David, J. R.: The Guillain-Barré syndrome and multiple sclerosis. In vitro cellular responses to nervous tissue antigens. New Eng. J. Med., 284:803, 1971.
73. Russell, D. S.: The nosological unity of acute hemorrhagic leucoencephalitis and acute disseminated encephalomyelitis. Brain, 78:369–376, 1955.
74. Scheinberg, L. C., Kies, M. W., and Alvord, E. C., Jr.: Research in demyelinating diseases. Ann. N.Y. Acad. Sci., 122:1–570, 1965.
75. Schneck, S. A.: Neurology and neuropathology of immunosuppressive therapy and acquired immunological deficiency. *In* Immunological Disorders of the Nervous System. Res. Publ. Ass. Nerv. Ment. Dis., 49:292–304, 1971.
76. Shaw, C., Alvord, E. C., Jr., Fahlberg, W. J., and Kies, M. W.: Adjuvant-antigen relationships in the production of experimental allergic encephalomyelitis in the guinea pig. J. Exper. Med., 115:169–179, 1962.
77. Siller, W. G.: Experimental allergic encephalomyelitis in the fowl. J. Path. Bact., 80:45–53, 1960.
78. Strauss, A. J. L., Van Der Geld, H. W. R., Kemp, P. G., Jr., Exum, E. D., and Goodman, H. O.: Immunological concomitants of myasthenia gravis. Ann. N.Y. Acad. Sci., 124:744–766, 1965.
79. Thomson, J. D., Austin, R. W., and Streetman, R. P.: The influence of chlorambucil on experimental allergic encephalomyelitis. Neurology, 13:505–511, 1963.
80. Thomas, L., Paterson, P. Y., and Smithwick, B.: Acute disseminated encephalomyelitis following immunization with homologous brain extracts. I. Studies on the role of a circulating antibody in the production of the condition in dogs. J. Exper. Med., 92:133–152, 1950.
81. Tourtellotte, W. W.: Cerebrospinal fluid immunoglobulins and the central nervous system as an immunological organ particularly in multiple sclerosis and subacute sclerosing panencephalitis. *In* Immunologic Disorders of the Nervous System. Res. Publ. Ass. Nerv. Ment. Dis., 49:112–147, 1971.
82. Vetters, J. M., Simpson, J. A., and Falkarde, A.: Experimental myasthenia gravis. Lancet, 2:28–31, 1969.
83. Van Reis, G., Liljestrand, A., and Matell, G.: Treatment of severe myasthenia gravis with large doses of ACTH. Ann. N.Y. Acad. Sci., 135:409–416, 1966.
84. Waksman, B. H., and Adams, R. D.: A comparative study of experimental allergic neuritis in the rabbit, guinea pig and mouse. J. Neuropath. Exper. Neurol., 15:293–333, 1956.
85. Waksman, B. H., and Morrison, L. R.: Tuberculin type sensitivity to spinal cord antigen in rabbits with isoallergic encephalomyelitis. J. Immunol., 66:421–444, 1951.
86. Waksman, B. H., Arbouys, S., and Arnason, B. G.: The use of specific lymphocyte antisera

to inhibit hypersensitive reactions of the delayed type. J. Exper. Med., *114*:997–1022, 1961.

86a.Warmolts, J. R., Engel, W. K., and Whitaker, J. N.: Alternate-day prednisone in a patient with myasthenia gravis. Lancet, 2:1198, 1970.

87. Wolf, A., Kabat, E. A., and Bezer, A. E.: The pathology of acute disseminated encephalomyelitis produced experimentally in the rhesus monkey and its resemblance to human demyelinating disease. J. Neuropath. Exper. Neurol., 6:333–357, 1947.

88. Wolfgram, F.: Macromolecular constituents of myelin. Ann. N.Y. Acad. Sci., *122*:104–115, 1965.

89. Whitaker, J. N., Hirano, A., Cook, S., and Dowling, P.: Circulating transformed lymphocytes in Guillain-Barré syndrome. Neurology, *19*:313, 1969.

Toronto General Hospital
Toronto, Ontario
Canada

Appraisal of Rheumatoid Arthritis as an Immune Complex Disease

I. Broder, M.D., M. B. Urowitz, M.D.,***
*and D. A. Gordon, M.D.****

There is considerable interest at the present time in the role of immune complexes in human disease. This subject is reviewed here, both in a general context and with specific reference to rheumatoid arthritis. The approach taken has been to describe immune complexes and the type of injury they may produce, to discuss the concept of immune complex disease in the context of experimental and naturally occurring models, and finally to examine rheumatoid arthritis from the viewpoint of an immune complex disease.

SOLUBLE AND INSOLUBLE IMMUNE COMPLEXES

Antigens, in general, possess multiple sites per molecule at which union with antibody may occur. Antibodies, depending on their immunoglobulin class, contain two or more sites per molecule at which union with antigen may occur. Therefore, the union of antigen with antibody may result in the formation of a spectrum of immune complexes, depending on the relative amounts of antigen and antibody which interact (Fig. 1). This spectrum is limited on one extreme by the complex which forms in high antibody excess, and on the other extreme by the complex which forms in high antigen excess. Between these two limits is a continuum, the central area of which consists of complexes having multiple cross-linkages between adjacent antigen and antibody molecules. From this zone of the continuum toward the limit of antibody excess, the immune complexes generally tend to be insoluble; complexes

From the Departments of Medicine, Pathology, and Pharmacology, Faculty of Medicine, University of Toronto

*Associate Professor of Medicine, University of Toronto; Medical Research Associate, Medical Research Council of Canada

**Associate, Department of Medicine, University of Toronto Rheumatic Disease Unit, The Wellesley Hospital, Toronto

***Assistant Professor of Medicine, University of Toronto Rheumatic Disease Unit, The Wellesley Hospital, Toronto

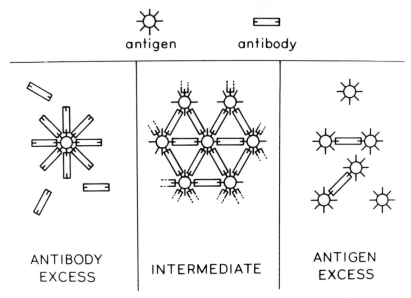

Figure 1. Varying composition of antigen-antibody complexes, depending on ratio of antigen and antibody in reaction mixture.

of this composition can elicit an Arthus reaction if formed under appropriate conditions (see below). From the central zone of the continuum towards the limit of antigen excess, the immune complexes become progressively more soluble; complexes of this composition have the capacity to release vasoactive amines and to produce vasculitis (see below).

Insoluble immune complexes produce an Arthus reaction through a mechanism which involves complement activation, chemotaxis of polymorphonuclear leukocytes, phagocytosis of immune precipitates, destruction of lysosomes, proteolytic enzyme release, and resultant tissue injury.[11] This process requires the formation of a large amount of immune precipitate in a localized site. Also, the antibody must be capable of activating the complement system. The morphologic highlights of the reaction include polymorphonuclear leukocyte infiltration, hemorrhage, and necrosis during the acute phase, followed after several hours[11] by the appearance of mononuclear cells. Chronic Arthus reactions have not been studied.

Soluble immune complexes cause vasoactive amine release and increased vascular permeability.[10, 37] The complexes then localize in the walls of blood vessels where they form deposits along the basement membrane and are associated with the appearance of acute vasculitis and glomerulitis.[13] The vasculitis, but not the glomerulitis, is complement dependent.[30] Tissue injury may be due to the release of proteolytic enzymes from polymorphonuclear leukocytes.[12, 26] It has not yet been established whether enzyme release is dependent on phagocytosis of soluble immune complexes by polymorphonuclear leukocytes.[26]

There are sufficient differences between the Arthus mechanism and the mechanism of injury by soluble immune complexes that it seems evident that the two represent distinct phenomena. The Arthus reaction appears to represent a local phenomenon, in which the antigen must diffuse from a depot to form a precipitate with antibody in the walls of adjacent blood vessels.[13] The presence of systemic immune precipitates seems to be relatively innocuous.[16] The Arthus reaction is inhibited in the absence of complement, as is the vasculitis of soluble immune complex disease.[14, 30] However, the glomerulitis of the latter system is not influenced by complement depletion.[14, 30] All aspects of soluble immune complex disease are inhibited by the combined use of histamine and serotonin antagonists, while the Arthus reaction is unchanged by the same treatment.[13, 37]

An individual who is immunized progresses through a sequence which corresponds to the spectrum of immune complexes described in Figure 1. When antibody production begins, there is a high ratio of antigen present, leading to formation of the complexes in extreme antigen excess. The ratio of antigen gradually falls as antibody production continues, traversing the spectrum toward the central zone and then into the zone of excess antibody. Eventually, the antigen disappears and only antibody persists.

Immune complex disease may become manifest when the individual encounters the zone of antigen excess. Fortunately, this type of disease does not occur with each immune response. Disease production is determined by factors which are not yet entirely understood. In experimental studies, immune complex disease was found in those animals which produced an intermediate level of antibody.[16] The high antibody producers, and the nonproducers, did not develop disease, suggesting that the velocity and amplitude of antibody production were important determinants.

ROLE OF IMMUNE COMPLEXES IN DISEASE

Experimental Studies

The main support for the role of immune complexes in disease has been obtained from studies of experimental serum sickness (reviewed by Cochrane and Dixon[13]). These studies have demonstrated that a single large dose of antigen was followed approximately 1 week later by the appearance of soluble immune complexes, and inflammatory tissue lesions of glomerulonephritis and widespread vasculitis. Associated with these events was a fall in serum complement. The renal lesions demonstrated a discontinuous precipitate in the subendothelial region of glomeruli containing antigen, gammaglobulin and complement. If no further antigen was given, the lesions began to resolve after several days. In some animals, repeated injections of antigen resulted in renal lesions resembling chronic glomerulonephritis.

The role of soluble immune complexes in producing the foregoing tissue lesions has been substantiated by studies in which soluble complexes were prepared in a test tube and injected into normal animals. This resulted in the accelerated appearance of vasculitis and glomerulitis.[45]

Naturally Occurring Animal Diseases

A number of spontaneously occurring diseases of animals appear to represent immune complex diseases. In Aleutian mink disease, lymphocytic choriomeningitis of mice, and the lupus-like disease of NZB mice, there is evidence that the disease is transmitted by a slow virus.[33, 48, 53, 58] Circulating soluble immune complexes, consisting of virus combined with non-neutralizing antibody, have been demonstrated.[54, 60] The soluble immune complexes, rather than the virus alone, are believed to be responsible for the induction of disease.[53, 58] These diseases have been associated with a variety of abnormalities, including vasculitis, glomerulonephritis, plasmacytosis, complement depletion, hypergammaglobulinemia, Coombs' positive hemolytic anemia, antinuclear antibodies, lupus erythematosus cells, and rheumatoid factor.[17, 32, 33, 46, 47, 54, 56, 59, 68, 74] The renal lesions exhibited glomerular subendothelial deposits containing gammaglobulin and complement.[29, 42, 54]

Naturally Occurring Human Diseases

It has been tempting to apply the foregoing information to the understanding of a number of naturally occurring human diseases. In human serum sickness, glomerulonephritis, and systemic lupus erythematosus, there is known to be a fall in serum complement during the acute phase.[23, 39, 50, 65, 66] One study of human serum sickness has provided indirect evidence suggesting the presence of immune complexes,[71] while another gave negative results.[4] Soluble immune complexes have not been demonstrated in the circulation of persons with acute glomerulonephritis,[2, 4] although the glomeruli do contain discontinuous deposits of gammaglobulin and complement, similar to experimental serum sickness.[49] Evidence is available in systemic lupus erythematosus, that immune complexes of DNA and anti-DNA form in the circulation and are responsible for the glomerular deposits and renal pathology found in this disease.[38, 40, 66, 69]

RHEUMATOID ARTHRITIS VIEWED AS AN IMMUNE COMPLEX DISEASE

Clinical Features

Polyarthritis is the hallmark of rheumatoid arthritis, but this is either not seen or is a minor feature of the foregoing animal and human diseases. On the other hand, the extra-articular features of rheumatoid arthritis, owing to vasculitis affecting a variety of sites, fit well with the picture of an immune complex disease. Glomerulitis appears to be the hallmark of immune complex diseases, but this is absent in rheumatoid arthritis. Thus, it would seem that the clinical features of rheumatoid arthritis are not entirely consistent with those of other conditions in which an immune complex mechanism is either suspected or proven.

Laboratory Features

RHEUMATOID FACTOR. The rheumatoid factors include both 7S and 19S immunoglobulins which have antibody specificity directed against determinants on the gammaglobulin molecule. Some of these determinants have been exposed either by physical aggregation[8, 55] or by immune complex formation.[18, 28] Thus, immune complexes may serve as the stimulus for rheumatoid factor formation.

Rheumatoid factor is detected in the serum of approximately 80 per cent of cases of definite or classical rheumatoid arthritis.[34] Also, persons who do not exhibit free rheumatoid factor in their serum may be found to have hidden rheumatoid factor.[1, 5] Therefore, in the majority of patients with rheumatoid arthritis, a stimulus for rheumatoid factor formation, possibly immune complexes, can be found.

COMPLEMENT. It was reported in 1964 that persons with rheumatoid arthritis exhibited synovial fluid complement levels which were disproportionately lowered relative to other joint fluid proteins.[27, 57] Subsequently, this was substantiated by many different workers. Ruddy and his associates have recently shown, in seropositive rheumatoid arthritis, that low total complement levels in synovial fluid were associated with a variable reduction in $C'1$ activity, marked depression of $C'4$ and $C'2$, and moderate depression of $C'3$.[63] It has also been shown that the catabolic rate of intra-articularly administered radioactive-labeled $C'3$ was greater than that of intravenously injected $C'3$.[63] These results were consistent with increased utilization of $C'3$ in the articular space.

On the other hand, many studies have shown that the serum complement levels are usually normal or elevated in rheumatoid arthritis.[19, 35, 72, 73] Mongan and his co-workers have shown that the serum complement in patients with seropositive rheumatoid arthritis was somewhat lower than in seronegative;[51] however, the complement levels were within normal limits in both instances. Franco and Schur have reported hypocomplementemia in 11 of 250 consecutive patients with rheumatoid arthritis.[21] These 11 patients had greater functional impairment, and more frequently exhibited positive latex tests and extra-articular manifestations of rheumatoid arthritis. Furthermore, in some patients with seropositive rheumatoid arthritis, systemic hypercatabolism of radioactively labelled $C'3$ has been demonstrated, suggesting increased systemic utilization of complement.[64, 75]

HISTOLOGIC FEATURES. Hollander and his associates demonstrated in 1965 the presence of IgG, IgM, and complement in the cytoplasmic inclusion granules of the neutrophils present in rheumatoid synovial fluid.[31, 61] They then reasoned that these neutrophils had phagocytosed immune complexes of rheumatoid factor and IgG. Similar inclusions have been found in cells present in the synovial membrane.[6, 20, 36, 62] The possibility that these inclusions may mark the presence of an Arthus reaction has been supported by the detection of lysosomal enzymes in rheumatoid synovial fluid.[76]

DEMONSTRATION OF COMPLEXES IN RHEUMATOID SERUM AND SYNOVIAL FLUID: BY ULTRACENTRIFUGATION. A number of ultracentrifugation studies of rheumatoid serum and synovial fluid have demonstrated the presence of high molecular weight components which dissociated at acid pH and consisted of IgG or IgM rheumatoid factor combined with IgG.[9, 22, 25, 41, 67, 77] The largest of the complexes formed a precipitate with IgM rheumatoid factor and with C'1q.[77] The amount of complex present in a given sample of synovial fluid correlated with the degree of depression of complement.[77] Similar complexes have been described in synovial tissue eluates.[52]

By Histamine-Releasing Activity.   A factor resembling a soluble immune complex (rheumatoid biologically active factor, or RBAF) has been detected in rheumatoid serum and synovial fluid by its capacity to release histamine from the perfused guinea-pig lung.[4] The RBAF contained IgG but had a molecular size considerably larger than IgG.[4] It did not contain IgM, IgA or C'3 and was not cryoprecipitable or associated with rheumatoid factor or complement fixing activity.[4, 7] Also, the RBAF did not correlate with complexes detected by ultracentrifugation.[4, 7]

In a prospective clinical study, the RBAF was found to correlate with the presence of a more accelerated and widespread form of rheumatoid disease.[24] A second assessment carried out in the same group of patients demonstrated that patients in whom the RBAF had disappeared were more markedly improved than the other patients being followed.[7]

By Complement Fixation.   Rheumatoid synovial fluid has also been found to contain a factor which exhibited complement fixing activity, was variably cryoprecipitable and sedimented as a high molecular weight material.[3, 44] With few exceptions, the cryoprecipitate contained DNA and IgG, with IgM or IgM and IgA also present in some instances. C'4 was also a common constituent but C'3 could not be demonstrated by direct means. Rheumatoid factor activity was associated with these complexes in about 60 per cent of cases.

UNANSWERED QUESTIONS

The foregoing describes insoluble immune complexes present in cells of rheumatoid synovium and synovial fluid, and also soluble immune complexes present in rheumatoid serum and synovial fluid. However, a number of questions remain to be answered. What is the relation between the insoluble and soluble immune complexes? What is the relation among the various soluble immune complexes described? If these are all immune complexes, what is the antigen? Does rheumatoid arthritis represent a chronic Arthus reaction? What is the relation of the complexes to clinical disease?

Relation Between Insoluble Immune Complexes and Soluble Immune Complexes Demonstrated by Different Methods

There are no known essential differences in composition between the insoluble intracellular complexes and the complexes demonstrated by ultracentrifugation and by complement fixation. However, each type of complex has not been studied by all of the same methods. The intracellular complexes contain C'3, which the others do not. This is not an essential difference, since complexes which bind C'3 promote immune adherence with resulting enhanced phagocytosis.

The complexes detected by histamine release differed from the others in showing no complement-fixing or rheumatoid factor activity, in not precipitating in the cold, in not containing IgM, and in bearing a random relationship with complexes demonstrable by ultracentrifugation. Therefore, it remains a possibility that different kinds of immune complexes, perhaps containing different antigens, may be present simultaneously in rheumatoid patients.

The intracellular insoluble complexes and some of the extracellular soluble complexes may coexist and may in fact represent the same antigen-antibody system. The difficulty then arises of explaining the simultaneous presence of soluble and insoluble complexes belonging to the same system. This could be explained, perhaps, on the basis that the soluble complexes contained nonprecipitating antibody. Alternatively, the individual may be exposed to varying levels of antigen and antibody, resulting at different times in the presence of excess antigen or excess antibody. As a third possibility, soluble complexes may become denatured following phagocytosis.[26]

What is the Antigen?

Certain of the complexes that have been described contain rheumatoid factor as the antibody and gamma-globulin as the antigen. However, this composition may not apply to all of the complexes. It is possible that some may contain as antigen, a virus or bacterial constituent, and thereby resemble the complexes present in certain naturally occurring animal diseases as Aleutian mink disease. The complement fixing complexes may contain DNA as the antigen.[43]

Relation of Rheumatoid Arthritis to an Arthus Reaction

Rheumatoid synovial fluid displays evidence of complement utilization, polymorphonuclear leukocytes which contain phagocytosed immune precipitates and free lysosomal enzymes. These findings provide strong circumstantial evidence for the presence of an Arthus reaction. The morphology of the synovial tissue reaction on the other hand is not that of an acute Arthus reaction, since mononuclear cells predominate and hemorrhage and necrosis are not striking features. However, mononuclear cells begin to appear in acute Arthus reactions after a period of several hours,[11] and the morphology of chronic Arthus reactions is not known. Therefore, it is not yet clear whether the mechanism of the arthritis is that of an Arthus reaction, or a soluble immune complex mechanism, or a process not yet defined. It is also not known whether the extra-articular features are due to the same mechanism as the arthritis.

This type of distinction may have practical significance in the search for new therapeutic approaches to rheumatoid arthritis. An effective anticomplement agent might be useful in suppressing all manifestations of an Arthus reaction or the vasculitis of soluble immune complex disease. On the other hand antihistamine or antiserotonin agents might be useful in suppressing all aspects of soluble immune complex disease. Although prototypes of the latter medications exist, they have not had clinical trials in rheumatoid arthritis. However, the possibility that rheumatoid arthritis may be an immunologic disease has already led to trials of immunosuppressive therapy, with promising results.[15, 70]

Relation of Complexes to Clinical Disease

The correlation between clinical features of rheumatoid arthritis and the presence of soluble complexes has been studied only in the case of the histamine-releasing factor. This factor has been described above to correlate with the level of rheumatoid disease activity. However, it has yet to be determined whether this or the other complexes are the cause or the result of rheumatoid disease.

CONCLUSION

The evidence for the role of immunologic mechanisms in the pathogenesis of rheumatoid arthritis has been reviewed. Although, there is some suggestion that an Arthus mechanism may be involved, the evidence is also consistent with a soluble immune complex mechanism. It is not yet possible to establish conclusively either mechanism to the exclusion of the other as the prime mediator of tissue injury in rheumatoid arthritis. Moreover, little is known at present about the involvement of other mechanisms, such as those mediated by sensitized lymphoid cells.

REFERENCES

1. Allen, J. C., and Kunkel, H. G.: Hidden rheumatoid factors with specificity for native γ-globulins. Arthritis Rheumat., 9:758, 1966.
2. Askenase, P. W., and Leonard, E. J.: C3 in high molecular weight complexes: separation from plasma of nephritic patients and normal subjects by a method that avoids in vitro artifacts. J. Immunol., 105:1578, 1970.
3. Barnett, E. V., Bluestone, R., Cracchiolo, A. III, Goldberg, L. S., Kantor, G. L., and McIntosh, R. M.: Cryoglobulinemia and disease. Ann. Intern. Med., 73:95, 1970.
4. Baumal, R., and Broder, I.: Studies into the occurrence of soluble antigen-antibody complexes in disease. III. Rheumatoid arthritis and other human diseases. Clin. Exper. Immunol., 3:555, 1968.
5. Bluestone, R., Goldberg, L. S., and Cracchiolo, A. III: Hidden rheumatoid factor in seronegative nodular rheumatoid arthritis. Lancet, 2:878, 1969.
6. Bonomo, L., Tursi, A., Trizio, D., Gillardi, U., and Dammacco, F.: Immune complexes in rheumatoid synovitis: A mixed staining immunofluorescence study. Immunology, 18:557, 1970.
7. Broder, I., Baumal, R., Gordon, D. A., Urowitz, M. B., and Shinder, E.: Immunoglobulin complexes in serum and synovial fluid of persons with rheumatoid arthritis. In Proceedings of the Fourth Canadian Conference on Research in the Rheumatic Diseases, University of Toronto Press, 1972.
8. Butler, V. P., Jr., and Vaughan, J. H.: The reaction of rheumatoid factor with animal γ-globulins: quantitative considerations. Immunology, 8:144, 1965.
9. Chodirker, W. B., and Tomasi, T. B., Jr.: Low-molecular-weight rheumatoid factor. J. Clin. Invest., 42:876, 1963.
10. Cochrane, C. G.: Studies on the localization of circulating antigen-antibody complexes and other macromolecules in vessels. 2. Pathogenetic and pharmacodynamic studies. J. Exper. Med., 118:503, 1963.
11. Cochrane, C. G.: The arthus phenomenon—a mechanism of tissue damage. Arthritis Rheumat., 10:392, 1967.
12. Cochrane, C. G. and Aikin, B. S.: Polymorphonuclear leukocytes in immunologic reactions. The destruction of vascular basement membrane in vivo and in vitro. J. Exper. Med., 124:733, 1966.
13. Cochrane, C. G., and Dixon, F. J.: Cell and tissue damage through antigen-antibody complexes. In Miescher, P. A., and Müller-Eberhard, H. J., eds.: Textbook of Immunopathology. New York, Grune and Stratton, 1968, vol. 1, p. 94.
14. Cochrane, C. G., Müller-Eberhard, H. J., and Aikin, B. S.: Depletion of plasma complement in vivo by a protein of cobra venom: Its effect on various immunologic reactions. J. Immunol., 105:55, 1970.

15. Co-operating Clinics Committee of the American Rheumatism Association. A controlled trial of cyclophosphamide in rheumatoid arthritis. New Eng. J. Med., 283:883, 1970.

16. Dixon, F. J., Feldman, J. D., and Vazquez, J. J.: Experimental glomerulonephritis. The pathogenesis of a laboratory model resembling the spectrum of human glomerulonephritis. J. Exper. Med., 113:899, 1961.

17. East, J., and Branca, M.: Autoimmune reactions and malignant changes in germ free New Zealand Black mice. Clin. Exper. Immunol., 4:621, 1969.

18. Edelman, G. M., Kunkel, H. G., and Franklin, E. C.: Interaction of rheumatoid factor with antigen-antibody complexes and aggregated γ-globulin. J. Exper. Med., 108:105, 1958.

19. Ellis, H. A., and Felix-Davies D.: Serum complement, rheumatoid factor and the serum proteins in rheumatoid disease and systemic lupus erythematosus. Ann. Rheumat. Dis., 18:215, 1959.

20. Fish, A. J., Michael, A. F., Gewurz, H., and Good, R. A.: Immunopathologic changes in rheumatoid arthritis synovium. Arthritis Rheumat., 9:267, 1966.

21. Franco, A., and Schur, P. H.: Hypocomplementemia in rheumatoid arthritis: Arthritis Rheumat., 14:231, 1971.

22. Franklin, E. C., Müller-Eberhard, H. J., Holman, H., and Kunkel, H. G.: An unusual protein component of high molecular weight in the serum of certain patients with rheumatoid arthritis. J. Exper. Med., 105:424, 1957.

23. Gewurz, H., Pickering, R. J., Good, R. A., and Mergenhagen, S. E.: Complement profile in acute glomerulonephritis, systemic lupus erythematosus and hypocomplementemic chronic glomerulonephritis. Contrasts and experimental correlations. Internat. Arch. Allerg., 34:557, 1968.

24. Gordon, D. A., Bell, D. A., Baumal, R., and Broder, I.: Studies into the occurrence of soluble antigen-antibody complexes in disease. IV. Correlation between the rheumatoid biologically active factor and clinical features of rheumatoid arthritis. Clin. Exper. Immunol., 5:57, 1969.

25. Hannestad, K.: Presence of aggregated γ-globulin in certain rheumatoid synovial effusions. Clin. Exper. Immunol., 2:511, 1967.

26. Hawkins, D., and Peeters, D.: The response of polymorphonuclear leukocytes to immune complexes in vitro. Lab. Invest., 24:483, 1971.

27. Hedberg, H., Nordin, A., Lindquist, A., and Afzelius, B.: Studies on the depressed hemolytic complement activity of synovial fluid in adult rheumatoid arthritis. Acta Med. Scand., 175:347, 1964.

28. Henney, C. S., and Stanworth, D. R.: The reactivity of rheumatoid factor with human γ-globulin. Immunology, 9:139, 1965.

29. Henson, J. B., Gorham, J. R., Padgett, G. A., and Davis, W. C.: Pathogenesis of the glomerular lesions in aleutian disease of mink. Arch. Path., 87:21, 1969.

30. Henson, P. M., and Cochrane, C. G.: Acute immune complex disease in rabbits. The role of complement and of a leukocyte-dependent release of vasoactive amines from platelets. J. Exper. Med., 133:554, 1971.

31. Hollander, J. L., McCarty, D. J., Astorga, G., and Castro Murillo, C.: Studies on the pathogenesis of rheumatoid joint inflammation. 1. The "R.A." cell and a working hypothesis. Ann. Intern. Med., 62:271, 1965.

32. Holmes, M. C., and Burnett, F. M.: Natural history of autoimmune disease in NZB mice. Comparison of humoral autoimmune manifestations. Ann. Int. Med., 59:265, 1963.

33. Karstad, L.: Aleutian disease. A slowly progressive viral infection of mink. In Current Topics in Microbiology and Immunology, New York, Springer-Verlag, 1967, vol. 40, p. 9.

34. Kellgren, J. H.: Epidemiology of rheumatoid arthritis. In Duthie, J. J. R., and Alexander, W. R. M., eds.: Rheumatic Diseases. Baltimore, Medical Monographs, 1968, p. 120.

35. Kellet, C. E.: Complement activity of the blood in rheumatism and certain allied disorders. Ann. Rheumat. Dis., 13:211, 1954.

36. Kinsella, T. D., Baum, J., and Ziff, M.: Immunofluorescent demonstration of an IgG-B$_{1c}$ complex in synovial lining cells of rheumatoid synovial membrane. Clin. Exper. Immunol., 4:265, 1969.

37. Kniker, W. T., and Cochrane, C. G.: The localization of circulating immune complexes in experimental serum sickness. The role of vasoactive amines and hydro-dynamic forces. J. Exper. Med., 127:119, 1968.

38. Koffler, D., and Kunkel, H. G.: Mechanisms of renal injury in systemic lupus erythematosus. Amer. J. Med., 45:165, 1968.

39. Kohler, P. F., and Ten Bensel, R.: Serial complement component alterations in acute glomerulonephritis and systemic lupus erythematosus. Clin. Exper. Immunol., 4:191, 1969.

40. Krishnan, C., and Kaplan, M. H.: Immunopathologic studies of systemic lupus erythematosus. II. Antinuclear reaction of γ-globulin eluted from homogenates and isolated glomeruli of kidneys from patients with lupus nephritis. J. Clin. Invest., 46:569, 1967.

41. Kunkel, H. G., Müller-Eberhard, H. J., Fudenberg, H. H., and Tomasi, T. B.: γ-globulin complexes in rheumatoid arthritis and certain other conditions: J. Clin. Invest., 40:117, 1961.

42. Lambert, P. H., and Dixon, F. J.: Pathogenesis of the glomerulonephritis of NZB/W mice. J. Exper. Med., 127:507, 1968.
43. Marcus, R. L., and Townes, A. S.: Partial dissociation of rheumatoid synovial fluid cryoprotein: micro complement fixation by IgG- or IgG and IgM-containing fractions and denatured calf thymus DNA. J. Immunol., 106:1499, 1971.
44. Marcus, R. L., and Townes, A. S.: The occurrence of cryoproteins in synovial fluid; the association of a complement-fixing activity in rheumatoid synovial fluid with cold-precipitable protein. J. Clin. Invest., 50:282, 1971.
45. McCluskey, R. T., Potter, J. L., Miller, F., and Benacerraf, G.: The pathologic effects of intravenously administered soluble antigen-antibody complexes. 1. Passive serum sickness in mice. J. Exper. Med., 111:181, 1960.
46. McGiven, A. R., and Ghose, R.: Antinuclear factor in NZB/NZW mice: incidence and in vitro effects. Clin. Exper. Immunol., 3:657, 1968.
47. McGiven, A. R., and Ironside, N. J.: Elution of antinuclear factor from renal lesions of NZB/NZW mice: Clin. Exper. Immunol., 3:665, 1968.
48. Mellors, R. C., and Chen Ya Huang: Immunopathology of NZB/BL mice. VI. Virus separable from spleen and pathogenic for swiss mice. J. Exper. Med., 126:53, 1967.
49. Michael, A. F., Jr., Drummond K. N., Good, R. A., and Vernier, R. L.: Acute poststreptococcal glomerulonephritis: immune deposit disease. J. Clin. Invest., 45:237, 1966.
50. Moll, F. C., Kirk, M., Schwab, L., Hown, C. van Z., Hall, T. C., and Janeway, C. A.: Experimental hypersensitivity: a study of the relationship of antibody production, serum complement activity and the development of pathologic lesions in response to single large injections of heterologous plasma protein: Amer. J. Dis. Child., 79:1130, 1950.
51. Mongan, E. S., Cass, R. M., Jacox, R. F., and Vaughan, J. H.: A study of the relation of seronegative and seropositive rheumatoid arthritis to each other and to necrotizing vasculitis. Amer. J. Med., 47:23, 1969.
52. Munthe, E., and Natvig, J. B.: Characterization of IgG complexes in eluates from rheumatoid tissue: Clin. Exper. Immunol., 8:249, 1971.
53. Oldstone, M. B. A., and Dixon, F. J.: Pathogenesis of chronic disease associated with persistent lymphocytic choriomeningitis viral infection. II. Relationship of the anti-lymphocytic choriomeningitis immune response to tissue injury in chronic lymphocytic choriomeningitis disease. J. Exper. Med.,131:1, 1970.
54. Oldstone, M. B. A., and Dixon, F. J.: Persistent lymphocytic choriomeningitis viral infection. III. Virus-anti-viral antibody complexes and associated chronic disease following transplacental infection. J. Immunol., 105:829, 1970.
55. Osterland, C. K., Harboe, M., and Kunkel, H. G.: Rheumatoid factor (7S and 19S types) reacting with different portions of the γ-globulin molecule. Arthritis Rheumat., 5:312, 1962.
56. Pan, I. C., Tsai, K. S., and Karstad, L.: Glomerulonephritis in Aleutian disease of mink: histological and immunofluorescence studies. J. Path., 101:119, 1970.
57. Pekin, T. J., and Zvaifler, N. J.: Hemolytic complement in synovial fluid. J. Clin. Invest., 43:1372, 1964.
58. Porter, D. D., and Larsen, A. E.: Virus-host interactions in Aleutian disease of mink. In Pollard, M., ed.: Perspectives in Virology VI. New York, Academic Press, 1968, p. 173.
59. Porter, D. D., Dixon, F. J., and Larsen, A. E.: The development of a myeloma-like condition in mink with Aleutian disease. Blood, 25:736, 1965.
60. Porter, D. D., and Larsen, A. E.: Aleutian disease of mink: Infectious virus-antibody complexes in the serum. Proc. Soc. Exper. Biol. Med., 126:680, 1967.
61. Rawson, A. J., Abelson, N. M., and Hollander, J. L.: Studies on the pathogenesis of rheumatoid joint inflammation. II. Intracytoplasmic particulate complexes in rheumatoid synovial fluids. Ann. Intern. Med., 62:281, 1965.
62. Rodman, W. S., Williams, R. C., Jr., Bilka, P. J., and Müller-Eberhard, H. J.: Immunofluorescent localization of the third and the fourth component complement in synovial tissue from patients with rheumatoid arthritis. J. Lab. Clin. Med., 69:141, 1967.
63. Ruddy S., Button, M. C., Schur, P. H., and Austen, K. F.: Complement components in synovial fluid: activation and fixation in seropositive rheumatoid arthritis. Ann. New York Acad. Sci., 168:161, 1969.
64. Ruddy, S., Müller-Eberhard, H. J., and Austen, K. F.: Direct measurement of intra-articular hypercatabolism of third complement component (C3) in rheumatoid arthritis (RA) and systemic lupus erythematosus (SLE). Arthritis Rheumat., 14:410, 1971.
65. Schur, P. H., and Austen, K. F.: Complement in human disease. Ann. Rev. Med., 19:1, 1968.
66. Schur, P. H., and Sandson, J.: Immunologic factors and clinical activity in lupus erythematosus. New Eng. J. Med., 278:533, 1968.
67. Schrohenloher, R. D.: Characterization of the γ-globulin complexes present in certain sera having high titers of anti γ-globulin activity. J. Clin. Invest., 45:501, 1966.
68. Tabel, H., and Ingram, D. G.: The immunoglobulins in Aleutian disease (viral plasmacytosis) of mink. Different types of hypergammaglobulinemias. Canad. J. Comp. Med., 34:329, 1970.

69. Tan, E. M., Schur, P. H., Carr, R. I., and Kunkel, H. G.: Deoxyribonucleic acid (DNA) and antibodies to DNA in the serum of patients with systemic lupus erythematosus. J. Clin. Invest., 45:1732, 1966.

70. Urowitz, M. B., Gordon, D. A., Smythe, H. A., Pruzanski, W., and Ogryzlo, M. A.: Azathioprine treatment of rheumatoid arthritis – a double-blind crossover study. Arthritis Rheumat., 14:419, 1971.

71. Vaughan, J. H., Barnett, E. V., and Leddy, J. P.: Serum sickness: Evidence in man of antigen-antibody complexes and free light chains in the circulation during the acute reaction. Ann. Int. Med., 67:596, 1967.

72. Vaughan, J. H., Bayles, T. B., and Favour, C. B.: Serum complement in rheumatoid arthritis. Amer. J. Med. Sci., 222:186, 1951.

73. Williams, R. C., Jr., and Law, D. H.: Serum complement in connective tissue disorders. J. Lab. Clin. Med., 52:273, 1958.

74. Williams, R. C., Jr., Russell, J. D., and Kenyon, A. J.: Anti-gamma-globulin factors and immunofluorescent studies in normal mink with Aleutian disease. Amer. J. Vet. Res., 27:1447, 1966.

75. Weinstein, A., Peters, K., Brown, D , and Bluestone, R.: Metabolism of the third component of complement (C3) in patients with rheumatoid arthritis. Proceedings of the Fourth Canadian Conference on Research in the Rheumatic Diseases, University of Toronto Press, 1972.

76. Weissmann, G.: Lysosomes and joint disease. Arthritis Rheumat., 9:834, 1966.

77. Winchester, R. J., Agnello, V., and Kunkel, H. G.: Gammaglobulin complexes in synovial fluids of patients with rheumatoid arthritis. Partial characterization and relationship to lowered complement levels. Clin. Exper. Immunol., 6:689, 1970.

Faculty of Medicine
University of Toronto
1 Spadina Crescent
Connaught Building
Toronto 179, Ontario
Canada

Chemical Mediators of the Vascular Phenomena of the Acute Inflammatory Reaction and of Immediate Hypersensitivity

*Henry Z. Movat, M.D., Ph.D., F.R.C.P.(C)**

Inflammation is the reaction of living tissue to injury, which comprises the series of changes of the terminal vascular bed, of the blood, and of the connective tissue which tend to eliminate the injurious agent and to repair the damaged tissue.

Immediate hypersensitivity reactions are acute inflammatory reactions (wheal and flare reaction, cutaneous anaphylaxis, the Arthus reaction, serum sickness), but they may manifest themselves as systemic reactions (anaphylactic shock) or reactions involving predominantly smooth muscle of an organ (asthma).

In discussing the chemical mediators I shall refer primarily to the acute inflammatory reaction, but the same mediators mediate also other processes such as smooth muscle contraction.

Today it is generally accepted that certain chemical mediators are of either cellular (mast cell, leukocytes) or of humoral (plasma) origin and that they can induce phenomena such as enhanced vascular permeability, leukocyte emigration, and smooth muscle contraction.

VASCULAR PHENOMENA OF ACUTE INFLAMMATION

Changes in the Blood Flow and the Formed Elements of the Blood

The changes which follow injury have been observed *in vivo* in many organs, but the best observations have been made on the microcirculation of the mesentery, by such pioneers as Cohnheim,[18] Illig,[37] and Zweifach.[131]

---

*Professor and Head, Division of Experimental Pathology, Faculty of Medicine, University of Toronto, Toronto, Canada.

Supported by the Medical Research Council of Canada (MT-1251), the Canadian Arthritis and Rheumatism Society, the Ontario Heart Foundation, and the Atkinson Charitable Foundation.

Soon after injury, changes occur in the terminal vascular bed or microcirculation. The terminal arterioles dilate and blood flows at a faster rate. The true capillaries open and blood flows through them. The post-capillary venules dilate and fill with rapidly flowing blood (hyperemia). During the early phase of hyperemia, vasomotion is still detectable, but later it completely subsides.

With mild injuries the vascular alterations do not progress beyond hyperemia. With moderate tissue injury, hyperemia is followed by a slow-ing of the blood. After severe injury, the blood flow comes to a standstill: stasis. Stasis may affect only a small portion of a vessel or a large area of the microcirculation. It is primarily the result of a severe vessel wall inju-ry, and is followed by rapid escape of fluid into the tissues and marked viscosity inside the lumen. While the red cells seem to have fused, tightly packed individual erythrocytes are recognizable by electron microscopy. With prolonged stasis, hemoglobin escapes from the red cells, some of which then resemble collapsed bags.[67]

If the inflammatory reaction is severe and hydrolytic enzymes are released, the vessel wall may be disrupted, followed by hemorrhage. The hemorrhage is probably due to enzymes derived from polymorphonuclear leukocytes, combined with a complete or partial occlusion of the vessels. The Arthus and Shwartzman reactions are good examples of severe acute inflammatory reactions in which thrombosis, in addition to hemorrhage, is a complicating factor.

Changes in the Blood-Tissue Barrier: Increase in Vascular Permeability and Exudation

The changes just described, but particularly the enhanced flow of blood through the fully open microcirculation, produce one of the cardi-nal signs of inflammation described by Celsus, rubor (redness). Another sign, tumor (swelling), is due to escape of plasma into the tissues: exuda-tion. Exudation requires (a) increase in blood flow, (b) increase in hydro-static pressure in the affected vessels, and (c) alterations of the vessel wall. Of these, the last is the most significant. Alterations in the vessel wall are followed by an increase in vessel permeability.

In the most common method used to detect increase in vascular per-meability, a dye such as Evans blue, injected intravenously complexes with plasma proteins (mainly albumin). When vessels in the affected area become permeable to plasma proteins, the dye escapes, discolors the tis-sues, and outlines the injured area in the skin. When inflammatory agents are tested in this manner, blue spots are obtained. The diameter and intensity of the blue spots can be measured and the intensity of the reaction ascertained in semiquantitative terms. For a more quantitative assay, Evans blue is injected with ^{125}I-labeled serum albumin and the degree of radioactivity is determined.[117] Colloidal particles, such as non-toxic colloidal carbon, have been used to determine the type of vessel in-volved during exudation.[19]

The ultrastructural basis of exudation was established with tracer particles. If an electron-dense tracer (colloidal carbon, saccharated iron oxide, thorium dioxide) is injected into an animal with an experimental inflammatory lesion, the circulating macromolecules escape from the postcapillary venule through gaps that form at the junction between two adjacent endothelial cells.[56, 57, 69, 70] Thus, exudation is due primarily to leakage between adjacent endothelial cells. Although such gaps occur almost exclusively in venules, some leakage occurs from capillaries after the skin has been heated for a time. It was believed for some time that leakage through capillaries was responsible for the so-called "delayed-prolonged" phase of exudation. However, venular leakage is the only form of exudation induced with known naturally occurring chemical mediators of inflammation. Capillary leakage probably represents direct injury of the vessel wall which affects the entire microcirculation, including capillaries, venules, terminal arterioles, and metarterioles.

MEDIATION OF THE VASCULAR PHENOMENA OF INFLAMMATION

Direct vs. Chemically Mediated Vascular Injury

Generations of physicians have been conditioned to think that microorganisms induce inflammation directly by elaborating various inflammatory agents. It is true that microorganisms are the most common causes of inflammatory disease, but the process by which inflammation is induced is mediated not by the parasite but by the host.

This can be demonstrated in the following simple experiment. Normal rabbits and rabbits made leukopenic (depleted of leukocytes with nitrogen mustard or an antileukocyte serum) are injected intradermally with a mixed bacterial culture. Next day the normal rabbits will have a well circumscribed inflammatory reaction with a small necrotic center, surrounded by a red swollen edematous area; the latter is surrounded by a red nonswollen halo or flare. The leukopenic rabbits will have no visible skin lesion but within a few days will die of septicemia. The normal rabbits show signs of repair and will eventually recover with a small residual scar. When the skin lesions of the normal rabbits are examined, one finds numerous polymorphonuclear leukocytes (neutrophils) that have ingested the bacteria. The bacteria are in phagolysosomes or digestive vacuoles, and some show signs of lysis. Many polymorphs are degranulated. In the skin of leukopenic animals, the bacteria have multiplied, lying free in the interstitial tissue.

Although chemical mediators are well recognized, most severe inflammatory lesions show some "direct" injury. Whether the lesion is caused by bacterial toxins or nonspecific trauma (e.g., heat), the center shows direct vascular injury and necrosis, peripherally there are varying degrees of vascular alterations, mediated, partly by direct injury and partly by chemical mediators, while at the extreme periphery the vascular events are produced entirely by chemical mediators.[67]

Two groups of criteria have been advanced to identify chemical mediators.[62]

Criteria supporting plausibility: (a) distribution of the mediator in various organs, tissues and species, (b) its availability and ability to become activated, (c) its ability to induce the vascular phenomena of acute inflammation and its potency in this respect, (d) the demonstration of natural inhibitors, and (e) the duration of its effect on the microcirculation.

Criteria proving mediation: (a) isolation of the chemical mediator at the time of its proposed action, (b) suppression of its effects by specific antagonists, and (c) depletion of the chemical mediator in the experimental animals and thereby inhibition of its action.

Several chemical mediators fulfil most of these criteria. With some mediators an occasional criterion has either not been fulfilled or for technical reasons could not be demonstrated.

Vasoactive Amines

The vasoactive amines, histamine (β-imidazolyl-ethylamine) and serotonin (5-hydroxytryptamine) are widely distributed throughout all tissues and species.[26] Both amines reproduce the vascular phenomena of inflammation when injected intradermally. Some animal species are particularly sensitive to histamine (guinea pig), others to serotonin (rat). Man is sensitive to histamine, but his sensitivity to serotonin has not yet been studied adequately. Both amines are effective in fractions of a microgram. Histamine is inactivated by the enzyme histaminase through oxidative deamination or by acetylation. Serotonin (5-hydroxytryptamine) is deaminated by amine oxidase to 5-hydroxyindole acetic acid.

The amines fulfil the criteria for mediation. When experimental pleurisy was induced in rats, histamine and serotonin could be isolated from the pleural exudate for the first 30 to 60 minutes, but not after that. Using specific antagonists such as antihistamine, BOL (bromolysergic acid diethylamine), the early phase of the pleural exudate could be suppressed.[112] Antagonists also suppressed the enhanced vascular permeability induced by local application of heat to the skin.[113, 127] These reactions cannot be elicited if the rats are depleted of their mast cells with repeated injections of compound 48/80, which causes mast cell degranulation.

Histamine and serotonin have been implicated in certain forms of local and systemic anaphylaxis.[13] In these forms of anaphylaxis the sensitizing antibody has been variously referred to as "anaphylactic," "homocytotropic," and "reagenic."[13] These antibodies belong to the immunoglobulin classes[9, 38] Ig_1 and IgE. This is an oversimplification of this complex field, which is difficult to describe in a few sentences. For an up to date report the reader is referred to the general discussion of a recent symposium.[8]

The immunologic release of amines and other chemical mediators from target cells represents a reaction which resembles secretion rather than a cytotoxic reaction. This is supported by morphologic findings;[36, 66, 71] the finding that there is no evidence of cell death, i.e. no potassium, lactic dehydrogenase, or ATP efflux when histamine is released;[45, 53] the observation that anaerobic glycolysis[64] and the activation of a serine esterase[6] are required for amine release; and finally, the fact that the cyclic adenosine 3',5'-monophosphate (AMP) system is involved in the release of histamine.[54]

Platelets, mast cells, and basophils form the main source of vasoactive amines in acute inflammation and anaphylactic reactions. Histamine and serotonin are released from human platelets when they phagocytose immune complexes.[74] This reaction does not require complement. However, histamine release from rabbit platelets by antigen-antibody complexes requires complement.[3, 28, 29, 33] A complement-independent immunologic mechanism of release of amines from platelets, involving IgE-sensitized leukocytes, antigen, and normal platelets has been described recently in a number of laboratories.[4, 5, 34, 106, 108] A soluble platelet activating factor has been demonstrated in this reaction. Its source was first thought to be the lymphocyte[106] or the monocyte,[34] but recent data indicate that it is the basophil leukocyte.[35, 109, 110] The release requires calcium, platelet energy metabolism, and serine esterases. The basophil leukocyte itself may be the source of histamine in both rabbit[110] and man.[38] Release of histamine from sensitized human leukocytes (probably basophils) is a process requiring energy. Good evidence has been accumulated in recent years that increase in cellular cyclic AMP levels prevents the release of histamine following antigenic challenge. This was demonstrable in vitro with isolated human leukocytes[54, 55] and lung fragments.[88]

The tissue mast cell is another source of vasoactive amines in many species.[65] Although histamine release has not been demonstrated, human mast cells sensitized with reagin became degranulated following antigenic challenge.[38] As with the platelet and leukocyte, the sensitized mast cell is not lysed following interaction with antigen but undergoes degranulation without evidence of cell death.[45] According to Uvnäs,[118, 119] histamine release from mast cells is a two-stage process. First there is degranulation of mast cells, and following exposure of the granules to the extracellular fluid, histamine is released from the granules by a cation exchange between granule histamine and extracellular sodium. As with platelets and basophils, the release of histamine from isolated mast cells is an active process. The biochemical sequence leading to release of histamine has been well studied after activation of the mast cells by a basic protein derived from neutrophil leukocytes[97] and after a complement-dependent antigen-antibody reaction.[98] Release of histamine requires first activation of an esterase, followed by a temperature-dependent state, which leads to the release of the amine through steps requiring divalent cations and energy.

As already stated, histamine – and in some species serotonin – fulfils most of the criteria proposed by Miles and Wilhelm.[62] It is widely distributed, readily available, induces the vascular phenomena of inflammation, is potent, has been isolated or demonstrated in tissue or inflammatory exudate, and is suppressible by specific antagonists, and its depletion is followed by negative inflammatory reactions, at least in some forms of acute inflammation.

Taken as a whole, these findings suggest that histamine and, in some species, serotonin mediate the early vascular phenomena, at least in some forms of acute inflammation.

Plasma Proteases (Esterases) and Polypeptides

Three complex systems – the kinin, the fibrinolytic, and the complement system – have been investigated as potential mediators of the vascular phenomena of inflammation. This intricate subject is complicated by the fact that the kinin, the fibrinolytic, and the blood-clotting systems are interrelated, and perhaps also the complement system.

Hageman factor (Factor XII),[102] when activated, initiates the activation of three systems:

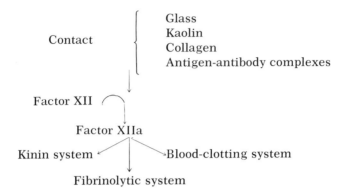

THE KININ SYSTEM. Evidence accumulated in the past decade suggests that, upon contact with certain "surface-active agents," Factor XII (Hageman factor) and Factor XI (plasma thromboplastin antecedent) are activated. Some believe that the two clotting factors form a complex (XIIa-XIa) – contact activation product – while others believe that Factor XIIa acts as an enzyme on Factor XI (substrate), converting it to Factor XIa.[101] Recently, it was possible to demonstrate that "contact activation product" is activated Factor XI, and contains little or no activated Factor XII.[92]

During activation of Factor XII, the kinin system is likewise activated. The mode of activation of the kinin system was controversial until recently. Many textbooks refer to a "globulin permeability factor" or "Pf/dil" (permeability factor dilute) first described by Miles, Wilhelm, and colleagues[128] when they diluted plasma in glass tubes. Because it could not be demonstrated when the dilution was made in siliconized glass or plastic test tubes, and because Factor XII becomes activated on contact with glass, it was assumed that Factor XII was responsible for the activation of Pf/dil.[58, 59] The exact mode of action of Pf/dil was not known, but circumstantial evidence seemed to indicate that it activates the kinin-forming enzyme, plasma kallikrein. Pf/dil had never been isolated in a functionally pure form, but it was shown to be moderately anionic, eluting with albumin during anion exchange chromatography.[7, 125]

In the past 2 years a highly anionic low molecular weight (30,000 to 36,000) permeability factor has been isolated in functionally pure form.[47, 68, 75, 78, 130] When the activator was added to purified prekallikrein, it converted it to the active enzyme (kallikrein), which hydrolyses arginine esters. It was shown that the enzyme obtained in this manner is kallikrein by adding it to kininogen (kinin-substrate) from which it liberated kinin. The activator has an isoelectric point of about 4.4, migrates in the albumin region by starch block or agar and as a prealbumin by polyacrylamide electrophoresis. It is now generally referred to as prekallikrein activator or PKA.[75]

The role of Factor XII in the activation of the kinin system was controversial until recently. As stated above, some believed that it acted on pro-Pf/dil, which then activated prekallikrein.[61] Others[83, 116] showed that when Factor XIIa was added to prekallikrein it induced its activation. Recent evidence indicates that the above mentioned PKA is a fragment of Factor XIIa.[47, 49, 77, 95, 111, 129] Upon massive contact exposure of plasma to celite almost all the Factor XIIa is converted to PKA.[93] The same effect can be obtained by exposing partially purified Factor XIIa to celite.[111] Factor XIIa can be converted to PKA also by trypsin[111, 129] and by plasmin.[14, 48]

The kinin liberated by plasma kallikrein is bradykinin (nonapeptide). Certain glands (pancreas, parotid) contain glandular kallikrein, which liberates lysyl-bradykinin (decapeptide) from kininogen. These two kinins were discovered independently by Rocha e Silva in Brazil[105] and by Werle in Germany.[126] A third kinin, consisting of 11 amino acids is methyonyl-lysyl-bradykinin.[107]

The kinin system fulfils almost all the criteria enumerated for potential chemical mediators: it is widely distributed, available, easy to activate, etc. Normally, a homeostasis exists between the activators and inhibitors of the system. Kinins are degraded by kininases (carboxypeptidases).[24] A natural inhibitor of kallikrein is a_2-macroglobulin,[32] a nonspecific inhibitor of many esterases (trypsin, thrombin, plasmin, elastase) C$\bar{1}$-inactivator (C′1-esterase inhibitor) is another inhibitor of kallikrein. It was first recognized as an inhibitor of the esterase derived from the first component of complement,[94] but subsequently, was found to inactivate many other esterases.[104] In addition to a_2-macroglobulin and C$\bar{1}$-inactivator, plasma contains a heat and acid stable polyvalent inhibitor, which inhibits also kallikrein.[115]

Many pathologic states represent either excess activation or inadequate inhibition of kinins. Kinins have been implicated in various forms of arthritis,[51, 60, 76] anaphylaxis,[12, 46] asthma,[1] wheal and flare reaction,[63] endotoxin shock,[25, 84] foreign body granuloma,[51a, 123] hereditary anioedema[21, 22] and pain.[2]

Kinins are the most potent inflammatory agents known; less than 0.1 microgram will enhance vascular permeability when injected intradermally and will cause pain when applied to a blister base. Smooth muscle contraction is induced by less than 0.1 nanogram (nanogram = mμg.).

THE FIBRINOLYTIC SYSTEM. The primary function of this system is to lyse blood clots. However, the active enzyme plasmin, derived from plasminogen, can induce the vascular phenomena of inflammation, although this action is primarily *via* the kinin system.

Plasminogen is activated by certain extrinsic "kinases" (e.g., streptokinase) or by intrinsic (tissue-derived) activators, e.g., urokinase, cytofibrinokinase.[31] Intrinsic activation of plasma requires Factor XII (Hageman factor), because this system, like the kinin system, cannot be activated in Factor XII-deficient plasma. Other less well defined substances ("Hageman factor cofactor") are likewise required.[85]

Plasmin may induce enhanced vascular permeability in three ways:

(a) by acting directly on kininogen, it liberates kinin;[14, 100] compared to the action of plasma kallikrein, this is a slow process and liberates relatively little kinin;[23] (b) by liberating PKA from Factor XIIa, which in turn acts on kininogen to form kinin as described above; (c) by cleaving off a vasoactive fragment from the third component (C3) of complement.[122]

THE COMPLEMENT SYSTEM. In 1910 Friedberger described a substance, "anaphylatoxin," which was generated when antigen-antibody complexes were added to guinea pig serum. When injected intravenously, such "toxic" serum produced more or less the signs and symptoms of anaphylactic shock. When injected intradermally it increased vascular permeability.

After Sir Henry Dale's discovery that "anaphylaxis" can be induced *in vitro* in serum-free tissue, the humoral "anaphylatoxin" theory of anaphylaxis fell into disrepute until some 10 years ago. In recent years great advances have been made in this field. We now know that, as suspected by Friedberger, complement is required for the generation of anaphylatoxin.[52] These discoveries started with the demonstration that the active esterase of the first component of complement (C1) enhances vascular permeability.[103] Subsequently, it was shown that $\overline{C1}$-activates the complement components C4,2,3 or C4, 2,3,5 and that a cleavage product of C3[20] or C5[44] is produced, referred to as C3a and C5a respectively. The fragment of C5a is believed to be identical to classical anaphylatoxin. These products can be generated also by incubating isolated and purified C3 or C5 with a cobra venom factor or trypsin. The subject was reviewed recently by Müller-Eberhard,[82] who also presented data on a natural inhibitor of anaphylatoxin.

Although complement is distributed throughout the body fluids and anaphylatoxin could conceivably be one of the natural mediators of inflammation, the role of these agents in the acute inflammatory reaction has not yet been tested.

Slow Reacting Substances

Slow-reacting substances (SRS) are defined as "those substances which slowly contract the guinea-pig ileum and are released from tissues or cells—as opposed to body fluids such as plasma—by any injury or potentially injurious stimulation."[121] Furthermore, according to Vogt the slow-reacting substances are not just released from stores, like for instance amines, but are formed *de novo*. Therefore, slow-reacting substances have to be extracted from treated tissues.

SRS-C was discovered by Feldberg and Kellaway.[27] It was obtained together with histamine when guinea pig lungs were perfused with cobra venom. It was noted that following the fast contraction of the guinea pig ileum, there was a slow relaxation. SRS-C was obtained also following incubation of lecithin with phospholipase A.[120] Today it is believed that most SRS-Cs are prostaglandins (PG); that venoms (containing phospholipase A) liberate PG precursors and, provided the converting enzyme system is present in the tissues, PG is formed.[121] A PG-like substance is released from phagocytosing neutrophil leukocytes.[73, 81]

SRS-A (slow reacting substance of anaphylaxis) was first encountered when Kellaway and Trethewie[50] perfused sensitized guinea pig lung with antigen. It too was released together with histamine. The latter could be inhibited with antihistamine and thereby it could be demonstrated that SRS-A causes both a slow contraction and a slow relaxation.[10, 11] SRS-A was demonstrated also in the peritoneal cavity of rats following antigen-antibody interaction.[91, 99, 114] The SRS-A obtained from rats induced a marked enhancement of vascular permeability when injected intradermally into guinea pigs, but had only a slight to moderate effect when injected in the homologous animal.[86] The SRS-A derived from guinea pig lung was mediated by a homocytotropic, gamma$_1$-antibody, that derived from rat peritoneal cavity by a heat-stable, complement-fixing antibody and required neutrophil leukocytes, but no mast cells.[86, 91, 114] More recently, it was demonstrated that SRS-A, in addition to histamine, may be released in the rat through a reaction requiring sensitization with homocytotropic (reagenic) antibody.[90] Also, a recent finding is the demonstration that human reagenic (γE) antibody is required for the release of SRS-A (in addition to histamine) from monkey[39] and human lung tissue.[88] Release of SRS-A from human lung was first demonstrated by Brocklehurst.[12] Like histamine release, release of SRS-A is inhibited by substances capable of increasing the intracellular levels of cyclic AMP.[39, 89]

Slow-reacting substances have been shown to be acidic, stable to boiling and at alkaline pH, labile at acid pH, insoluble in ethanol, propanol, and chloroform, but soluble in water, 80 per cent methanol, or ethanol. They are dialyzable, with a molecular weight of from 900 to 1150. SRSs readily adsorb to protein. They are not affected by proteolytic enzymes. By thin layer chromatography an Rf-value of 0.6 was found for most SRSs.[12, 15, 87]

Neutrophil Leukocyte Lysosomes

As already stated, certain forms of acute inflammation, namely those associated with phagocytosis, can be suppressed almost completely when experimental animals are rendered neutropenic.[16, 72, 79] Examples of such reactions are the Arthus reaction and serum sickness[16] and systemic aggregate anaphylaxis.[80]

In the phagocytosing neutrophil leukocytes of such inflammatory reactions, the ingested substances (bacteria, antigen-antibody precipitates) are found in digestive vacuoles, together with fragments of granules or lysosomes. As the lesions progress, more and more of the infiltrating leukocytes undergo such changes and become degranulated.

To study the chemical mediators released by the phagocytosing cells, the *in vivo* happenings can be imitated in *in vitro* experiments. Neutrophil leukocytes were incubated with or without phagocytosible material, such as antigen-antibody precipitates. After incubation the cells were spun out, the pellet was examined morphologically, and the supernatant was examined for its ability to enhance vascular permeability and for its physicochemical properties. A smear of the pellet showed leukocytes aggregating around clumps of antigen-antibody precipitates. Fluorescein-labeled antigen demonstrated fluorescent precipitates within the leukocytes. By electron microscopy, one could detect digestive vacuoles containing antigen-antibody precipitates and fragments of granules, just like in the *in vivo* experiments. When injected intradermally, the supernatant or ambient fluid (in which both Ag-Ab precipitates and leukocytes had been incubated) enhanced vascular permeability, and produced changes in the endothelium identical to those seen with other mediators. In high concentration, the supernatant produced thrombosis and hemorrhage, associated with necrosis of the vessel wall.[73, 81]

To date, the principal chemical mediators isolated from neutrophil leukocytes are cationic or basic proteins of low molecular weight (6000-12,000) present in the lysosomes.[42, 96] Of the four basic proteins recovered from rabbit neutrophil leukocyte granules, one (band 2) disrupted rat mast cells and released histamine from these cells.[96] However, it is uncertain whether this happens in the homologous animal (rabbit) from which mast cells cannot be isolated.

In addition to the basic proteins, the phagocytosing polymorphonuclear leukocytes release other mediators. Acid proteases or cathepsins of rabbit lysosomes degrade many proteins at acid pH, including basement membrane.[17, 124] Cathepsins also release kinin from kininogen, but this is an even slower process than the release due to plasmin.[30, 72] Human neutrophil leukocytes contain a neutral protease that digests elastin, collagen, and basement membrane, enhances vessel permeability, and causes hemorrhage when injected intradermally.[41, 43]

Neutrophil leukocyte lysosomes fulfil most of the criteria for a natural chemical mediator. Leukocytes are found throughout the body and their release can readily be induced by phagocytosis, but also by other means (endotoxin, streptolysin). They can be depleted (leukopenia) experimentally with nitrogen mustard or a specific antileukocyte serum. Inflammatory reactions associated with phagocytosis of the etiologic agent (e.g. bacteria, antigen-antibody precipitates) and degranulation of the polymorphonuclear leukocytes cannot be elicited in neutropenic animals.

CONCLUDING REMARKS

There is good evidence today that the vascular phenomena of acute inflammation and certain hypersensitivity reactions are mediated by chemical mediators derived from cells and plasma. Of these, the best studied is histamine, which seems to play a definite role in some forms of acute inflammation and anaphylaxis. It derives from various cells, namely mast cells, basophils, and platelets. Histamine has a transient effect and has been demonstrated only in the early phase of acute inflammatory reactions. While histamine has a transient effect, the kinin and complement systems – both plasma-derived – may play a role in the delayed phase of acute inflammatory reactions. The vascular phenomena of certain inflammatory reactions, which may culminate in thrombosis, hemorrhage and necrosis, are quite definitely mediated by neutrophil leukocytes. The mediators are released from the lysosomes of these cells.

REFERENCES

1. Abe, K., Watanabe, N., Kumagai, N., Mouri, T., Seki, T., and Yoshinaga, K.: Circulating kinin in patients with bronchial asthma. Experientia, 23:626, 1967.
2. Armstrong, D., Jepson, J. B., Keele, C. A., and Steward, J. W.: Pain-producing substance in human inflammatory exudates and plasma. J. Physiol., 135:350, 1957.
3. Barbaro, J. F.: The release of histamine from rabbit platelets by means of antigen-antibody precipitates. II. The role of plasma in the release of histamine. J. Immunol., 86:377, 1961.
4. Barbaro, J. F., and Schoenbechler, M. J.: The nature of the reaction of antigen with lymphocytes from rabbits infected with Schistosoma mansoni on the release of histamine from rabbit platelets. J. Immunol., 104:1124, 1970.
5. Barbaro, J. F., and Zvaifler, N. J.: Antigen-induced histamine release from platelets of rabbits producing homologous PCA antibody. Proc. Soc. Exper. Biol. Med., 122:1245, 1966.
6. Becker, E. L., and Austen, K. F.: A comparison of the specificity of inhibition by phosphonate esters of the first component of complement and the antigen-induced release of histamine from guinea pig lung. J. Exper. Med., 120:491, 1964.
7. Becker, E. L., and Kagen, L.: The permeability globulins of human serum and the biochemical mechanism of hereditary angioneurotic edema. Ann. N.Y. Acad. Sci., 116:866, 1964.
8. Benacerraf, B.: General discussion. In Austen, K. F., and Becker, E. L., eds.: Biochemistry of the Acute Allergic Reactions. Philadelphia, F. A. Davis Company, in press.
9. Bloch, K. J.: The stable homocytotropic antibodies of guinea pig, mouse and rat: A review and some recent developments. In Austen, K. F., and Becker, E. L., eds.: Biochemistry of the Acute Allergic Reactions. Philadelphia, F. A. Davis Company, in press.
10. Brocklehurst, W. E.: The release of histamine and formation of a slow-reacting substance (SRS-A) during anaphylactic shock. J. Physiol., 151:416, 1960.
11. Brocklehurst, W. E.: Slow-reacting substance and related compounds. Progr. Allergy, 6:539, 1962.
12. Brocklehurst, W. E., and Lahiri, S. C.: Formation and destruction of bradykinin through anaphylaxis. J. Physiol., 165:39, 1962.
13. Broder, I.: Anaphylaxis. In Movat, H. Z., ed.: Inflammation, Immunity and Hypersensitivity. New York, Harper and Row, 1971.
14. Burrowes, C. E., Movat, H. Z., and Soltay, M. J.: The kinin system of human plasma. VI. The action of plasmin. Proc. Soc. Exper. Biol. Med., 139:959, 1971.
15. Chakravarty, N.: The occurrence of a lipid-soluble smooth-muscle stimulating principle ("SRS") in anaphylactic reaction. Acta Physiol. Scand., 48:167, 1960.
16. Cochrane, C. G.: Immunologic tissue injury mediated by neutrophilic leukocytes. Adv. Immunol., 9:97, 1968.
17. Cochrane, C. G., and Aikin, B. S.: Polymorphonuclear leukocytes in immunologic reactions: The destruction of vascular basement membrane in vivo and in vitro. J. Exper. Med., 124:733, 1966.
18. Cohnheim, J.: Lectures on General Pathology. London, New Sydenham Society, 1971.
19. Cotran, R. S., and Majno, G.: A light and electron microscopic analysis of vascular injury. Ann. N.Y. Acad. Sci., 116:750, 1964.
20. Dias da Silva, W., and Lepow, I. H.: Complement as a mediator of inflammation. II. Biological properties of anaphylatoxin prepared with purified components of human complement. J. Exper. Med., 125:921, 1967.
21. Donaldson, V. H.: Mechanism of activation of C'1 esterase in hereditary angioneurotic edema plasma in vitro. The role of Hageman factor, a clot-promoting agent. J. Exper. Med., 127:411, 1968.
22. Donaldson, V. H., Ratnoff, O. D., Dias da Silva, W., and Rosen, F. S.: Permeability-increasing activity in hereditary angioneurotic edema. II. Mechanism of formation and partial characterization. J. Clin. Invest., 48:642, 1969.
23. Eisen, V., and Vogt, W.: Plasma kininogenase and their activators. In Erdös, E. G., ed.: Handbook of Experimental Pharmacology. New York, Springer-Verlag, vol. 25, 1970.
24. Erdös, E. G.: Hypotensive peptides: Bradykinin, kallidin, and eledoisin. Adv. Pharmacol., 4:1, 1966.
25. Erdös, E. G., and Miwa, I.: Effect of endotoxin shock on the plasma kallikrein-kinin-system of the rabbit. Fed. Proc., 27:92, 1968.
26. Feldberg, W.: Distribution of histamine in the body. In Wolstenholme, G. E. W., and O'Conner, C. M., ed.: Ciba Foundation Symposium on Histamine. London, Churchill, 1956.
27. Feldberg, W., and Kellaway, C. H.: Liberation of histamine and formation of lysolecithin-like substances by cobra venom. J. Physiol., 94:187, 1938.

28. Gocke, D. J., and Osler, A. G.: *In vitro* damage of rabbit platelets by an unrelated antigen-antibody reaction. I. General characteristics of the reaction. J. Immunol., 94:236, 1965.
29. Gocke, D. J., and Osler, A. G.: In vitro damage of rabbit platelets by an unrelated antigen-antibody reaction. II. Studies of the plasma requirements. J. Immunol., 94:247, 1965.
30. Greenbaum, L., and Kim, K. S.: The kinin-forming and kininase activities of rabbit polymorphonuclear leucocytes. Brit. J. Pharmacol., 29:238, 1967.
31. Hamberg, U.: The fibrinolytic activation mechanism in human plasma. Proc. Roy. Soc. B., 173:293, 1969.
32. Harpel, P. C.: Human plasma alpha 2-macroglobulin. An inhibitor of plasma kallikrein. J. Exper. Med., 132:329, 1970.
33. Henson, P. M.: Mechanism of release of constituents from rabbit platelets by antigen-antibody complexes and complement. I. Lytic and nonlytic reactions. J. Immunol., 105:476, 1970.
34. Henson, P. M.: Release of vasoactive amines from rabbit platelets induced by sensitized mononuclear leukocytes and antigen. J. Exper. Med., 131:287, 1970.
35. Henson, P. M., and Benveniste, J.: Antibody-leukocyte-platelet interactions. *In* Austen, K. F., and Becker, E. L., eds.: Biochemistry of the Acute Allergic Reactions. Philadelphia, F. A. Davis Company, in press.
36. Humphrey, J. H., Austen, K. F., and Rapp, H. J.: *In vitro* studies of reversed anaphylaxis with rat mast cells. Immunology, 6:226, 1963.
37. Illig, L.: Die terminale Strombahn. New York, Springer-Verlag, 1961.
38. Ishizaka, K., and Ishizaka, T.: IgE immunoglobulins of human and monkey. *In* Austen, K. F., and Becker, E. L., eds.: Biochemistry of the Acute Allergic Reactions. Philadelphia, F. A. Davis Company, in press.
39. Ishizaka, K., Ishizaka, T., Orange, R. P., and Austen, K. F.: Pharmacologic inhibition of the antigen-induced release of histamine and slow-reacting substance of anaphylaxis (SRS-A) from monkey lung tissues mediated by human IgE. J. Immunol., 106:1267, 1971.
40. Jahreiss, R., and Habermann, E.: *In vitro* investigations on some components of the kinin system (kininogen, serum kallikrein, Hageman factor), and their interaction. *In* Sicuteri, F., Rocha e Silva, M., and Back, N., eds.: Bradykinin and Related Kinins – Cardiovascular, Biochemical and Neuro-Actions. New York, Plenum Press, 1970.
41. Janoff, A.: Mediators of tissue damage in leukocyte lysosomes. X. Further studies on human granulocyte elastase. Lab. Invest., 22:228, 1970.
42. Janoff, A., Schaefer, S., Scherer, J., and Bean, M. A.: Mediators of inflammation in leukocyte lysosomes. II. Mechanism of action of lysosomal cationic protein upon vascular permeability in the rat. J. Exper. Med., 122:841, 1965.
43. Janoff, A., and Zeligs, J. G.: Vascular injury and lysis of basement membrane by neutral proteases of human leukocytes. Science, 161:702, 1968.
44. Jensen, J.: Anaphylatoxin in its relation to the complement system. Science, 155:1122, 1967.
45. Johnson, A. R., and Moran, N. C.: The selective release of histamine from rat mast cells. *In* Movat, H. Z., ed.: Cellular and Humoral Mechanisms in Anaphylaxis and Allergy. New York, S. Karger, 1969.
46. Jonasson, O., and Becker, E. L.: Release of kallikrein from guinea pig lung during anaphylaxis. J. Exper. Med., 123:509, 1966.
47. Kaplan, A. P., and Austen, K. F.: A prealbumin activator of prekallikrein. J. Immunol., 105:802, 1970.
48. Kaplan, A. P., and Austen, K. F.: A prealbumin activator of prekallikrein. II. Derivation of activators of prekallikrein from active Hageman factor by digestions with plasmin. J. Exper. Med., 133:696, 1971.
49. Kaplan, A. P., and Austen, K. F.: Immunologic activation of the bradykinin-forming system in man. *In* Austen, K. F., and Becker, E. L., eds.: Biochemistry of the Acute Allergic Reactions. Philadelphia, F. A. Davis Company, in press.
50. Kellaway, C. H., and Trethewie, E. G.: The liberation of slow reacting smooth muscle stimulating substance in anaphylaxis. Quart. J. Exper. Physiol., 30:121, 1940.
51. Kellermeyer, R. W., and Breckenridge, R. T.: The inflammatory process in acute gouty arthritis. I. Activation of Hageman factor by sodium urate crystals. J. Lab. Clin. Med., 65:307, 1965.
51a. Kellermeyer, R. W., and Warren, K. S.: The role of chemical mediators in the inflammatory response induced by foreign bodies: Comparison with the schistosome egg granuloma. J. Exper. Med., 131:21, 1970.
52. Lepow, I. H., Dias da Silva, W., and Patrick, R. A.: Biologically active components of complement. *In* Movat, H. Z., ed.: Cellular and Humoral Mechanisms in Anaphylaxis and Allergy. New York, S. Karger, 1969.
53. Lichtenstein, L. M.: Mechanism of allergic histamine release from human leukocytes. *In* Austen, K. F., and Becker, E. L., eds.: Biochemistry of the Acute Allergic Reactions. Philadelphia, F. A. Davis Company, 1968.

54. Lichtenstein, L. M.: Characteristics of leukocytic histamine release by antigen and by anti-immunoglobulin and anticellular antibodies. *In* Movat, H. Z., ed.: Cellular and Humoral Mechanisms in Anaphylaxis and Allergy. New York, S. Karger, 1969.

55. Lichtenstein, L. M., and Bourne, H. R.: Inhibition of allergic histamine release by histamine and other agents which stimulate adenylcyclase. *In* Austen, K. F., and Becker, E. L., eds.: Biochemistry of the Acute Allergic Reaction. Philadelphia, F. A. Davis Company, in press.

56. Majno, G., and Palade, G. E.: Studies on inflammation. I. The effect of histamine and serotonin on vascular permeability: An electron microscopic study. J. Biophys. Biochem. Cytol., *11*:57, 1961.

57. Marchesi, V. T.: The passage of colloidal carbon through inflamed endothelium. Proc. Roy. Soc. (B)., *156*:550, 1962.

58. Margolis, J.: Activation of plasma by contact with glass: Evidence for a common reaction which releases plasma kinins and initiates coagulation. J. Physiol., *144*:1, 1958.

59. Margolis, J.: Quantitative studies of kinin-releasing enzymes in plasma. *In* Erdös, E. G., Back, N., Sicuteri, F., and Wilde, A. F., eds.: Hypotensive Peptides. New York, Springer-Verlag, 1966.

60. Melmon, K. L., Webster, M. E., Goldfinger, S. E., and Seegmiller, J. E.: The presence of a kinin in inflammatory synovial effusion from arthritides of varying etiologies. Arthritis Rheumat., *10*:13, 1967.

61. Miles, A. A.: Large molecular substances as mediators of the inflammatory reaction. Ann. N.Y. Acad. Sci., *116*:855, 1964.

62. Miles, A. A., and Wilhelm, D. L.: The activation of endogenous substances including pathological increase in capillary permeability. *In* Stoner, H. B., ed.: The Biochemical Response to Injury. Oxford, Blackwell, 1960.

63. Michel, B., Russell, II, Th., Winkelmann, R. K., and Gleich, G. J.: Release of kinins from site of wheal-and-flare allergic skin reactions. Int. Arch. Allergy, *39*:616, 1970.

64. Mongar, J. L., and Schild, H. O.: Cellular mechanisms in anaphylaxis. Physiol. Rev., *42*:226, 1962.

65. Mota, I.: Release of histamine from mast cells. *In* Eichler, O., Farah, A., and Rocha e Silva, M., eds.: Handbook of Experimental Pharmacology. New York, Springer-Verlag, vol. 18, 1966.

66. Mota, I., and Vugman, I.: Effects of anaphylactic shock and compound 48/80 on the mast cells of the guinea pig lung. Nature, *177*:427, 1956.

67. Movat, H. Z.: The acute inflammatory reaction. *In* Movat, H. Z., ed.: Inflammation, Immunity and Hypersensitivity. New York, Harper and Row, 1971.

68. Movat, H. Z., DiLorenzo, N. L., and Treloar, M. P.: Activation of the plasma kinin system by antigen-antibody aggregates. II. Isolation of permeability-enhancing and kinin-releasing fractions from activated guinea pig serum. Lab. Invest., *19*:201, 1968.

69. Movat, H. Z., and Fernando, N. V. P.: The earliest changes in acute normergic and allergic inflammation. *In* Breese, S. S., ed.: Proceedings, Fifth International Congress on Electron Microscopy. New York, Academic Press, 1962.

70. Movat, H. Z., and Fernando, N. V. P.: Acute Inflammation. I. The earliest fine structural changes at the blood tissue barrier. Lab. Invest., *12*:895, 1963.

71. Movat, H. Z., Lovett, C. A., and Taichman, N. S.: Demonstration of antigen on the surface of sensitized rat mast cells. Nature, *212*:851, 1966.

72. Movat, H. Z., Macmorine, D. R. L., Takeuchi, Y., and Burrowes, C. E.: Chemical mediators released by PMN-leukocytes during phagocytosis of Ag-Ab complexes. *In* Movat, H. Z., ed.: Cellular and Humoral Mechanisms in Anaphylaxis and Allergy. New York, S. Karger, 1969.

73. Movat, H. Z., Macmorine, D. R. L., and Takeuchi, Y.: The role of PMN-leukocyte lysosomes in tissue injury, inflammation and hypersensitivity. VIII. Mode of action and properties of vascular permeability factors released by PMN-leukocytes during *in vitro* phagocytosis. Int. Arch. Allergy, *40*:218, 1971.

74. Movat, H. Z., Mustard, J. F., Taichman, N. S., and Uriuhara, T.: Platelet aggregation and release of ADP, serotonin and histamine associated with phagocytosis of antigen-antibody complexes. Proc. Soc. Exper. Biol. Med., *120*:232, 1965.

75. Movat, H. Z., Poon, M.-C., and Takeuchi, Y.: The kinin system of human plasma. I. Isolation of a low molecular weight activator of prekallikrein. Int. Arch. Allergy, *40*:89, 1971.

76. Movat, H. Z., Russell, M. L., and Gordon, D. A.: The nature and properties of kinin-forming substances in synovial fluid in rheumatoid arthritis. Proceedings of the Fourth Canadian Conference in the Rheumatic Diseases. Toronto, University of Toronto Press, 1971.

77. Movat, H. Z., Soltay, M. J., and Özge-Anwar, A. H.: The relationship between the plasma kinin system and the contact phase of blood coagulation in man. *In* Back, N., and Sicuteri, F., eds.: Vasoactive Polypeptides. New York, Plenum Press, in press.

78. Movat, H. Z., Treloar, M. P., and Takeuchi, Y.: A small molecular weight permeability

factor in guinea pig serum: adsorption to antigen-antibody aggregates. J. Immunol., 103:875, 1969.

79. Movat, H. Z., Udaka, K., and Takeuchi, Y.: Polymorphonuclear leukocyte lysosomes and vascular injury. Thromb. Diath. Haemorrh., Suppl., 40:211, 1970.

80. Movat, H. Z., Uriuhara, T., Taichman, N. S., Rowsell, H. C., and Mustard, J. F.: The role of PMN-leucocyte lysosomes in tissue injury, inflammation and hypersensitivity. VI. The participation of the PMN-leucocyte and the blood platelet in systemic aggregate anaphylaxis. Immunology, 14:637, 1968.

81. Movat, H. Z., Uriuhara, T., Takeuchi, Y., and Macmorine, D. R. L.: The role of PMN-leukocyte lysosomes in tissue injury, inflammation and hypersensitivity. VII. Liberation of vascular permeability factors from PMN-leukocytes during *in vitro* phagocytosis. Int. Arch. Allergy, 40:197, 1971.

82. Müller-Eberhard, H. J., and Vallota, E. H.: Formation and inactivation of anaphylatoxins. *In* Austen, K. F., and Becker, E. L., eds.: Biochemistry of the Acute Allergic Reactions. Philadelphia, F. A. Davis Company, in press.

83. Nagasawa, S., Takahashi, H., Koida, M., Suzuki, T., and Schoenmakers, J. G. G.: Partial purification of bovine plasma kallikreinogen, its activation by Hageman factor. Biophys. Biochem. Res. Com., 32:644, 1968.

84. Nies, A. S., Forsyth, R. P., Williams, H. E., and Melmon, K. L.: Contribution of kinins to endotoxin shock in unanesthetized Rhesus monkeys. Circulation Res., 22:155, 1968.

85. Ogston, D., Ogston, C. M., Ratnoff, O. D., and Forbes, C. D.: Studies on a complex mechanism for the activation of plasminogen by kaolin and by chloroform: The participation of Hageman factor and additional co-factors. J. Clin. Invest., 48:1789, 1969.

86. Orange, R. P., and Austen, K. F.: Slow-reacting substance of anaphylaxis in the rat. *In* Movat, H. Z., ed.: Cellular and Humoral Mechanisms in Anaphylaxis and Allergy. Basel and New York, S. Karger, 1969.

87. Orange, R. P., and Austen, K. F.: Immunological release of chemical mediators of immediate type hypersensitivity from human lung. *In* Amos, B., ed.: Progress in Immunology. First International Congress of Immunology. New York, Academic Press, in press.

88. Orange, R. P., Austen, W. G., and Austen, K. F.: The immunological release of histamine and slow-reacting substance of anaphylaxis from human lung. I. Modulation by agents influencing cellular levels of cyclic 3',5' adenosine monophosphate. J. Exper. Med., 134:1363, 1971.

89. Orange, R. P., Kaliner, M. A., and Austen, K. F.: The immunological release of histamine and slow-reacting substance of anaphylaxis from human lung. III. Biochemical control mechanism involved in the immunologic release of the chemical mediators. *In* Austen, K. F., and Becker, E. L., eds.: Biochemistry of the Acute Allergic Reactions. Philadelphia, F. A. Davis Company, in press.

90. Orange, R. P., Stechschulte, D. J., and Austen, K. F.: Immunochemical and biologic properties of rat IgE. II. Capacity to mediate the immunologic release of histamine and slow-reacting substance of anaphylaxis (SRS-A). J. Immunol., 105:1087, 1970.

91. Orange, R. P., Valentine, M. D., and Austen, K. F.: Antigen-induced release of slow-reacting substance of anaphylaxis (SRS-A^{rat}) in rats prepared with homologous antibody. J. Exper. Med., 127:767, 1968.

92. Özge-Anwar, A. H., Movat, H. Z., and Scott, J. G.: The human plasma kinin system. II. Contact activation of plasma prekallikrein and Factor XI in Factor XII-deficient plasma. Proc. Soc. Exper. Biol Med., 138:330, 1971.

93. Özge-Anwar, A. H., Movat, H. Z., and Scott, J. G.: The kinin system of human plasma. IV. The interrelationship between the contact phase of blood coagulation and the plasma kinin system. Thromb. Diath. Haemorrh., in press.

94. Pensky, J. L., Levy, R., and Lepow, I. H.: Partial purification of serum inhibitor of C'1 esterase. J. Biol. Chem., 236:1674, 1961.

95. Poon, M.-C.: The human plasma kinin system. Dissertation. School of Graduate Studies, University of Toronto, 1970.

96. Ranadive, N. S., and Cochrane, C. G.: Isolation and characterization of permeability factors from rabbit neutrophils. J. Exper. Med., 128:605, 1968.

97. Ranadive, N. S., and Cochrane, C. G.: Mechanism of histamine release from mast cells by cationic protein (band 2) from neutrophil lysosomes. J. Immunol., 106:506, 1971.

98. Ranadive, N. S., and Muir, J. D.: Similarity in the mechanism of histamine release induced by cationic protein from neutrophils and by complement-dependent Ag-Ab reaction. Int. Arch. Allergy, in press.

99. Rapp, H. J.: The release of a slow-reacting substance (SRS) in the peritoneal cavity of rats by antigen-antibody interaction. J. Physiol., 158:35P, 1961.

100. Ratnoff, O. D.: Increased vascular permeability induced by human plasmin. J. Exper. Med., 122:905, 1965.

101. Ratnoff, O. D.: The biology and pathology of the initial steps of blood coagulation. Prog. Hematol., 5:204, 1966.

102. Ratnoff, O. D., and Calopy, J. E.: A familial hemorrhagic trait associated with a deficiency of a clot-promoting fraction of plasma. J. Clin. Invest., 34:602, 1955.
103. Ratnoff, O. D., and Lepow, I. H.: Complement as a mediator of inflammation: Enhancement of vascular permeability by purified C′1 esterase. J. Exper. Med., 118:681, 1963.
104. Ratnoff, O. D., Pensky, J., Ogston, D., and Naff, G. B.: The inhibition of plasmin, plasma kallikrein, plasma permeability factor, and the C′1 sub-component of the first component of complement by serum C′1 esterase inhibitor. J. Exper. Med., 129:315, 1969.
105. Rocha e Silva, M., Beraldo, W. T., and Rosenfeld, G.: Bradykinin, a hypotensive and smooth muscle stimulating factor released from plasma globulin by snake venom and by trypsin. Amer. J. Physiol., 156:261, 1949.
106. Schoenbechler, M. J., and Barbaro, J. F.: The requirement for sensitized lymphocytes in one form of antigen-induced histamine release from rabbit platelets. Proc. Nat. Acad. Sci., 60:1247, 1968.
107. Schröder, E.: Üeber Peptidsynthesen: Synthese von Methionyl-Lysyl-Bradykinin, einem Kinin aus Rinderblut. Experientia, 20:39, 1964.
108. Siraganian, R. P., and Osler, A. G.: Antigenic release of histamine from rabbit leukocytes. J. Immunol., 104:1340, 1970.
109. Siraganian, R. P., and Osler, A. G.: Destruction of rabbit platelets in the allergic response of sensitized leukocytes. I. Demonstration of a fluid phase intermediate. J. Immunol., 100:1244, 1971.
110. Siraganian, R. P., and Osler, A. G.: Destruction of rabbit platelets in the allergic response of sensitized leukocytes. II. Evidence for basophil involvement. J. Immunol., 100:1252, 1971.
111. Soltay, M. J., Movat, H. Z., and Özge-Anwar, A. H.: The kinin system of human plasma. V. The probable derivation of prekallikrein activator from activated Hageman factor. Proc. Soc. Exp. Biol. Med., 139:952, 1971.
112. Spector, W. G., and Willoughby, D. A.: The demonstration of the role of mediators in turpentine pleurisy in rats by experimental suppression of the inflammatory changes. J. Path. Bact., 77:1, 1959.
113. Spector, W. G., and Willoughby, D. A.: Experimental suppression of the acute inflammatory changes of thermal injury. J. Path. Bact., 78:121, 1959.
114. Stechschulte, D. J., Austen, K. F., and Bloch, K. J.: Antibodies involved in antigen-induced release of slow-reacting substance of anaphylaxis (SRS-A) in the guinea pig and rat. J. Exp. Med., 127:127, 1967.
115. Takeuchi, Y., and Movat, H. Z.: Conversion of activated Hageman factor (Factor XIIa) of the guinea pig to prekallikrein activator and inhibition of the formed kallikrein by a natural plasma inhibitor. Eur. J. Immunol., in press.
116. Temme, H., Jahreiss, R., Habermann, E., and Zilliken, F.: Aktivierung von Gerinnungs- und Kinin-system durch eine Plasmaesterase (Hageman-Factor). Reinigung und Wirkungsbedingungen. Hoppe-Seyler's Z. Physiol. Chem., 350:519, 1969.
117. Udaka, K., Takeuchi, Y., and Movat, H. Z.: Simple method for quantitation of enhanced vascular permeability. Proc. Soc. Exper. Biol. Med., 133:1384, 1970.
118. Uvnäs, B.: Metabolic and non-metabolic processes in the mechanism of histamine release from mast cells. In Austen, K. F., and Becker, E. L., eds.: Biochemistry of the Acute Allergic Reactions. Philadelphia, F. A. Davis Company, 1968.
119. Uvnäs, B.: Quantitative correlation between degranulation and histamine release in mast cells. In Austen, K. F., and Becker, E. L., eds.: Biochemistry of the Acute Allergic Reactions. Philadelphia, F. A. Davis Company, in press.
120. Vogt, W.: Pharmacologically active substances formed in egg yolk by cobra venom. J. Physiol., 136:131, 1957.
121. Vogt, W.: Slow-reacting substances. In Movat, H. Z., ed.: Cellular and Humoral Mechanisms in Anaphylaxis and Allergy. New York, S. Karger, 1969.
122. Ward, P. A.: A plasmin-split fragment of C′3 as a new chemotactic factor. J. Exper. Med., 126:189, 1967.
123. Warren, K. S., and Kellemeyer, R. W.: Foreign body granulomas as response to chemical mediators of inflammation. J. Clin. Invest., 47:99a, 1968.
124. Wasi, S., Murray, R. K., Macmorine, D. R. L., and Movat, H. Z.: The role of PMN-leukocytes in tissue injury, inflammation and hypersensitivity. II. Studies on the proteolytic activity of PMN-leukocyte lysosomes of the rabbit. Brit. J. Exper. Path., 47:411, 1966.
125. Webster, M. E.: Human plasma kallikrein, its activation and pathological role. Fed. Proc., 27:84, 1968.
126. Werle, E., and Berek, U.: Zur Kenntnis des Kallikreins. Angew. Chem., 60A:53, 1948.
127. Wilhelm, D. L., and Mason, B.: Vascular permeability changes in inflammation: The role of endogenous permeability factors in mild thermal injury. Brit. J. Exper. Path., 41:487, 1960.
128. Wilhelm, D. L., Miles, A. A., and Mackay, M. E.: Enzyme-like globulins from the serum reproducing the vascular phenomena of inflammation. II. Isolation and properties of the permeability factor and its inhibition. Brit. J. Exper. Path., 36:82, 1955.

129. Wuepper, K. D., and Cochrane, C. G.: Isolation and mechanism of activation of components of the plasma kinin-forming system. *In* Austen, K. F., and Becker, E. L., eds.: Biochemistry of the Acute Allergic Reactions. Philadelphia, F. A. Davis Company, in press.
130. Wuepper, K. D., Tucker, E. S. III., and Cochrane, C. G.: Plasma kinin system: proenzyme components. J. Immunol., *105*:307, 1970.
131. Zweifach, B. W.: Functional Behaviour of the Microcirculation. Springfield, Illinois, Charles C Thomas, 1961.

Division of Experimental Pathology
University of Toronto
Medical Sciences Building
Toronto, Ontario
Canada

Genetics and Regulation of Immunoglobulin Allotypes

Stanislaw Dubiski, M.D., Ph.D *

Antibody formation, one of the main functions of the immune apparatus has been the subject of extensive research during the past few years. An impressive volume of information with regard to the structure of antibody molecules has been gathered and many attempts have been made to explain the mechanism of the genetic control of antibody synthesis and antibody variability. One of the main difficulties of research in this area is the vast heterogeneity of immunoglobulin molecules in terms of their *antibody-combining sites*. In the following discussion we will ignore this heterogeneity and will confine our discussion to a limited number of genetic markers of immunoglobulin molecules, known as *allotypes* or *allotypic specificities*. The heterogeneity of antibody molecules in terms of their genetic markers is considerably smaller than the heterogeneity in terms of antibody-combining sites. This approach may, therefore, enable us to reach some conclusions, which could help to understand the overall genetic control of antibody synthesis.

Immunoglobulin molecules, like other proteins, are potentially antigenic; consequently, immunization with immunoglobulins of a foreign species will, obviously, lead to the formation of antibody directed against the immunoglobulins used as an immunizing antigen. Isoimmunization (i.e., immunization with immunoglobulins from an individual of the same species) may also lead to antibody production. Isoimmunization of rabbits with rabbit serum was attempted in the early days of immunology by Schütze[120] and resulted in the formation of precipitating antibodies. The antigen was a serum protein, but it was not characterized any further.

More recently, isoantigens of rabbit serum were rediscovered.[37, 103, 104] The method of immunization as well as the properties of the isoantigen made it clear that the antigenic protein was an immunoglobulin.

*Associate Professor, Departments of Pathological Chemistry and Medicine, University of Toronto; Head, Laboratory of Immunology, The Toronto Western Hospital, Toronto, Ontario, Canada.

Research supported by The Medical Research Council of Canada, Grant No. MT-1580.

The typical procedure involves immunizing a rabbit D (D = donor) with soluble or particulate antigen (e.g., protein solution or suspension of bacterial cells). Next, the antiserum raised in D is allowed to form immune complexes (precipitates or agglutinates) with the homologous antigen; these complexes are washed and injected into another rabbit, R (R = recipient). Whole normal serum[25] or purified immunoglobulins[134] of D can also be used for immunization, but this procedure is less effective than the immunization with immune complexes. Furthermore, inadequate purification may result in the formation of additional antibodies directed to serum proteins, other than immunoglobulins.

If the individual D contained an antigenic determinant not present in R, this immunization should result in formation of antibody, reacting with D, and with serum of any other rabbit, whose immunoglobulins carry a determinant, identical with that present in D. In other words, the immune serum R can be used as a reagent for detecting D and can divide a rabbit population into two groups: D+ and D−, respectively possessing or lacking the determinant in question.

Oudin[104, 105] proposed the term "allotypy" for this phenomenon. Consequently, an antigenic specificity detected by the immune serum is called "allotypic specificity." The exciting possibility that allotypic specificities may be of hereditary character[37] was fully confirmed by subsequent studies.[26, 31, 40, 41, 94−96, 106, 108] These studies also resulted in finding and characterizing many more allotypic specificities. Allotypy has been described in several species other than the rabbit, including man and mouse. By far the largest number of specificities is known in man. So far, all except a few of them (InV and Am), are localized on heavy chains of the IgG. Readers interested in the details of human allotypy are referred to the excellent and comprehensive book by Grubb.[57] In the mouse, most specificities thus far described are localized on the Fc portion of the heavy chains.[34, 59, 60, 61, 69, 84] and will not be very useful for our considerations. Edelman and Gottlieb[46] have described in the mouse a genetically determined allotypic variant localized in the variable region of the heavy chain. It will be interesting to see if the genetic control of this marker conforms to the general hypothesis outlined later in this article.

Our discussion will therefore center mainly around rabbit allotypes. As a basis for this discussion, Table 1 gives a summary of the present knowledge of allotypy in the rabbit.

Both heavy and light chains of all major rabbit immunoglobulin classes contain allotypic specificities. For the kappa (κ) light chains only one locus has, so far, been described. The four allotypic specificities of the kappa chains are controlled by genes which seem to be true alleles.[22, 40, 68, 92, 108] High concentration of kappa chains in rabbit serum and the fact that the specificities localized on these chains are strong isoantigens makes these specificities excellent markers of immunoglobulins. However, in using these markers one has to remember that these specificities share a number of antigenic determinants (subspecificities) which can cause cross-reactions between antisera and various nonhomologous specificities.[39, 105] The lambda chains constitute a minor proportion of rabbit light chains; the existence of these chains in the rabbit has only recently been reported.[3] Allotypic specificities of the chains are Ac7 and Ac21.[26, 55, 87, 141, 142] Their genetics is not clear, however, they seem to be controlled at two closely linked loci (or one complex locus),[55, 88] and consequently may not be true alleles.

The allotypes of heavy chains present a very complex situation. Each class of heavy chains has a number of class-specific allotypic markers. For the gamma-chain there are four recently described but relatively well-established markers: A11, A12[71, 94−96, 115, 117] and A14, A15[2, 31, 32, 79] as well as less known A8 and A10.[58] The mu-chains seem to carry at least one, perhaps two or more class-specific markers (Ms6, Ms4).[70] The last group of class-specific allotypes are localized on IgA molecules. It has been claimed that the c1 marker is localized on alpha-chains, probably on the Fc portion.[98] This has still to be confirmed by independent investigations. Other IgA markers, the *Af* group, are under the control of a complex locus, with five allotypic markers occurring in pheno-groups.[17, 18, 23] The relationship between *Af* and the c1 is not known. The still uncertain molecular localization of the *Af* specificities remains a particularly tantalizing problem, in view of the fact that the *Af* locus may be linked with the *Aa* locus.[83]

Besides class-specific, Fc allotypes, a group of variable region-allo-typic specificities (*Aa*) has long been known.[22, 65, 108] Todd[138] reported the presence of these specificities on IgG and IgM molecules. It was difficult to reconcile this observation with any plausible hypothesis explaining the genetic control of antibody synthesis. The validity of this observation, named the "Todd phenomenon" was successfully verified[50, 72, 73, 82, 122, 133, 136, 139] many times. The original report described the presence of *Aa* allotypes on gamma- and mu-chains; later, the validity of this finding was confirmed and extended to the alpha and epsilon classes of heavy chains. The genetic mechanism proposed for the Todd phenomenon will be discussed later.

The status of the recently described A31 marker is still uncertain.[21] It is located on a minor proportion of H-chains, the so-called "a-negative" chains (the "a-negative" chains do not carry the specificities of the *Aa* group). More information about the A31 specificity, as well as about "a-negative" chains will be essential for testing the validity of the genetic hypothesis discussed later in this article.

THE STRUCTURAL BASIS OF ALLOTYPY

It can reasonably be assumed that allotypic differences reflect differences in amino acid sequences of immunoglobulin polypeptide chains. In the rabbit direct and unequivocal evidence has, so far, been obtained for the *Ad*[115] and *Ae*[2] allotypes. In man, such evidence is available for the light chain allotypes, InV[1, 52, 100, 137] and for some of the Gm allotypes.[57, 113] Other rabbit specificities (*Aa* and *Ab*) were also found to be correlated with characteristic amino acid composition or sequences.[51, 77, 117, 131, 147, 148] In these cases, however, comparison between the sequences characteristic for various allotypes, suggests substitutions at more than one position. This may either be purely coincidental, a result of the presence of another allotypic specificity,[116] of individual or subclass variations in sequence, or of the presence of multiple subspecificities within each allotypic specificity (e.g., in the A*b* group).[39]

Correlation of a given allotypic specificity with a single amino acid

Table 1. *Allotypic Markers of Rabbit Immunoglobulins*

SYSTEM OR GROUP	SPECIFICITIES	MOLECULAR LOCALIZATION AND PROPERTIES	ALLELES	RELATION TO OTHER SYSTEMS	REFERENCES
Ab	Ab4, Ab5, Ab6, Ab9	Kappa chain; possess shared sub-specificities causing cross-reactions	$A_b^4, A_b^5, A_b^6, A_b^9$	No close linkage with any other system	3, 10, 22, 26, 36, 40–42, 65, 68, 84, 88, 105, 106, 108
Ac	Ac7, Ac21	Lambda chain	A_c^7, A_c^{21} may not be alleles	No close linkage with Ab	26, 55, 87, 88, 101, 141, 142
Aa	Aa1, Aa2, Aa3	All Ig classes (IgG, IgM, IgA, IgE) H-chain, variable part	A_a^1, A_a^2, A_a^3	Closely linked with Ad, Ae	22, 26, 36, 41, 42, 50, 65, 68, 72, 73, 77, 78, 82, 97, 99, 105, 106, 112, 114, 122, 133, 135, 136, 138, 139, 148
	A31+, A31−	IgG, H-chain, Fd (variable ? part) other Ig classes? Found on so-called "a-negative" molecules.	Genetics unknown	?	6, 21, 24, 27, 75, 134
Ad	Ad11, Ad12	IgG, Fc part; Methionine-threonine inter-change at the position amino-terminal and adjacent to the inter-H-chain bond in the hinge region.	A_d^{11}, A_d^{12}	Closely linked with Aa, Ae	71, 94–96, 114, 115

Ae	Ae14, Ae15	IgG, Fc part; Threonine-alanine interchange at position 309	A_e^{14}, A_e^{15}	Closely linked with Aa, Ad	2, 31, 32, 79
	A8, A10	IgG, Fc part; associated with A1, i.e. only A1-positive animals can have these specificities	?	?	58
Ms	Ms4	Igm, μ-chain, (Fc?)	?	Probably linked with Aa, Ad, Ae	66, 70
	Ms6	IgM, μ-chain, (Fc?)	?	Probably linked with Aa, Ad, Ae	70
	Ms5	IgM; may be identical or associated with Ms4	?	?	66, 70
	Ms1	IgM; associated with A3, i.e. only A3-positive animals are Ms1-positive	?	?	66, 67, 70
	Ms3	IgM; associated with A4, i.e. only A4+ animals can be Ms3+	?	?	66, 70
	Ms2	IgM	?	?	70, 121
	c1	IgA, Fc?	?	?	98
Af	Af1, Af2, Af3, Af4, Af5	IgA	$A_f^{1,5}$, $A_f^{2,4}$ $A_f^{3,4}$	May be linked with Aa	17, 18, 23, 83

substitution does not mean, however, that a single amino acid residue can act as an antigenic determinant. When an immunoglobulin molecule or its fragments are broken down to smaller peptides, allotypic activity (i.e., the ability to combine with antiallotype antibody) disappears.[9] It appears, therefore, likely that the primary structure of a polypeptide chain determines surface configurations and that these configurations in turn, function as allotypic determinants.[135]

Immunoglobulin molecules are built symmetrically, i.e., the two antibody combining sites have identical specificity and each pair of polypeptide chains has identical structure. This also applies to allotypic structure and is true, even in a heterozygous animal which, as a whole, synthesizes two allotypic variants of a given chain.[107] One can easily appreciate the biological importance of the symmetrical structure of immunoglobulin molecules. Production of such symmetrical units is assured by keeping the various assembly lines in physical separation: each immunoglobulin-producing cell is highly specialized and is committed to the synthesis of only one allotypic specificity.[110] This aspect of antibody formation will be discussed later in more detail.

GENETIC CONTROL OF HEAVY CHAIN ALLOTYPIC SPECIFICITIES

Each group of allotypic specificities, when considered in isolation from the others, conforms to the simple Mendelian rules of inheritance. However, these simple genetic mechanisms do not adequately explain either the linkage relationships between the class-specific allotypes and the specificities of the Aa group, or the Todd phenomenon. It was clear that some "unorthodox" mechanisms would have to be found to account for these phenomena.

One of these "unorthodox" solutions was the proposed two-loci control of the heavy chain.[31, 32] The same mechanism was proposed on the basis of structural studies.[76, 78, 143, 144] This concept was later confirmed by the observation of a crossing-over between the Aa and Ae[86] and between Aa and Ad genes.[93] However, this two-loci control mechanism was only a partial solution since it did not explain the Todd phenomenon. Moreover, it did not reconcile the rabbit situation with the situation described for man and mouse. In these species the Todd phenomenon has not been observed, i.e., no genetic markers shared by several immunoglobulin classes or subclasses have been found. In man, a concept of a series of closely linked loci, each controlling one immunoglobulin class or subclass has been proposed.[57]

Similarly, in mouse, Herzenberg and Warner[59, 60] put forward a hypothesis of a chromosome region, containing several distinct loci, each locus coding for the structure of the heavy chain of one of the immunoglobulin classes or subclasses. This hypothesis was based on a very interesting observation of a nonhomologous crossing-over between chromosomal regions controlling two different immunoglobulin subclasses (IgG_{2a} and IgG_{2b}). A myeloma protein induced in a heterozygous mouse carried one marker specific for IgG$_{2a}$ and another marker, specific for IgG$_{2b}$ sub-class. These markers were originally controlled by two genes *in repulsion.* Similar linkage relationships have not been observed in the rabbit, since the genetics of the mu and alpha chain markers have not yet been studied.

Clearly the overall genetic hypothesis dealing with the control of immunoglobulin synthesis should:

1. Explain the Todd phenomenon.

2. Take into account the linkage between the variable and constant (*Aa* and *Ad-e*) markers in the rabbit, as well as anticipate an analogous phenomenon in man and mouse and reconcile it with the linkage between various heavy chain genes observed in these species.

3. Take into account the linkage between constant gene markers in man and mouse, as well as anticipate an analogous phenomenon in the rabbit and reconcile it with the variable-constant (*Aa - Ad-e*) linkage, observed in this species.

4. Have a potential for extrapolation; i.e., it should provide a plausible explanation for the heterogeneity of antibody-combining sites and for the genetic control of this heterogeneity.

Assuming that the situation in the rabbit is similar to the situation in man and mouse (and vice versa), we have one variable gene linked to a number of constant genes, which are also linked to each other. From this group of closely linked genes only one variable and one constant gene contribute to the synthesis of any single chain. The constant genes can, therefore, be visualized as situated in *parallel,* rather than in *tandem.* When "reading" proceeds from the variable to the constant region, at one point a decision must be made, which of the many parallel genes should be "read."

A hypothesis, according to which closely linked genes are arranged in parallel and alternative "reading" of one of them depends on a "switching mechanism", has been proposed by Smithies[132] and its modification is represented in Figure 1. So far, in our considerations we left out the A 31 specificity which seems to be a marker of the variable part of the heavy chain, alternative to the *Aa* markers.[75] The "*a-negative*" heavy chains apparently carry the *Ae* specificities.[21] To integrate this information into the proposed scheme, it would be necessary to postulate *two* variable genes in parallel; either of these two variable genes would be able to link with any of the 4 c-genes. Furthermore, all 6 genes would be closely linked.

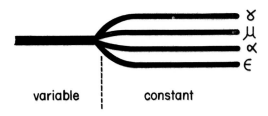

Figure 1. Illustration of the complex linkage relationship between genes controlling H-chain structure.

The modified hypothesis is represented in Figure 2. It has some predictive values which are listed below:

1. All constant, class-specific H-chain markers must be controlled by closely linked loci.
2. Each c-locus must be closely linked with both variable loci (*Aa* and "a-negative").
3. Specificities carried by the *"a-negative"* variable portion should be present in association with all heavy chain classes, i.e., the Todd phenomenon should also apply to the *"a-negative"* markers.

GENETIC CONTROL OF THE LIGHT-CHAIN ALLOTYPES

Can a similar mechanism control the synthesis of the light chains? Neither the kappa nor lambda chain allotypic specificities have been localized on variable or constant portions of the light chain. The complex locus controlling the two lambda-chain specificities, A7 and A21, may well be two closely linked loci, one controlling the v-portion, the other the c-portion of the lambda-chain. All kappa-chain specificities appear to be controlled by true alleles. However, immunochemically these specificities are complex structures, which have several shared subspecificities. This suggests multiple amino acid substitutions. It cannot be excluded that these substitutions are located on different parts of the light chains and that each part of the light chain is controlled by separate, but closely linked locus. More detailed structural and genetic studies should clarify these uncertainties.

A SERIES OF CLOSELY LINKED GENES CONTROLLING THE SYNTHESIS OF THE HEAVY CHAINS

Can the information on the genetic control of allotypic specificities be used to explain the genetic control of antibody specificities? Coming

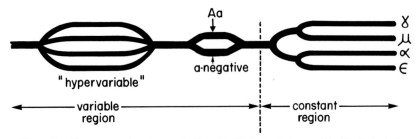

Figure 2.   Chromosomal region controlling the H-chain allotypes. "Reading" starts from the N-terminal and the "hypervariable" region, controlling the specificity of the antibody combining site. Then it proceeds through the switch, selecting the "variable" allotypic region and finally selects the constant gene. In the concept proposed by Smithies[132] the v-gene allotypic markers are located to the left of the region coding for antibody combining site. In this figure, to simplify the discussion and to focus it on allotypic markers, the v-allotypic and c-allotypic regions were placed next to each other, with the "hypervariable" region at the N-terminus. Which of these two alternatives represents the true situation can be answered only by structural studies.

back to the hypothesis proposed by Smithies,[132] one can imagine several "hypervariable" genes arranged in parallel (Fig. 2). The "reading" of the DNA molecule may start at some point, common to all these genes, then go through a switching mechanism, selecting one of these genes and resulting in a particular sequence of the antibody combining site. It would then go through a switch, selecting between *Aa* and *"a-negative"* specificities, and finally selecting one of the constant region genes. Alternatively, the reading may start from the "variable" part and then proceed to the "hypervariable." Appropriate structural studies should determine which of these possible arrangements is true.

THE ROLE OF SOMATIC RECOMBINATIONS IN THE GENERATION OF ANTIBODY HETEROGENEITY

It has been postulated that somatic recombination is the major mechanism responsible for generating antibody diversity.[45] This hypothesis can be directly tested using the heavy chain allotypic markers. Allotypic composition of heavy chains has been tested in animals which were double heterozygotes at the *Aa* and *Ae* or *Aa* and *Ad* loci. It was found that the majority of molecules contain markers contributed by the genes *in coupling* and only a small proportion of molecules contained markers determined by genes *in repulsion*.[80] These molecules, which apparently are "recombinant" molecules are released by "recombinant" cells, which can be detected by fluorescent staining.[111] The proportion of "recombinant" molecules and the frequency of "recombinant" cells is approximately 1 per cent. It seems likely that the origin of such molecules is the result of somatic recombinations, but at such low frequency it is unlikely that this mechanism could be responsible for substantially contributing to the generation of antibody heterogeneity. It cannot, however, be excluded that similar, and perhaps more frequent, recombinations occur between the "hypervariable" and the "variable" regions.

ARE ALLOTYPIC GENES STRUCTURAL OR REGULATORY GENES?

The entire preceding discussion was based on the assumption that the allotypic genes are structural genes. Although, this is a generally accepted view, there are a few isolated experiments which do not support this contention and seem to indicate that the allotypic genes are, in fact, regulatory genes, which control the *expression* of some structural genes which are always present, but which can express themselves only in the presence of the appropriate regulatory gene.

Rivat, Gilbert, and Ropartz[119] maintained isolated human peripheral blood lymphocytes in culture for up to 96 hours and were able to detect, in some supernatants, allotypic (Gm) specificities which were not present in the serum of the lymphocyte donors. The interpretation suggested by the authors is that the structural genes were under control of regulatory genes and that this control was lost in tissue culture, allowing the expression of previously unexpressed genes.

Bell and Dray[5] incubated extracts of lymph node cells from immunized rabbits with spleen cells from unimmunized animals. Extracts from immunized cells induced antibody production by the normal spleen cells. The light-chain allotypes of the antibody produced in this way was of the same specificity as the allotype of the donor of the extracts and not of the donor of the spleen cells. The authors claim that the RNA contained in the extracts either functioned as a messenger for the synthesis of the donor-type antibody or, if the structural information for both allotypes was present in the normal spleen cells, the RNA extracts might have affected the hypothetical regulatory genes. It is difficult to express any opinion for or against these possibilities until more experimental evidence is available.

DO ALLOTYPES HAVE ANY SELECTIVE VALUE?

In the above discussion on the genetics of the antibody response, the allotypic specificities were employed as markers of immunoglobulin chains and their respective genes. The mechanism which was proposed as the genetic mechanism controlling antibody synthesis *involves* allotypes, but it does not *explain* their biological function. Do allotypic specificities have any biological function and, if so, do they have any selective value? The results of recent family studies showed highly significant deviations in the frequencies of A_b^4/A_b^5 and A_b^5/A_b^5 from the expected frequencies of these genotypes.[92] These data could be taken as an indication that the gene A_b^5 is being selected against.

There are also observations which show that there is selective coupling between the A_a and A_{d-e} genes.[39] The gene A_e^{14} was found *in coupling* only with A_a^1 and A_a^2 and not with A_a^3. There is no such selective coupling of A_e^{15}. This phenomenon may be due to different frequencies of recombination between different pairs of genes, but it is also possible that there is a selection against individuals, in which the genes A_a^3 and A_e^{14} *are in coupling*.

Through what mechanisms can a selective advantage or disadvantage operate? Allotypic specificities do not contribute directly to the structure of the antibody-combining site, but a given allotypic specificity may change the folding of a polypeptide chain, perhaps increasing the avidity of the antibody. If any of the allotypic specificities had indeed such properties, one would expect them to be fairly specific, i.e. to increase the avidity of only a small proportion of antibodies, directed to a small group of antigens. Finding such an antigen, even among a limited number of environmental antigens, would be a formidable task.

CELLULAR ASPECTS OF ANTIBODY FORMATION

The observations discussed above seem to suggest that allotypes do indeed have some selective value, but they do not suggest any feasible experimental approach to this problem. Such an approach may, however, be coming from another area of research: from the study on the regulation of *expression* of allotypic genes.

In general, molecules are twice as concentrated in homozygotes as in heterozygotes, if their inheritance is codominant and under the control of a single gene.[35] There are striking departures from the gene-dose relationship in the proportion of molecules carrying different allotypic markers. When we consider the specificities of the kappa chain, we will invariably find that in any heterozygous combination the proportion of A4 molecules is always *greater* than 50 per cent.[11, 12, 24] Conversely, in any heterozygous combination involving A9, the proportion of these molecules will always be *less* than 50 per cent.[10–12] By looking at phenotypic expression of all four A_b genes in all possible heterozygous combinations, it has been possible to arrive at the following "hierarchy" or "pecking order" of phenotypic expression: A4 > A6 > A5 > A9.[13, 14, 33] A similar hierarchy seems to exist within the Aa locus: A1 > A2[79] (the position of A3 in this hierarchy is uncertain). Moreover, a similar hierarchy seems to exist at the class (kappa > lambda)[3, 10, 88] or sub-class (Aa > "a-negative")[75] levels.

It is interesting to note that the position in the "pecking order" of a given Aa gene, determines also the degree of expression of a constant region gene, which is *in coupling* with the Aa gene. In a double heterozygote $A_a{}^1/A_a{}^2$; $A_e{}^{14}/A_e{}^{15}$ the $A_e{}^{14}$ gene may be expressed on 80 per cent of the molecules if it is linked with the $A_a{}^1$ gene, but the same $A_e{}^{14}$ gene, if linked with $A_a{}^2$ will only be expressed on 20 per cent of the molecules.[79]

Phenotypic expression of allotypic genes may be altered experimentally. A spectacular method of altering this expression is provided by "allotypic suppression".[20, 29, 30, 43, 44, 85] To induce allotypic suppression, newborn rabbits are injected with antibody to their allotypic specificities. Since immunoglobulins acquired from the mother may interfere with the induction of suppression, the antibody injected should usually be directed to the allotypic specificity of the paternal type, which is absent from the mother. By this method, phenotypic expression of one of the alleles can be affected for the entire life of the animal. Expression of the other allele will simultaneously increase to compensate for the suppression. By special procedures (induction of allotypic suppression in the mother[28, 29] or by zygote transfer,[19, 141]) allotypic suppression can be induced in homozygous rabbits. Here, the loss of the product of one locus is compensated for by an increased production of the product of another locus. If expression of the A_b locus is suppressed, it is compensated for by the increased production of lambda chain,[3, 28] if suppression of the heavy chain A_a locus was induced, the compensatory mechanism will increase the synthesis of "a-negative" chains.[75]

Another mechanism controlling the expression of allotypic genes is the feed-back control.[30, 38] Feed-back control can be demonstrated if the concentration of the product of one allele is increased several times. As a result, the expression of the allele in question will be substantially reduced with the effects still visible after several weeks.

Phenotypic expression and its regulation must be intimately related to the process of cell differentiation. During this process the preproductive immunocompetent cells which initially seem to be multipotent[56] become highly specialized. Fully differentiated, specialized productive cells are committed to the synthesis of only *one* type of combining site[89] and *one* allotypic specificity.[109, 110] It is believed that this is accomplished by *de-repression,* or activation of one of the two homologous chromosomes present in each cell. Through the mechanism known as "allelic exclusion," the productive cell becomes functionally haploid. It seems that one of the main functions of the allelic exclusion is the prevention of random association of chains. Such randomly associated immunoglobulin molecules could be devoid of most of their antibody-binding capacity.

In the light of the above discussion it becomes clear that the unequal expression of allotypic genes must be exercised by a non-random process of chromosome activation. There seems to be a general consensus that this activation and the consequent allelic exclusion are initiated by the contact of a pre-productive cell with an antigen. It is assumed that an antigen attaches itself to specific receptors which are present on the cell surface. This event triggers the process of cell differentiation leading to antibody synthesis. The structure of cellular receptors, responsible for these events, has been the subject of extensive studies. These receptors appear to possess antibody combining sites, Fab and Fc portion, heavy and light chains, allotypic specificities etc.[56, 130] The evidence for this structure is based on the reaction of immunocompetent cells upon exposure to antisera directed against various parts of an immunoglobulin molecule,[54, 102, 123–128, 149] on combination of cells with antigen in form of red cells (rosette formation), or bacterial cells (bacterial adherence test)[90, 91] and finally on specific retention of cells on immunoabsorbents.[64, 129, 140, 145, 146] In the light of these experiments it can be assumed, although there is no direct evidence for this assumption, that each receptor is a *complete antibody molecule.* It is only logical to assume further that the antibody produced by a given cell, will be identical in its specificity and allotype, with the antibody-like receptor, the triggering of which initiated the antibody production.

If *activation* of cellular receptors initiates antibody formation and determines allotypic specificity of the antibody produced, *allotypic suppression* must be induced by *deactivation* of these receptors. Such deactivation can be exercised by several mechanisms: (1) *destruction* of receptors by complement-mediated death of cells with which the anti-allotype antibody has combined; (2) *blocking* of receptor sites, so that antigen cannot combine with them — "blindfolding"; or (3) an *"inadequate signal"* which follows combination between receptor and anti-allotype antibody (rather than antigen) and which would result in abortive and nonproductive differentiation. Experimental evidence does not entirely exclude the first possibility. Although suppression can be induced in C5-deficient mice,[16] one cannot rule out a by-pass in complement activation sequence which does not require C5. The decision between the remaining two possibilities, i.e. "blindfolding" and "inadequate signal," remains a task for the future.

We will now consider the possible role of cellular receptors in enforcing the "pecking order." This problem was approached experimentally by Chou, Cinader, and Dubiski[15] who used a modification of the Jerne plaque assay and were able to enumerate cells making IgG antibody to sheep red cells and to determine the allotypic specificity of antibody made by each of these cells. Specificities of the kappa-chain were used as the allotypic markers. It was first established that in all rabbits, both homozygous and heterozygous, the average total number of plaque-forming cells were the same. It can be taken to indicate that neither is there any obvious correlation between allotypic specificities and the ability to make antibody, nor are the heterozygotes any better antibody-producers than homozygotes.

Next, the proportions of A4 and A5 plaques were determined (a) in animals immunized with sheep red cells conjugated with various haptens,* in order to change the electric charge of the immunizing antigen; (cells from these animals were tested with unconjugated sheep red cells), (b) in animals immunized with dinitrophenyl-conjugated human gamma globulin (cells were assayed with dinitrophenyl-conjugated sheep red cells) and (c) in animals immunized with sheep red cells, whose spleen cells were tested for cross-reactivity with goat red cells. In none of the animals did the degree of predominance of A4 over A5 differ from the predominance observed previously in circulating immunoglobulins of normal rabbits or in plaque-forming cells after immunization with sheep red cells. The above results indicate that there are no allotype-correlated differences in the specificity and affinity spectra of cellular receptors. It was then proposed that the position in the "pecking order" of various allotypic genes reflects the relative numbers of cellular receptors, carrying the respective allotypic specificities. If this were the case, one could expect that the allotypic composition of the antibodies, would reflect the allotypic composition of the cellular receptor, only after antigenic stimulation, sufficient to trigger a large number of receptors and to induce formation of a fairly large number of cell clones. Clearly, if only a small number of clones were induced as a result of a weak antigenic stimulation, the allotypic composition of the antibody will not reflect the allotypic composition of cellular receptors.†

Experimental results were in full agreement with this prediction: A^4/A^5 heterozygous rabbits were given 1, 2, and 10 injections of sheep red cells, and the percentages of cells making antibodies of A4 and A5 allotypic specificity were compared. After 1 injection, half of the animals made monoallotypic response, a proportion of them made pure A4 response, and a small number made an A5 response. After 2 injections, no animals made pure A5 response and after 10 injections there were no rabbits which made a monoallotypic response. The percentages of cells making A4 in the last group showed very little heterogeneity and did not differ significantly from the proportions found in rabbits immunized with other antigens and haptens. These observations show that the increasing number of plaque-forming cells during prolonged immunization is not only due to clonal expansion, but is also due to new cell recruitment.

---

*Para-amino-benzene arsonic acid, para-amino-benzene sulphonic acid, and tri-methyl-ammonium-azo benzene.

†This situation can be compared to tossing a coin. After a large number of tosses, the observed frequency of heads and tails will be very close to 50 per cent. However, after only one toss, the frequency of heads may be 100 per cent, and tails 0 per cent, or vice versa. Increasing the number of tosses in each trial, will bring the observed frequencies closer and closer to the expected value of 50 per cent.

The experiments discussed above indicate that the departure from the simple gene-dose relationship occurs at the level of receptor-carrying cell and is most likely due to unequal numbers of receptors of different allotypic specificities. Such an interpretation may perhaps provide an explanation for some of the reports by other workers, who described antibodies in which the proportion of various allotypes deviated from the average values.[1, 5, 81, 118] Some observations, however, cannot be interpreted in this way. It was recently described by Krause and his colleagues[7, 8, 47-49, 62, 63, 74] that immunization of rabbits with streptococcal carbohydrate results sometimes in a formation of high concentration of virtually monoclonal antibodies. In such animals, even a prolonged immunization did not result in the increase of the heterogeneity, i.e., in the recruitment of new cells and formation of new clones. Here, an entirely new mechanism will have to be visualized: either a very efficient blocking of the formation of new clones or a "locking in" of the proliferation of one clone, the latter strongly suggesting analogy with the myeloma. One can hope that with more experimental data, the mechanism of this phenomenon will be better understood.

In summary, evidence was presented that antibody synthesis is controlled at two different levels, the structural level and the regulatory level. Control at the first level is exercised by a complex of structural genes at closely linked loci; the control at the second level is exercised by generating antibody-like cell-surface receptors. Combination of these receptors with antigen leads to antibody formation. Allotypic specificities are expressed on these receptors in unequal proportions. The mechanism responsible for the unequal distribution of allotypic specificities on these receptors remains unknown.

ACKNOWLEDGEMENTS

The author wishes to thank Dr. B. Cinader and Dr. A. M. Kaplan for helpful discussion.

REFERENCES

1. Allen, J. G., Kunkel, H. G., and Kabat, E. A.: Studies on human antibodies. II. Distribution of genetic factors. J. Exper. Med., 119:453, 1964.
2. Appella, E., Chersi, A., Mage, R. G., and Dubiski, S.: Structural basis of the A14 and A15 allotypic specificities in rabbit immunoglobulin G. Proc. Nat. Acad. Sci., 68:1341-1345, 1971.
3. Appella, E., Mage, R. G., Dubiski, S., and Reisfeld, R. A.: Chemical and immunochemical evidence for different classes of rabbit light polypeptide chains. Proc. Nat. Acad. Sci., 60:975-981, 1968.
4. Baglioni, C., Zonta, L. A., Cioli, D., and Carbonara, A.: Allelic antigenic factor InV (a) of the light chains of human immunoglobulins: chemical basis. Science, 152:1517-1519, 1966.
5. Bell, C., Dray, S.: Conversion of non-immune rabbit spleen cells by ribonucleic acid of lymphoid cells from an immunized rabbit to produce IgG antibody of foreign light chain allotype. J. Immunol., 105:541-556, 1970.
6. Bornstein, P., and Oudin, J.: A study of rabbit gamma-globulin allotypy by means of heteroimmunizations. J. Exper. Med., 120:655-676, 1964.
7. Braun, D. G., Eichman, K., and Krause, R. M.: Rabbit antibodies to streptococcal carbohydrates. Influence of primary and secondary immunization and of possible genetic factors on the antibody response. J. Exper. Med., 129:809, 1969.

8. Braun, D. G., and Krause, R. M.: The individual antigenic specificity of antibodies to streptococcal carbohydrates. J. Exper. Med., 128:969, 1968.

9. Burton, R. M., and Deutsch, H. F.: The structure of Fc-fragment from IgG-globulin of known allotypic specificity. Immunochemistry, 7:145, 1970.

10. Carbonara, A. O., Tosi, R. M., Mancini, G., and Luzzati, A. L.: Further immunochemical studies on Ab9 specificity in homozygous rabbits. Boll. Inst. Sieroter. Milan, 48:154–159, 1969.

11. Chou, C.-T., Cinader, B., and Dubiski, S.: Allotypic specificity and hemolytic capacity of antibodies produced by single cells. Int. Arch. Allergy, 32:583–616, 1967.

12. Chou, C.-T., Cinader, B., and Dubiski, S.: Quantitative studies of antibody production by plaque-forming cells. The in vitro inhibition and enhancement of plaque formation by antibody directed against allotypic specificities determined by the Ab locus. Cold Spring Harb. Symp. Quant. Biol., 22:317–331, 1967.

13. Chou, C.-T., Cinader, B., and Dubiski, S.: Allotypic specificity in productive, pre-productive and progenitor cells. In Franěk, F., and Shugar, D., eds.: FEBS Symposium. New York, Academic Press, 15:133–168, 1969.

14. Chou, C.-T., Cinader, B., and Dubiski, S.: Allotypy as a probe. In Peeters, H., ed.: Protides of the Biological Fluids. Proceedings of the 17th Colloquium., New York, Pergamon Press, 1970, pp. 189–203.

15. Chou, C.-T., Cinader, B., and Dubiski, S.: The effect of antigen and the mode of immunization on the allotypic distribution of enhanceable plaque-forming antibodies. Submitted for publication.

16. Cinader, B., and Dubiski, S.: Suppression of allotypic specificities in animals with a complement defect and in animals with a complete hemolytic complement system. J. Immunol., 101:1236–1242, 1968.

17. Conway, T. P., Dray, S., and Lichter, E.: Identification and genetic control of three rabbit IgA immunoglobulin allotypes. J. Immunol., 102:544–554, 1969.

18. Conway, T. P., Dray, S., and Lichter, E.: Identification and genetic control of the f4 and f5 rabbit IgA immunoglobulin allotypes – phenogroups at the f locus. J. Immunol., 103:662–667, 1969.

19. David, G. S., and Todd, C. W.: Suppression of heavy and light chain allotypic expression in homozygous rabbit through embryo transfer. Proc. Nat. Acad. Sci., 62:860, 1969.

20. Dray, S.: Effect of maternal isoantibodies on the quantitative expression of the allelic genes controlling gamma-globulin allotypic specificity. Nature, 195:785, 1962.

21. Dray, S.: Personal communication, 1971.

22. Dray, S., Dubiski, S., Kelus, A., Lennox, E. S., and Oudin, J.: A notation for allotypy. Nature, 195:785–786, 1962.

23. Dray, S., Lichter, E., and Conway, T. P.: Genetic control of rabbit IgA immunoglobulins. In Peeters, H., ed.: Protides of the Biological Fluids. Proceedings of the 17th Colloquium. New York, Pergamon Press, 1970, pp. 131–136.

24. Dray, S., and Nisonoff, A.: Contribution of allelic genes $A_b{}^4$ and $A_b{}^5$ to formation of rabbit 7S gamma-globulins. Proc. Soc. Exper. Biol. Med., 113:20–26, 1963.

25. Dray, S., and Young, G. O.: Differences in the antigenic components of sera of individual rabbits as shown by induced isoprecipitins. J. Immunol., 81:142–149, 1958.

26. Dray, S., Young, G. O., and Gerald, L.: Immunochemical identification and genetics of rabbit gamma-globulin allotypes. J. Immunol., 91:403–415, 1963.

27. Dray, S., Young, G. O., and Nisonoff, A.: Distribution of allotypic specificities among rabbit gamma-globulin molecules genetically defined at two loci. Nature, 199:52–55, 1963.

28. Dubiski, S.: Suppression of the synthesis of allotypically defined immunoglobulins and compensation by another subclass of immunoglobulin. Nature, 214:1365, 1967.

29. Dubiski, S.: Suppression of allotypically defined immunoglobulins in rabbits. Cold Spring Harb. Symp. Quant. Biol., 22:311–316, 1967.

30. Dubiski, S.: Regulation of the synthesis of allotypically defined immunoglobulins. In Cinader, B., ed.: Regulation of Antibody Response. Springfield, Illinois, Charles C Thomas, 1968, pp. 182–203.

31. Dubiski, S.: Immunochemistry and genetics of a "new" allotypic specificity of rabbit IgG immunoglobulins: Recombination in somatic cells. J. Immunol., 103:120–128, 1969.

32. Dubiski, S.: Does antibody synthesis involve somatic recombination? In Peeters, H., ed.: Protides of the Biological Fluids. Proceedings of the 17th Colloquium, New York, Pergamon Press, 1970, pp. 117–124.

33. Dubiski, S., Chou, C.-T., and Cinader, B.: Allotypic specificity as a marker of cells and cell receptors. In Cellular Intractions in the Immune Response, Second International Convocation Immunol., Buffalo, New York 1970, Basel, S. Karger, 1971, pp. 140–152.

34. Dubiski, S., and Cinader, B.: A new allotypic specificity in the mouse (Mu A2). Nature, 197:705, 1962.

35. Dubiski, S., and Cinader, B.: Gene dosage effect on the serum concentration of a complement component, MuB1. Proc. Soc. Exper. Biol. Med., 122:775–778, 1966.

36. Dubiski, S., Dubiska, A., Skalba, D., and Kelus, A.: Antigenic structure of rabbit gamma-globulin. Immunol., 4:236–242, 1961.

37. Dubiski, S., Dudziak, Z., Skalba, D., and Dubiska, A.: Serum groups in rabbits. Immunol., 2:84–92, 1959.
38. Dubiski, S., and Fradette, K.: The feed-back mechanism in immunoglobulin synthesis. Proc. Soc. Exper. Biol. Med., 122:126–130, 1966.
39. Dubiski, S., and Good, P. W.: Manuscript in preparation.
40. Dubiski, S., and Muller, P. J.: A "new" allotypic specificity (A9) of rabbit immunoglobulin. Nature, 214:696, 1967.
41. Dubiski, S., Rapacz, J., and Dubiska, A.: Heredity of rabbit gamma-globulin iso-antigens. Acta Genet., 12:136–155, 1962.
42. Dubiski, S., Skalba, D., Dubiska, A., and Kelus, A.: Iso-antigens of rabbit gamma-globulins. Nature, 184:1811, 1959.
43. Dubiski, S., and Swierczynska, A.: Allotypic suppression in rabbits; operational characterization of the target cells. Int. Arch. Allergy, 40:1–18, 1971.
44. Dubiski, S., and Swierczynska, Z.: Allotypic suppression in rabbits: operational characterization of the target cells. In Grubb, R., and Samuelsson, G., eds.: Human Anti-human Gamma Globulins. New York, Pergamon Press, 1971, pp. 39–56.
45. Edelman, G. M., and Gally, J. A.: Somatic recombination of duplicated genes: an hypothesis on the origin of antibody diversity. Proc. Nat. Acad. Sci., 57:353–358, 1967.
46. Edelman, G. M., and Gottlieb, P. D.: A genetic marker in the variable region of light chains of mouse immunoglobulins. Proc. Nat. Acad. Sci., 67:1192–1199, 1970.
47. Eichman, K., Braun, D. G., Feizi, T., and Krause, R. M.: The emergence of antibodies with either identical or unrelated individual antigenic specificity during repeated immunizations with streptococcal vaccine. J. Exper. Med., 131:1169–1189, 1970.
48. Eichman, K., Braun, D. G., and Krause, R. M.: Influence of genetic factors on the magnitude and the heterogeneity of the immune response in the rabbit. J. Exper. Med., 134:48–65, 1971.
49. Eichman, K., and Kindt, T. J.: The inheritance of individual antigenic specificities of rabbit antibodies to streptococcus carbohydrates. J. Exper. Med., 134:532–552, 1971.
50. Feinstein, A.: Character and allotypy of an immune globulin in rabbit colostrum. Nature, 199:1197–1199, 1963.
51. Fleischman, J. B.: A partial amino acid sequence in the heavy chain of a rabbit antibody to group C streptococcal carbohydrate. Biochemistry, 10:2753–2761, 1971.
52. Frangione, B., Franklin, E. C., Fudenberg, H. H., and Koshland, M. E.: Structural studies of human IgG myeloma proteins of different antigenic subgroups and genetic specificities. J. Exper. Med., 124:715–732, 1966.
53. Gell, P. G. H.: Allotypes and antibodies. In Cinader, B., ed.: Regulation of Antibody Response. Springfield, Illinois, Charles C Thomas, 1968, pp. 204–211.
54. Gell, P. G. H., and Sell, S.: Studies on rabbit lymphocytes in vitro. II. Induction of blast transformation with antiserum to six IgG allotypes and summation with mixture of antisera to different allotypes. J. Exper. Med., 122:813, 1965.
55. Gilman-Sachs, E., Mage, R. G., Young, G. O., Alexander, C. O., and Dray, S.: Identification and genetic control of two rabbit immunoglobulin allotypes at a second light chain locus, the c locus. J. Immunol., 103:1159–1167, 1969.
56. Greaves, M. F.: The expression of immunoglobulin determinants on the surface of antigen-binding lymphoid cells in mice. Europ. J. Immunol., 1:186–194, 195–201, 1971.
57. Grubb, R.: The genetic markers of human immunoglobulins. In Molecular Biology Biochemistry and Biophysics, vol. 9. New York, Springer-Verlag, 1970.
58. Hamers, R., and Hamers-Casterman, C.: Evidence for the presence of the Fc allotypic marker As8 and the Fd allotypic marker As1 in the same molecules of rabbit IgG. Cold Spring Harb. Symp. Quant. Biol., 32:129–132, 1967.
59. Herzenberg, L. A.: A chromosome region for gamma$_{2a}$ and beta$_{2a}$ globulin H-chain isoantigens in the mouse. Cold Spring Harb. Symp. Quant. Biol., 29:455–462, 1964.
60. Herzenberg, L. A., and Warner, N. L.: Genetic control of mouse immunoglobulins. In Cinader, B., ed.: Regulation of Antibody Response. Springfield, Illinois, Charles C Thomas, 1968, pp. 322–348.
61. Herzenberg, L. A., Warner, N. L., and Herzenberg, L. A.: Immunoglobulin isoantigens in the mouse. I. Genetics and cross reactions of the gamma$_{2a}$-isoantigens controlled by the IgI locus. J. Exper. Med., 121:415–438, 1965.
62. Hood, L., Eichman, K., Lackland, H., Krause, R. M., and Ohms, J. J.: Rabbit antibody light chains and gene evolution. Nature, 228:1040–1044, 1970.
63. Hood, L., Lackland, H., Eichman, K., Kindt, T. J., Braun, D. G., and Krause, R. M.: Amino acid sequence restriction in rabbit antibody light chains. Proc. Nat. Acad. Sci., 63:890–896, 1969.
64. Inman, G. K., and Dintzis, H. M.: Derivation of cross-linked polyacrylomide beads. Controlled introduction of functional groups for the preparation of special purpose, biochemical adsorbents. Biochemistry, 8:4074–4082, 1969.
65. Kelus, A. S.: Gamma-globulin allotypes in the rabbit. Biochem. J., 88:4P, 1963.

66. Kelus, A. S.: Rabbit allotypic markers as a model for molecular immunology. *In* Killander, J., ed.: Gamma Globulins. Proceedings of the Third Nobel Symposium, Stockholm, Almquist and Wiksell, 1967, pp. 329–339.
67. Kelus, A. S., and Gell, P. G. H.: An allotypic determinant specific to rabbit macroglobulin. Nature, 206:313–314, 1965.
68. Kelus, A. S., and Gell, P. G. H.: Immunoglobulin allotypes of experimental animals. Prog. Allergy, 11:141–184, 1967.
69. Kelus, A., and Moor-Jankowski, J. K.: An iso-antigen (γBA) of mouse γ-globulin present inbred strains. Nature, 191:1405–1406, 1961.
70. Kelus, A. S., and Pernis, B.: Allotypic markers of rabbit IgM: European J. Immunol., 1:123–132, 1971.
71. Kindt, T. J., Mandy, W. J., and Todd, C. W.: Association of allotypic specificities of group *a* with allotypic specificities A11 and A12 in rabbit immunoglobulin. Biochemistry, 9:2028–2032, 1970.
72. Kindt, T. J., Steward, M. W., and Todd, C. W.: Allotypic markers on rabbit IgA. Biochem. Biophys. Res. Commun., 31:9–15, 1968.
73. Kindt, T. J., and Todd, C. W.: Heavy and light chain allotypic markers on rabbit homocytotropic antibody. J. Exper. Med., 130:859–866, 1969.
74. Kindt, T. J., Todd, C. W., Eichman, K., and Krause, R. M.: Allotype exclusion in uniform rabbit antibody to streptococcal carbohydrate. J. Exper. Med., 131:343–352, 1970.
75. Knight, K. L., Gilman-Sachs, A., Fields, R., and Dray, S.: Allotypic determinants on the Fab fragment of rabbit *Aa* locus negative IgG-immunoglobulin. J. Immunol., 106:761–767, 1971.
76. Köhler, H., Shimizu, A., Paul, C., Moore, V., and Putnam. F. W.: Three variable gene pools common to IgM, IgG and IgA immunoglobulins. Nature, 227:1318–1320, 1970.
77. Koshland, M. E.: Location of specificity and allotypic amino acid residues in antibody Fd fragments. Cold Spring Harbor Symp. Quant. Biol., 32:119–127, 1967.
78. Koshland, M. E., David, I. J., and Fujita, N. J.: Evidence for multiple gene control of a simple polypeptide chain: the heavy chain of rabbit immunoglobulin. Proc. Nat. Acad. Sci., 63:1274–1281, 1969.
79. Landucci-Tosi, S., Mage, R. G., and Dubiski, S.: Distribution of allotypic specificities A1, A2, A14 and A15 among immunoglobulin G molecules. J. Immunol., 104:641–647, 1970.
80. Landucci-Tosi, S., and Tosi, R. M.: The proportion of recombinant IgG molecules in rabbits doubly heterozygous for *a* and *e* allotypic specificities. To be submitted for publication.
81. Lark, C. A., Eisen, H. N., and Dray, S.: Distribution of allelic allotypes among IgG globulins and purified anti-hapten antibodies from the same rabbit. J. Immunol., 95:104, 1965.
82. Lichter, E. A.: Rabbit IgA and IgM immunoglobulins with allotypic specificities controlled by the *a* locus. J. Immunol., 98:139–142, 1967.
83. Lichter, E.: Personal communication, 1970.
84. Lieberman, R., and Dray, S.: Five allelic genes at the *Asa* locus which control gamma-globulin allotypic specificities in mice. J. Immunol., 93:584–594, 1964.
85. Mage, R., and Dray, S.: Persistent altered phenotypic expression of allelic IgG-immoglobulin allotypes in heterozygous rabbits exposed to isoantibodies in fetal and neonatal life. J. Immunol., 95:525–535, 1965.
86. Mage, R. G., Young-Cooper, G. O., and Alexander, C.: Genetic control of variable and constant regions of immunoglobulin heavy chains. Nature – New Biol., 230:63, 1971.
87. Mage, R. G., Young, G. O., and Reisfeld, R. A.: The association of the *c*7 allotype of rabbits with some light polypeptide chains which lack *b* locus allotypy. J. Immunol., 101:617, 1968.
88. Mage, R. G., Young, G. O., Rejnek, J., Reisfeld, R. A., Dubiski, S., and Appella, E.: The quantitative expression, genetics and chemistry of allotypes, types and subtypes of rabbit light polypeptide chains. *In* Peeters, H., ed.: Protides of the Biological Fluids. Proceedings of the 17th Colloquium. New York, Pergamon Press, 1970, pp. 215–223.
89. Mäkelä, O.: The specificity of antibodies produced by single cell. Cold Spring Harb. Symp. Quant. Biol., 22:423–430, 1967.
90. Mäkelä, O., and Nossal, G. J. U.: Bacterial adherence: a method for detecting antibody production in single cells. J. Immunol., 87:447, 1961.
91. Mäkelä, O., and Nossal, G. J. U.: Studies on antibody-producing capacity of single cells by bacterial adherence and immobilization. J. Immunol., 87:457, 1961.
92. Mancini, G., Carbonara, A. O., Tosi, R. M., and Luzzati, A. L.: An immunogenetic study of the Ab9 allotypic specificity in rabbit. Boll. Inst. Sieroter. Milan, 48:142–153, 1969.
93. Mandy, W. J.: Personal communication, 1971.
94. Mandy, W. J., and Todd, C. W.: Allotypy of rabbit immunoglobulin: an agglutinating specificity. Vox Sang., 14:264–270, 1968.

95. Mandy, W. J., and Todd, C. W.: Characterization of allotype A11 in rabbits: a specificity detected by agglutination. Immunochem., 6:811–823, 1969.
96. Mandy, W. J., and Todd, C. W.: Rabbit immunoglobulin allotype A12: A new agglutinating specificity. Biochem. Genet., 4:59:71, 1970.
97. Marrack, J. R., Richards, C. B., and Kelus, A.: Antigenic specificity of hydrolysis products of gamma-globulins. In Peeters, H., ed.: Protides of the Biological Fluids. Proceedings of the 9th Colloquium. Amsterdam, Elsevier, 1962, pp. 200–206.
98. Masuda, T., Kuribayashi, K., and Hanaoka, M.: A new allotypic antigen of rabbit collostral IgA immunoglobulin. J. Immunol., 102:1156–1162, 1969.
99. Micheli, A., Mage, R. G., and Reisfeld, R. A.: Direct demonstration and quantitation of Aa1, Aa2, and Aa3 allotypic specificities on Fd fragments of rabbit immunoglobulin G. J. Immunol., 100:604–611, 1968.
100. Milstein, C.: Variations in amino acid sequence near the disulphide bridge of Bence-Jones proteins. Nature, 209:370–373, 1966.
101. Nisonoff, A., and Thorbecke, G. J.: Immunochemistry. Ann. Rev. Biochem., 33:355, 1964.
102. Nota, N. R., Liacopoulos-Briot, M., Stiffel, C., and Biozzi, G.: L'immunocytoadhérence: une méthode simple et quantitative pour l'étude "in vitro" des cellules productrices d'anticorps. Acad. Sci., Paris, 259:1277, 1964.
103. Oudin, J.: Réaction de précipitation spécifique entre des sérums d'animaux de même espéce. Acad. Sci., Paris, 242:2489–2490, 1956.
104. Oudin, J.: L'"allotypie" de certains antigènes protéidiques du sérum. Acad. Sci., Paris, 242:2606–2608, 1956.
105. Oudin, J.: Allotypy of rabbit serum proteins. I. Immunochemical analysis leading to the individualization of seven main allotypes. J. Exper. Med., 112:107–124, 1960.
106. Oudin, J.: Allotypy of rabbit serum proteins. II. Relationships between various allotypes: their common antigenic specificity, their distribution in a sample population, genetic implications. J. Exper. Med., 112:125–142, 1960.
107. Oudin, J.: On the associated state of rabbit allotypes, the existence of rabbit antibody molecules against two allotypes, and the dissociation of human gamma-globulin antigens into smaller molecules. Biochem. Biophys. Res. Commun., 5:358–361, 1961.
108. Oudin, J.: Genetic regulation of immunoglobulin synthesis. J. Cell. Physiol., 67:(Suppl. 1): 77–108, 1966.
109. Pernis, B.: Relationship between the heterogeneity of immunoglobulin and the differentiation of plasma cells. Cold Spring Harb. Symp. Quant. Biol., 22:333–341, 1967.
110. Pernis, B., Chiappino, G., Kelus, A. S., and Gell, P. G. H.: Cellular localization of immunoglobulins with different allotypic specificities in rabbit lymphoid tissues. J. Exper. Med., 122:853–876, 1965.
111. Pernis, B., Dubiski, S., Mandy, U. J., and Todd, C. W.: A study of heavy chain variable and constant region allotypes in single rabbit plasma cells. Submitted for publication.
112. Pernis, B., Torrigiani, G., Amante, L., Kelus, A. S., and Cebra, J. J.: Identical markers of heavy polypeptide chains present in different immunoglobulin classes. Immunol., 14:445–451, 1968.
113. Pink, R., Wang, A-C., and Fudenberg, H. H.: Antibody variability. Ann. Rev. Med., 22:145–170, 1971.
114. Prahl, J. W., Mandy, W. J., David, G. S., Steward, M. W., and Todd, C. W.: Participation of allotypic markers in rabbit immunoglobulin classes. In Peeters, H., ed.: Protides of the Biological Fluids. Proceedings of the 17th Colloquium, New York, Pergamon Press, 1970, pp. 125–130.
115. Prahl, J. W., Mandy, W. J., and Todd, C. W.: The molecular determinants of the A11 and A12 allotypic specificities in rabbit immunoglobulin. Biochemistry, 8:4935–4940, 1969.
116. Prahl, J. W., and Porter, R. R.: Allotype-related sequence variation of the heavy chain of rabbit immunoglobulin G. Biochem. J., 107:753–763, 1968.
117. Reisfeld, R. A., Dray, S., and Nisonoff, A.: Differences in amino-acid composition of rabbit IgG-immunoglobulin light polypeptide chain controlled by allelic genes. Immunochemistry, 2:155–167, 1965.
118. Rieder, R. F., and Oudin, J.: Studies on the relationship of allotypic specificities to antibody specificities in the rabbit. J. Exper. Med., 118:627, 1963.
119. Rivat, L., Gilbert, D., and Ropartz, C.: The genes of the Gm system, are they structural genes? In Peeters, H., ed.: Protides of the Biological Fluids. Proceedings of the 17th Colloquium. New York, Pergamon Press, 1970, pp. 223–237.
120. Schütze, A.: Specifische serumreaktion, Isopräcipitin. Deutsche Med. Wschr., 29:4, 1902.
121. Sell, S.: Immunoglobulin M allotypes of the rabbit: Identification of a second specificity. Science, 153:641–643, 1966.
122. Sell, S.: Isolation and characterization of rabbit collostral IgA. Immunochemistry, 4:49–55, 1967.

123. Sell, S.: Studies on rabbit lymphocytes in vitro. V. The induction of blast transformation with sheep antisera to rabbit Ig subunits. J. Exper. Med., 125:289, 1967.
124. Sell, S.: Studies on rabbit lymphocytes in vitro. VI. The induction of blast transformation with sheep antisera to IgA and IgM. J. Exper. Med., 125:393, 1967.
125. Sell, S.: Studies on rabbit lymphocytes in vitro. VII. The induction of blast transformation with the F(ab')₂ and Fab fragments of sheep antibody to rabbit IgG. J. Immunol., 98:786, 1967.
126. Sell, S., and Asofsky, R.: Lymphocytes and immunoglobulins. Progr. Allergy, 12:86, 1968.
127. Sell, S., and Gell, P. G. H.: Studies on rabbit lymphocytes in vitro. I. Stimulation of blast transformation with an anti-allotype serum. J. Exper. Med., 122:423, 1965.
128. Sell, S., and Gell, P. G. H.: Studies on rabbit lymphocytes in vitro. IV. Blast transformation of the lymphocytes from newborn rabbit induced by anti-allotype similar to a paternal IgG allotype not present in the serum of the lymphocyte donors. J. Exper. Med., 122:923, 1965.
129. Singhal, S. K., and Wigzell, H.: In vitro induction of specific unresponsiveness of immunologically reactive, normal bone marrow cells. J. Exper. Med., 131:149, 1970.
130. Singhal, S. K., and Wigzell, H.: Cognition and recognition of antigen by cell associated receptors. Progr. Allergy, 1971, in press.
131. Small, P. A., Jr., Reisfeld, R. A., and Dray, S.: Peptide maps of rabbit IgG immunoglobulin heavy chains controlled by allelic genes. J. Molec. Biol., 16:328-333, 1966.
132. Smithies, O.: Pathways through networks of branched DNA. Science, 169:882-883, 1970.
133. Stemke, G. W.: Allotypic specificities of A- and B- chains of rabbit gamma-globulin. Science, 145:403-405, 1964.
134. Stemke, G. W.: A study of soluble complexes and uncombined material in antigen-antibody reactions involving allotypic specificities of purified rabbit gamma-globulin. Immunochem., 2:359-377, 1965.
135. Stemke, G. W.: Rabbit immunoglobulin allotypy: the physicochemical nature of a- group determinants. Canadian J. Biochem., 49:1257-1263, 1971.
136. Stemke, G. W., and Fischer, R. S.: Rabbit 19S antibodies with allotypic specificities of the a- locus group. Science, 150:1298-1303, 1965.
137. Thorpe, N. O., and Deutsch, H. F.: Studies on pepsin produced subunits of human IgG-globulins, II. Immunochem., 3:329-337, 1966.
138. Todd, C. W.: Allotypy in rabbit 19S protein. Biochem. Biophys. Res. Commun., 11:170-175, 1963.
139. Todd, C. W., and Inman, F. P.: Comparison of the allotypic combining sites on H-chains of rabbit IgG and IgM. Immunochemistry, 4:407-417, 1967.
140. Truffabachi, P., and Wofsy, L.: Specific separation of cells on affinity columns. Proc. Nat. Acad. Sci., 66:685-692, 1970.
141. Vince, J. L., Hunt, W., and Dray, S.: Zygote transfer to facilitate altered expression of immunoglobulin light chain phenotypes in homozygous rabbits. Proc. Soc. Exper. Biol. Med., 130:730-733, 1969.
142. Vince, J. L., Hunt, W. L., and Dray, S.: Contribution of the b and c light chain loci to the composition of rabbit IgG-immunoglobulins. J. Immunol., 104:38-44, 1970.
143. Wang, A. C., Pink, J. R. L., Fudenberg, H. H., and Ohms, J.: A variable region subclass of heavy chains common to immunoglobulins G, A, and M and characterized by an unblocked amino-terminal residue. Proc. Nat. Acad. Sci., 66:657-663, 1970.
144. Wang, A. C., Wilson, S. K., Hopper, J. E., Fudenberg, H. H., and Nisonoff, A.: Evidence for control of synthesis of the variable regions of the heavy chains of immunoglobulins G and M by the same gene. Proc. Nat. Acad. Sci., 66:337-343, 1970.
145. Wigzell, H.: Use of humoral or cell bound antibody to achieve depression of immunological activity. Antibiot. Chemother., 15:82, 1969.
146. Wigzell, H., and Anderson, B.: Cell separation on antigen coated columns. Elimination of high-rate antibody forming cells and immunological memory cells. J. Exper. Med., 129:23, 1969.
147. Wilkinson, J. M.: Alpha-chains of immunoglobulin A from rabbits of different allotype: composition and N-terminal sequence. Nature, 223:616-617, 1969.
148. Wilkinson, J. M.: Variation in the N-terminal sequence of heavy chains of immunoglobulin G from rabbits of different allotype. Biochem. J., 112:173-185, 1969.
149. Zaalberg, O. B.: A simple method for detecting antibody-forming cells. Nature, 202:1231, 1964.

1 Spadina Crescent
Toronto 179, Ontario
Canada

Index

Note: Page numbers of symposium and article titles are in **boldface** type.

577

THIS VOLUME MAY CIRCULATE FOR 1 WEEK.
Renewals May Be Made In Person Or By Phone:
x 5300; from outside 472-5300

DATE DUE	DATE RETURNED

ONE WEEK SERIAL

99622

FIRST CLASS
PERMIT NO. 101
PHILADELPHIA, PA.

BUSINESS REPLY MAIL
NO POSTAGE STAMP NECESSARY IF MAILED IN UNITED STATES

POSTAGE WILL BE PAID BY

W. B. Saunders Company

West Washington Square
Philadelphia, Pa. 19105

Time for a periodical checkup!

☐ HUMAN PATHOLOGY
Quarterly, $18.50 per year

☐ MEDICAL CLINICS
Bimonthly, $21 per year

☐ SURGICAL CLINICS
Bimonthly, $21 per year

☐ PEDIATRIC CLINICS
Quarterly, $18 per year

☐ RADIOLOGIC CLINICS
3 issues, $20 per year

☐ OTOLARYNGOLOGIC CLINICS
3 issues, $22 per year

☐ ORTHOPEDIC CLINICS
3 issues, $22.50 per year

☐ DENTAL CLINICS
Quarterly, $20 per year

☐ NURSING CLINICS
Quarterly, $12 per year

☐ VETERINARY CLINICS
3 issues, $22 per year

**3 new Clinics
with an international outlook**

☐ GASTROENTEROLOGY CLINICS
3 issues, $30 per year

☐ HEMATOLOGY CLINICS
3 issues, $30 per year

☐ ENDOCRINOLOGY & METABOLISM
CLINICS, 3 issues, $30 per year

Check over this list of Saunders periodicals. Thousands of your colleagues rely on the widely acclaimed *Clinics of North America* to keep them abreast of new developments. Each hardbound, illustrated issue focuses on a specific topic of current interest and concern. Use this convenient card to order the periodicals of interest to you.

Name_____

Address_____

City_____State_____ZIP_____

On the move?

Make sure that your subscription to Saunders periodicals goes with you. Fill in and mail the attached card today. Please be sure to include your new zip code. Allow one month for your change of address to be processed.

As of__/__/__send my "Clinics" issues to my new address given below.

Name_____

NEW ADDRESS_____

City_____State_____ZIP_____

OLD ADDRESS_____

City_____State_____ZIP_____

☐ MEDICAL CLINICS

☐ SURGICAL CLINICS

☐ PEDIATRIC CLINICS

☐ OTOLARYNGOLOGIC CLINICS

☐ RADIOLOGIC CLINICS

☐ ORTHOPEDIC CLINICS

☐ DENTAL CLINICS

☐ NURSING CLINICS

☐ VETERINARY CLINICS